The Management of Malignant Disease Series

General Editor: Professor M. J. Peckham

Titles now published

Forthcoming titles

The Prevention of Cancer

Edited by Michael Alderson MD, FFCM

Professor of Epidemiology, Institute of Cancer Research, London University

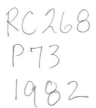

Edward Arnold

© Edward Arnold (Publishers) Ltd 1982

First published 1982
by Edward Arnold (Publishers) Ltd
41 Bedford Square, London WC1B 3DQ

British Library Cataloguing in Publication Data
The Prevention of cancer.—(The Management of
    malignant disease series, ISSN 0144-8692; 4)
    1. Cancer—Prevention
    I. Alderson, Michael II. Series
    616.99'4052   RC268

ISBN 0-7131-4401-7

Filmset in 10/11pt Baskerville and printed in Great Britain by
Butler and Tanner Ltd, Frome and London

Contributors

Michael Alderson MD, FFCM
Professor of Epidemiology, Institute of Cancer Research, London University

Michael Calnan PhD
Division of Epidemiology, Institute of Cancer Research, London University

Jocelyn Chamberlain FFCM
Acting Head, Division of Epidemiology, Institute of Cancer Research, London University

Joan M Davies PhD
Division of Epidemiology, Institute of Cancer Research, London University

Preface

All the authors of this book were on the scientific staff of the Division of Epidemiology, Institute of Cancer Research, London when it was planned and written. The four authors combine a range of disciplines; they have worked in a wide variety of different fields, including (a) varying numbers of years on research, including into the aetiology of cancer, and (b) involvement with the practical issues of cancer control.

The book describes the extent of the cancer problem, presents information on the causes of cancer, and provides a critical assessment of the steps that may be taken to reduce the toll from this disease. The emphasis is upon steps which may be pursued now, on the basis of presently available evidence. Many of the issues involved are complex and where no realistic control programme can be advocated the research required as a basis for future action is indicated.

The intention was that the book should be of interest to: those involved in cancer control as health administrators and planners, health educators, epidemiologists, academic social scientists involved in research and teaching on Social Sciences in Medicine, and clinicians (particularly those interested in early detection of cancer). Though written by four UK authors, the text should be of equal interest in other countries—though the extent of the cancer problem and the causes differ.

The authors would like to thank their colleagues for discussing various points that arose in clarifying views on the prevention of cancer; particular thanks are due to members of ASH who helped with some issues of smoking. A review such as this places a heavy load on library facilities and thanks are due to Mrs Sue Dobby, librarian at the Institute of Cancer Research. It is a pleasure to acknowledge the help given, not only with typing, by our secretaries: Mrs D. Folkes, Mrs S. Skeet, Miss J. Miller, and Mrs T. Bagley.

December 1981   M. R. Alderson

Contents

1

Introduction

Michael Alderson

The scope of this book

The book, as indicated by its title, deals with various ways of preventing cancer. It has embodied a review of present information on the causes of cancer and critical assessment of the steps that may be taken to reduce the toll from this disease.

A brief section follows which explains the various levels of prevention and those that specifically come within the scope of the book.

The next chapter deals briefly with the available information on the extent of the cancer problem, looking particularly at trends in mortality of cancer in England and Wales. This is followed by a review of the causes of cancer; this is only to set the scene for consideration of various steps in prevention and an extensive literature on aetiology has been compressed into a short review.

Chapter 4 discusses lay and professional beliefs and feelings about cancer; it is felt that an understanding of these is a first step in any satisfactory campaign of cancer control. The next two chapters deal with the role of central government and industry in preventing cancer. Chapter 7 covers various non-governmental approaches to cancer prevention; smoking and alcohol being selected for special treatment as examples of actual hazards.

Chapters 8 and 9 review screening, beginning with theoretical and practical aspects; evaluation of various methods is discussed. The specific methods of screening for cancer of the lung, breast, colorectum, stomach, bladder, cervix, choriocarcinoma, skin, testis and prostate are critically reviewed.

The final chapter is concerned with patient and professional delay in achieving treatment for symptomatic cancer; this indicates the steps that may be taken to reduce this to an absolute minimum.

The levels of prevention

Control of any disease may be achieved by (i) primary prevention, which aims at removing the causative agent; (ii) secondary prevention, which has the general aim of improving the results from therapy, partly by early detection; or (iii) tertiary prevention, which covers the care directed at general support and alleviation of the problems associated with disease. In slightly more specific terms for cancer control, these activities imply (i) primary prevention through the avoidance of genetic transmission of cancer risk, or the removal or reduction of exposure of individuals to known carcinogens, or (perhaps) the use of therapy which will 'block' the action of carcinogens; (ii) secondary prevention involving the early detection of disease either through the screening of the population to detect precursor lesions (such as in-situ carcinoma of the cervix) or the detection of 'early' cancer (as with the screening for localized cancer of the breast)—rather different are the steps that may be taken to ensure that any patient with fresh signs or symptoms of cancer does not delay before seeking medical advice and, once this step has been taken, that diagnosis occurs without any delay; (iii) the issues of tertiary prevention involving quite different concepts, and solutions; an example of this is the care of the terminally ill—with the reduction in pain, discomfort and worry that can come with appropriate treatment. This subject has already been dealt with in a companion volume in this series (Saunders, 1978). Other aspects of tertiary prevention are not dealt with in this book, which is restricted to the consideration of methods of primary and secondary prevention.

The emphasis of the book is upon steps which may be pursued now, on the basis of presently available evidence. Many of the issues involved are complex and where no realistic control programme can be advocated, the research required as a basis for future action is indicated.

Reference

Saunders, Cicely M. (ed.) (1978). *The Management of Terminal Disease*. The Management of Malignant Disease Series, Vol. 1. Ed. by M. J. Peckham and R. L. Carter. Edward Arnold, London.

2

The extent of the cancer problem

Michael Alderson

This chapter presents data for England and Wales for the latest period available and also a number of time trends for the major part of this century. These are to indicate the extent of the cancer problem and in particular whether malignancies of specific sites are becoming more or less common. Some limited data on international material are provided and also some data for England and Wales on survival from malignancy.

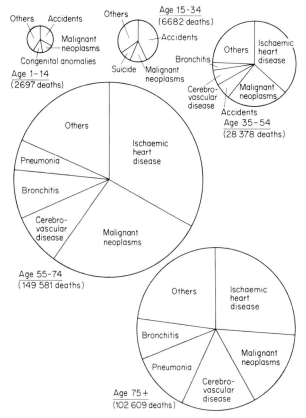

Fig. 2.1 Main causes of mortality for males at different ages in England and Wales, 1973.

3

England and Wales: current data

Approximately 20 per cent of the deaths in England and Wales in any year are due to malignant disease. The actual toll from malignancy varies with both age and sex. This is indicated in broad terms in Figs. 2.1 and 2.2. These show the main causes of mortality at five different ages in males and then in females in England and Wales in 1973. For males in each of the five age groups that are identified, malignant disease is the second commonest cause of death. A rather different picture is demonstrated for females; in three of the five age groups, malignant disease is the commonest cause of death (from ages 15–74). It then drops in order of importance in those aged 75 and over, becoming the fourth commonest cause of death.

Turning attention now to the specific sites of malignancy involved, Tables 2.1 and 2.2 show the numbers of deaths from different malignancies in males and females and the cumulative percentage of all malignancies site by site. Again, there are major differences between the sexes; lung cancer is the commonest cause of death in males, accounting for a horrifying 39.2 per cent of malignant neoplasm deaths. For females it is the second cause and at the moment only adds 12.8 per cent to the toll from malignancy. Because of the sex-specific malignancies being

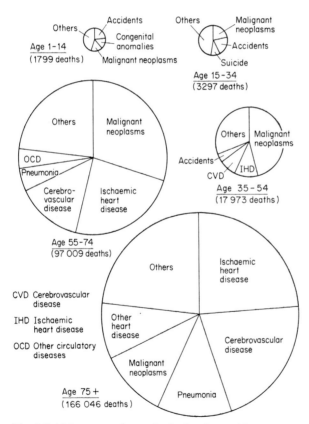

Fig. 2.2 Main causes of mortality for females at different ages in England and Wales, 1973.

Table 2.1 Neoplasms: numbers of deaths and cumulative percentage of deaths from various sites, males (England and Wales, 1978)

Site	Number of deaths	Cumulative percentage
1 Lung	26 925	39.2
2 Stomach	6 698	48.9
3 Prostate	4 730	55.8
4 Large intestine	4 324	62.1
5 Rectum	3 202	66.8
6 Pancreas	3 008	71.2
7 Bladder	2 951	75.5
8 Oesophagus	2 085	78.5
9 Leukaemia	1 832	81.2
10 Brain tumours	1 761	83.7
11 Liver and gall bladder	1 318	85.6
12 Kidneys and suprarenals	1 095	87.2
13 Multiple myeloma	758	88.3
14 Larynx	649	89.3
15 Other neoplasms of lymphoid tissue	635	90.2
16 Skin excluding scrotum	605	91.1
17 Lymphosarcoma	532	91.9
18 Hodgkin's disease	398	92.4
19 Bones	395	93.0
20 Pharynx	319	93.5
21 Mouth and tonsils	272	93.9
22 Testes	233	94.2
23 Tongue	209	94.5
24 Connective and other soft tissue	202	94.8
25 Myelofibrosis	124	95.0
26 Thyroid	109	95.2
27 Small intestine	104	95.3
28 Penis	95	95.4
29 Breast	92	95.6
30 Salivary gland	89	95.7
31 Eye	76	95.8
32 Polycythaemia vera	69	95.9
33 Lip	38	96.0
34 Other (including site unspecified, benign, or nature unspecified)	2 765	100.0
All neoplasms	68 697	

relatively common in both males and females, the ordering of some of the other sites also varies between the sexes.

England and Wales: trends in deaths from neoplasms

As a general background to consideration of the major trends, Figs. 2.3 and 2.4 show the mortality rates for males and females at three points during the present century—1911–15, 1941–45 and 1971–75. These curves are thus separated by periods of thirty years. There is a marked contrast between the figures for males and females; for the latter there is very little difference in the distribution of the curve until the very elderly. However, for the males the 1941–45 curve is higher from age 50, and higher again for the same age from 1971–75; there is a very marked increase in the rate for those over 70 years of age. (The specific site

Table 2.2 Neoplasms: numbers of deaths and cumulative percentage of deaths from various sites, females (England and Wales, 1978)

	Site	Number of deaths	Cumulative percentage
1	Breast	11 915	20.1
2	Lung	7 606	32.9
3	Large intestine	6 057	43.1
4	Stomach	4 799	51.2
5	Ovaries and fallopian tubes	3 784	57.6
6	Rectum	2 847	62.4
7	Pancreas	2 692	66.9
8	Uterus, cervix	2 153	68.9
9	Oesophagus	1 623	73.3
10	Uterus, others	1 567	75.9
11	Leukaemia	1 540	78.5
12	Liver and gall bladder	1 327	80.8
13	Bladder	1 318	83.0
14	Brain tumours	1 312	85.2
15	Multiple myeloma	732	86.4
16	Kidneys and suprarenals	658	87.6
17	Skin	653	88.7
18	Other neoplasms of lymphoid tissue	525	89.5
19	Vulva and vagina	472	90.3
20	Lymphosarcoma	430	91.1
21	Bones	305	91.6
22	Thyroid	283	92.1
23	Hodgkin's disease	268	92.5
24	Pharynx	235	92.9
25	Larynx	189	93.2
26	Mouth and tonsils	163	93.5
27	Connective and other soft tissue	156	93.8
28	Tongue	125	94.0
29	Myelofibrosis	114	94.2
30	Small intestine	102	94.3
31	Eye	93	94.5
32	Polycythaemia vera	64	94.6
33	Salivary gland	59	94.7
34	Lip	9	94.7
35	Other (including site unspecified, benign, or nature unspecified)	3 136	100.0
	All neoplasms	59 311	

responsible for this difference between the sexes is identified in subsequent graphs as lung cancer.) Another way of looking at the overall trends is to consider the percentage of all deaths at different ages that have been accounted for by neoplasm. Such data are demonstrated in the next two figures (Figs. 2.5 and 2.6). For the same calendar periods these show the percentage of all deaths by age for males and then females. Both curves show a bimodal distribution with a peak in children and a peak in the middle-aged; each shows a considerable rise in the percentage of all deaths accounted for by neoplasm. This is a reflection, not so much of an increase in neoplasms, as a decrease in other causes of death such as infectious disease. The two figures show differences, with a more pronounced rise in the proportion of deaths from malignancy in females aged 30–60. This is a reflection of the relative toll from ischaemic heart disease and breast cancer in the two sexes.

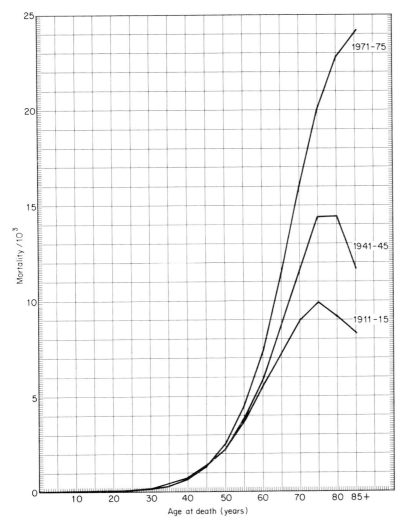

Fig. 2.3 All neoplasms: mortality rates for males by age at death in England and Wales, 1911–15, 1941–45, 1971–75.

Trends by site of malignancy

Pairs of graphs are now provided which cover the main groups of sites involved in malignancy. The number of specific sites on each graph varies, depending on the appropriate aggregation in the broad group. The pairs of graphs show the trends in mortality rate for males and then females for the major part of this century. For ease of presentation, the data for all these series of graphs are restricted to the age group 65–69; the rates are all presented on a three-cycle log scale, so that the slopes of the curves can be compared within one graph and also from one graph to another.

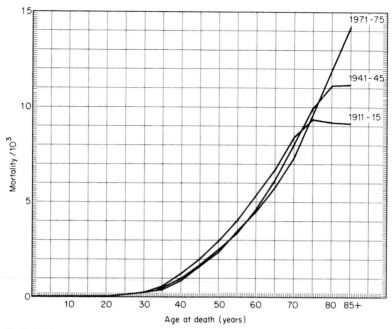

Fig 2.4 All neoplasms: mortality rates for females by age at death in England and Wales, 1911–15, 1941–45, 1971–75.

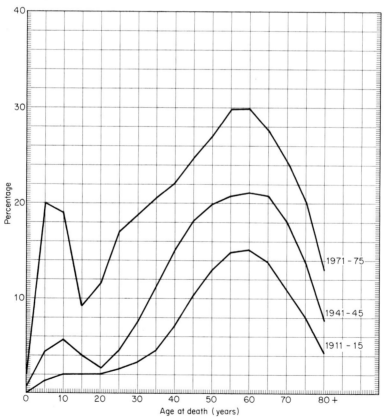

Fig. 2.5 All neoplasms: deaths as a percentage of deaths from all causes for males by age at death in England and Wales, 1911–15, 1941–45, 1971–75.

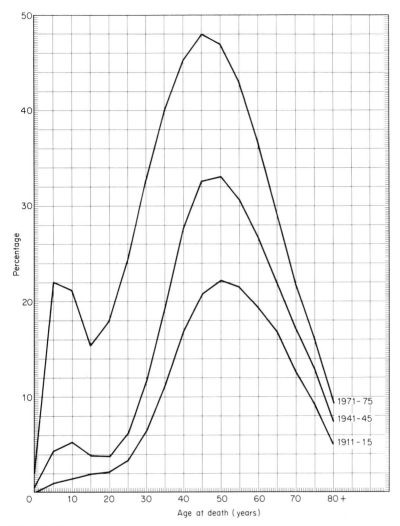

Fig. 2.6 All neoplasms: deaths as a percentage of deaths from all causes for females by age at death in England and Wales, 1911–15, 1941–45, 1971–75.

Figure 2.7 presents data for the alimentary tract for males. In general, the alterations in the rates have been similar for both sexes. Stomach, intestines and rectum all show a decline for both sexes, though there is a slight suggestion that this has slowed in the recent years, particularly for intestinal cancers. Very different is the curve for pancreas which shows an increase throughout the century for both sexes. Intermediate between these are the curves for oesophagus which show a degree of undulation, though the rates appear to be climbing for both sexes over the past thirty years. Similarly, the rates for liver and gall bladder have decreased throughout the major proportion of this century, but again show cessation of the fall or even a modest rise in the males.

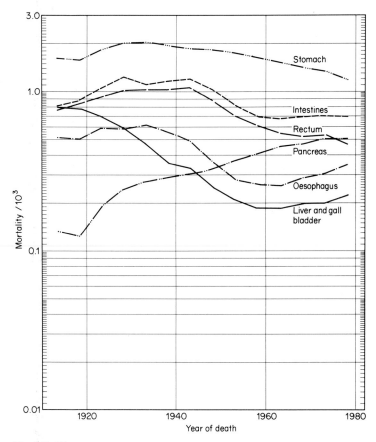

Fig. 2.7 Alimentary cancers: mortality rates for specific sites for males aged 65–69 years, England and Wales, 1911–78.

The next graph (Fig. 2.8) shows the trends for respiratory cancer for females. The overall picture is a horrifying rise in the lung cancer rates for both males and females. For males, the rates for larynx, pharynx, and mouth and tonsil showed a rise at the earlier part of the century and then a decline from about the early 1930s which appears to persist up until the latest date. For the females, the rates are slightly different, showing no appreciable increase or decrease throughout the century.

The next pair of graphs really require separate consideration as they show genito-urinary cancers for males and females. Figure 2.9 shows bladder, kidney and suprarenal, and two sex-specific cancers—prostates and testis. The testis curve (which is based on the lowest number of deaths) shows no appreciable trend in mortality rates throughout the century; however, this is an example where selection of one age group provides a very incomplete picture, as the trends in the younger age groups have shown an increase in testicular cancer. Prostate cancer appeared to show a rise at the earlier part of the century, but no appreciable change since the 1940s. Kidney and suprarenal and bladder cancer both show a

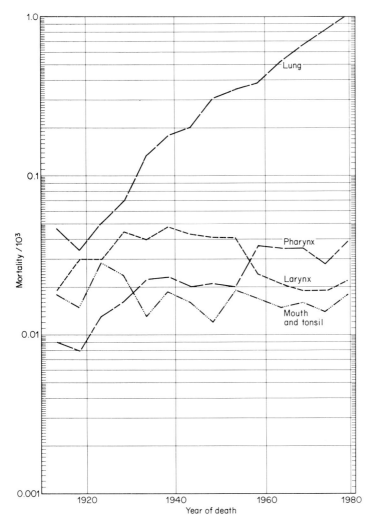

Fig. 2.8 Respiratory cancers: mortality rates for specific sites for females aged 65–69 years, England and Wales, 1911–78.

rise during this century, which is more marked for the kidney than for the bladder. The female data (Fig. 2.10) provide, of course, very different sex-specific sites; for the bladder and kidney the trends are comparable, with a modest rise at both of these sites which is slightly greater for kidney than for bladder. Data are only available throughout the century for uterus as a whole and this shows a steady fall in mortality throughout the period. This is more than balanced by a steady increase in mortality from ovarian cancer. Data were only available from the early 1940s for cervical cancer and the remainder of the uterus; these indicate a modest fall at both sites throughout a forty-year period. Cancer of the breast shows a very slight increase in mortality, which has occurred throughout the century.

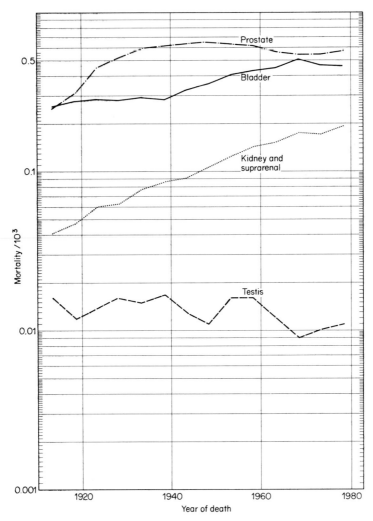

Fig. 2.9 Genito-urinary cancers: mortality rates for specific sites for males aged 65–69 years in England and Wales, 1911–78.

Figure 2.11 shows the trends in mortality rates for females from haematopoietic and lymphatic neoplasms. Data are only available throughout the century for leukaemia as a whole and Hodgkin's disease. Both these show rises for either sex, which is more marked for leukaemia than for Hodgkin's disease. Data are available for more specific sub-groups of other neoplasms in the broad category for the past twenty years. These appear to show an increase in all forms of these neoplasms, though some are based on small numbers. The lymphosarcoma and reticulum cell sarcoma trends show an increase and then a decrease with the latest data, whilst multiple myeloma, polycythaemia vera and other neoplasms of lymphoid tissue show relatively steady increases (after allowing for the small numbers of deaths).

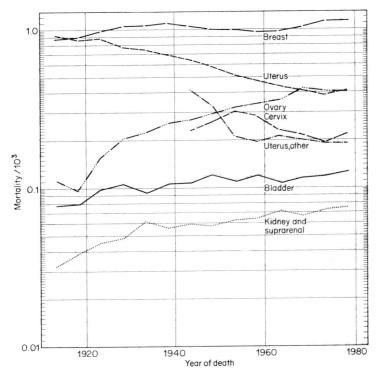

Fig. 2.10 Genito-urinary cancers: mortality rates for specific sites for females aged 65–69 years in England and Wales, 1911–78.

Figure 2.12 presents some miscellaneous sites that do not fit into any of the preceding groups of sites. Data are available throughout the century for skin cancer (excluding scrotal cancer in males) and for both sexes this shows a steady decrease. Melanoma was separately identified in the national statistics from the 1950s and for both sexes there is an appreciable rise in mortality data. There was no major variation for deaths from bone tumours other than of the jaw for the early part of the century, but there was some decline in the last thirty years (this may seem a peculiar exclusion of jaw, but is due to the classification used in the earlier part of the century). In contrast, tumours of the brain showed no appreciable variation in the first thirty years but a fairly steady rise from 1940 onwards. The graph also presents data for scrotal cancer, the rates having decreased appreciably throughout the century.

A rather different way of reviewing the overall change in malignancy for the different sites is to calculate the percentage change in the age-specific rates for the different sexes for a specific age group. Again the age group 65–69 has been used; for many sites this is an age group at which there is a relatively large number of deaths and thus fairly stable age-specific rates. Table 2.3 shows the data for male death rates; the various sites have been listed in International Classification of Diseases (ICD) order. The age-specific rate for 1926–30 is provided and then the latest available rate for 1978. The percentage changes in the rates are then presented in the table. There is an horrific rise in lung cancer, but for the majority

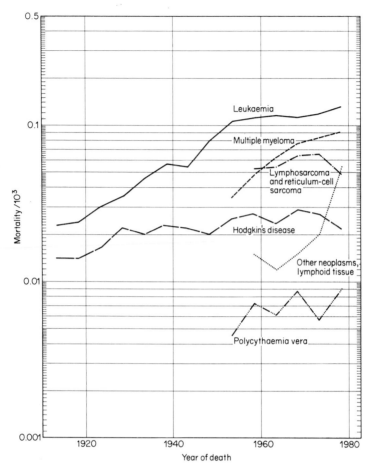

Fig. 2.11 Haematopoietic and lymphatic neoplasms: mortality rates for specific neoplasms for females aged 65–69 years in England and Wales, 1911–78.

of other sites there is a decrease, the exceptions being pancreas, breast (of course based on very small numbers), prostate, bladder, kidney and suprarenal, brain tumours, Hodgkin's disease and leukaemia. For females, comparable data are not presented though lung cancer also shows the most marked change—a change that is out of all proportion to any of the other variations that have occurred. There is an appreciable increase in the mortality from cancer of the pharynx, oesophagus, and pancreas; a very small increase in cancer of the breast, ovary, bladder, kidney, brain tumour, and leukaemia. The general patterns are thus similar for the different sexes, despite the relative importance of sex-specific cancers.

International data

Obviously in a brief review such as this it is not possible to provide an adequate range of data to demonstrate the variation in malignancy across the world and the trends site by site. Limited data are presented in Table 2.4; this has ranked a

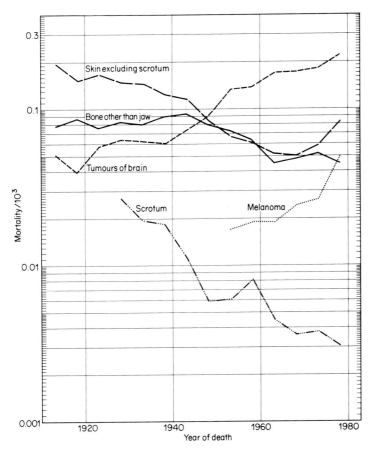

Fig. 2.12 Other neoplasms: mortality rates for various sites for males aged 65–69 years in England and Wales, 1911–78.

number of populations throughout the world in order of age-adjusted malignancy for 'all sites except skin cancer' for males. These data are based on the publication of Waterhouse *et al.* (1976). The table is based on selection for sixteen localities with varying populations; sometimes the registry material has been presented for the entire population in the locality (such as Saarland), whilst other material is restricted to a sub-group of the population (such as Blacks in Bulawayo). The final column in the table shows more than a twofold scatter in adjusted rates for males for all sites; there is a similar scatter for females, but very different ranking in the localities. For the selected sites, the relative variation from the locality with the highest to lowest rate is considerably greater (for example, lip cancer in males varies from 16.4 for Sascatchewan to 0.1 for Osaka). For each separate site the variation is different, both for males and for females. The locality with the highest rate for males may be quite different for that having the highest rate for females for a specific site; similarly, there is a difference in the ranking of the localities from site to site. These data are presented just to indicate the variation that exists across the world at the present time as far as registration data are concerned.

Table 2.3 Malignant disease: mortality rates for various sites for males aged 65–69 in England and Wales in 1926–30 and 1978, and percentage change in the rates

Site	1926–30	1978	Percentage change
Lip	0.088	0.004	− 95
Tongue	0.422	0.022	− 95
Mouth and tonsils	0.264	0.041	− 84
Pharynx	0.166	0.053	− 54
Oesophagus	0.584	0.345	− 41
Stomach	2.009	1.168	− 42
Intestines	1.225	0.691	− 44
Rectum	1.018	0.465	− 54
Liver and gall bladder	0.599	0.227	− 62
Pancreas	0.245	0.500	+ 104
Larynx	0.301	0.103	− 66
Lung and pleura	0.169	4.988	+2851
Bones	0.244	0.053	− 78
Skin excluding scrotum	0.149	0.086	− 42
Breast	0.014	0.019	+ 36
Prostate	0.524	0.578	+ 10
Testes	0.016	0.011	− 31
Penis and scrotum	0.075	0.015	− 80
Bladder	0.280	0.466	+ 66
Kidneys and suprarenals	0.063	0.192	+ 205
Brain tumours	0.064	0.222	+ 247
Thyroid	na	0.022	—
Hodgkin's disease	0.034	0.042	+ 24
Leukaemia	0.042	0.220	+ 424

No attempt is made here to present data on trends in incidence or mortality comparable to the material that has been reviewed above for England and Wales. Where variation in the international trends has been relevant to consideration of the aetiology of malignancy, this is specifically discussed in the next chapter on cause of malignancy.

Survival from malignancy

Table 2.5 contains the latest survival data for England and Wales (OPCS, 1980). The material is listed in ICD order of site, and shows for males and females the numbers of each cancer registered in 1971–73, and then the one- and five-year relative survival. The relative survival is the actual survival adjusted for the expected mortality from all causes in the follow-up period, after taking into account the age distribution and sex of the patients registered with cancer and the population age/sex mortality rates for the same calendar period.

It can readily be seen that the five-year survival varies considerably from site to site. Liver cancer has the worst results with less than 3 per cent alive after five years, closely followed by pancreas (less than 4 per cent), and lung (less than 8 per cent). At the other extreme, skin cancer other than melanoma has about 100 per cent survival, whilst all the female gynaecological sites have good results. It must be emphasized that the table does not include data for every site; those involving relatively few patients or with imprecisely defined sites have been

Table 2.4 Malignant disease of various sites: age-adjusted incidence for 16 localities throughout the world by sex, 1969–73

Area/population	Lip	Oesophagus		Large intestine	Lung	Breast	Ovary	Prostate	Kidney	Lympho-sarcoma	All sites	(except skin)
	Male	Male	Female	Male	Male	Female	Female	Male	Male	Male	Male	Female
Bulawayo (Black)	0.1	63.8	2.2	7.0	70.7	13.8	8.1	32.3	1.2	1.7	345.9	147.4
Hawaii (Hawaiian)	0.0	8.0	1.6	14.1	71.3	66.2	11.6	19.8	6.8	6.7	288.2	272.1
Alameda (White)	4.0	3.6	1.5	25.3	55.5	76.1	13.5	40.4	7.1	8.1	277.7	267.8
Saarland	1.3	4.9	1.0	15.5	67.7	50.6	9.3	21.1	6.0	2.4	257.6	234.5
Ayrshire	2.9	5.9	1.9	16.6	68.8	50.1	9.9	19.2	6.1	2.7	242.3	172.2
Saskatchewan	16.4	2.5	0.7	17.8	35.6	62.8	11.0	39.0	8.5	5.3	237.0	204.8
Norway (Urban)	2.7	4.0	0.8	15.0	33.0	49.6	15.0	36.3	8.6	3.3	228.0	199.9
Denmark	4.8	3.1	1.4	16.2	40.2	49.1	15.1	21.8	7.2	2.8	216.3	219.1
Israel (Europe/US born)	2.0	2.6	2.0	12.9	30.3	60.8	14.7	12.6	7.2	7.3	209.9	236.8
Osaka	0.1	9.7	2.9	6.3	23.5	12.1	2.8	2.7	2.0	2.6	207.1	142.6
Cracow	7.6	3.0	0.7	6.0	45.7	19.6	9.1	8.0	3.6	1.8	196.8	143.1
Zaragoza	8.0	4.0	0.8	6.5	23.5	30.6	3.6	17.7	3.6	2.7	186.0	133.2
Puerto Rico	1.5	14.8	5.4	6.0	15.4	25.4	5.3	21.4	2.2	1.7	174.0	146.7
Cuba	2.6	5.7	2.4	6.9	44.7	28.0	4.6	18.0	1.6	2.3	169.9	147.0
New Mexico (Spanish)	0.8	2.2	1.1	8.7	16.7	32.4	10.4	34.3	5.0	1.9	157.9	177.1
Bombay	0.3	15.2	10.8	4.6	13.5	20.1	4.8	8.0	1.2	1.6	141.0	120.5

Table 2.5 Malignant disease: number of registrations and relative percentage survival at 1 and 5 years by sex and site, for patients diagnosed in England and Wales (1971–73)

Site	Sex	Number	Percentage relative survival	
			1 year	5 years
Oesophagus	M	5 033	17	6
	F	3 983	19	8
Stomach	M	19 619	19	7
	F	12 938	19	7
Large intestine except rectum	M	14 564	47	30
	F	19 703	45	29
Rectum and rectosigmoid junction	M	13 003	56	31
	F	10 537	55	33
Liver and intrahepatic bile ducts, specified	M	1 056	7	2
as primary	F	680	8	3
Pancreas	M	7 051	10	4
	F	6 071	10	3
Larynx	M	3 890	81	64
	F	725	76	57
Trachea, bronchus and lung	M	71 710	20	8
	F	16 461	18	7
Malignant melanoma of skin	M	1 253	76	48
	F	2 587	90	69
Other malignant neoplasm of skin	M	25 817	98	99
	F	22 814	99	100
Breast	F	57 232	84	57
Cervix uteri, excluding *in-situ*	F	11 965	76	83
Other malignant neoplasm of uterus	F	10 341	79	66
Ovary, fallopian tube and broad ligament	F	11 472	46	25
Prostate	M	17 943	67	36
Testis	M	1 981	80	67
Bladder	M	16 172	71	54
	F	5 629	61	47
Brain	M	3 717	27	15
	F	2 620	28	16
Thyroid gland	M	511	61	50
	F	1 368	60	53
Lymphosarcoma and reticulum-cell sar-	M	2 785	51	30
coma	F	2 435	50	32
Hodgkins disease	M	2 546	73	56
	F	1 581	73	57
Lymphatic leukaemia	M	2 560	60	30
	F	1 741	60	34
Myeloid leukaemia	M	2 314	28	8
	F	2 140	27	6

excluded. In marked contrast to the site variation, for any given site the results for either sex are remarkably similar.

No figures are given for all malignancies. This is deliberate, as the variation is so great from site to site that the overall survival will depend to a great extent upon the case mix involved.

Considerable attention was paid in a previous section (see p. 7) to the trends in mortality. Incidence data are available for England and Wales from 1961; however, though some results of survival have been published there are major problems in trying to interpret the trends. The efficiency of registration has altered with change in the proportion of patients registered after death; the method of follow-up has altered from local enquiry at hospital level to linkage to mortality records at national level; the method of calculating the survival has changed. These points directly affect the quality of the data; in addition, without valid information about the stage distribution of the patients attending for treatment it is extremely difficult to determine whether there has been an improvement in survival *per se* or a change in the stage distribution (and thus prognosis). In contrast to the limitation of national data, periodic reports from clinical studies have reported improving results from innovations in treatment.

Conclusions

The material presented here provides a somewhat cursory look at the extent of the cancer problem; in particular, very limited international data are included. The point of having this chapter is that it may serve as a background to subsequent text on prevention—by helping to differentiate the common from the rare sites of malignancy, those that are increasing or decreasing in frequency, and ones which presently respond well or poorly to medical care. Other things being equal (such as the feasibility of action), it is suggested that effort on prevention will be best directed to cancers that are common, which have increasing incidence (or mortality), and which respond poorly to treatment. Brief as the international data are, they are sufficient to emphasize that plans for cancer control will require quite different lines of action in different countries.

A very different concept is the use of routine mortality statistics to serve as a source of hunches when considering the aetiology of various cancers. This issue is beyond the scope of the present chapter, but is relevant to some of the topics discussed in the following chapter.

References

Office of Population Censuses and Surveys (OPCS) (1980). *Cancer Statistics: Survival 1971– 73 Registrations, England and Wales*. HMSO, London.

Waterhouse, J., Muir, C., Correa, P. and Powell, J. (1976). *Cancer Incidence in Five Continents*, Vol. III. International Agency for Research in Cancer, Lyon.

3

The causes of cancer

Michael Alderson

Organization of the material on aetiology

As a preliminary to discussing the prevention of cancer it is necessary to consider what is known about the causes of cancers. A rather brief review of the knowledge that presently exists on the causes of malignant disease is provided. When action on the primary prevention of cancer is to be planned, it will usually be in relation to the specific agent concerned, rather than from the axis of the site of malignancy involved. Exactly the opposite applies when considering early detection campaigns; this will usually begin with consideration of the particular site of malignancy, and then only take into account the known factors that permit division of the total population into sub-groups at various degrees of risk. Obviously it would have been possible to order the epidemiological reviews of aetiological material either by cause or by site; for a variety of reasons the latter approach has been selected for the present chapter. Either approach may lead to duplication of material, as a number of known carcinogens each involve several sites of malignancy. This occurs in the following review, but has been accompanied by liberal cross-references, the first mention of a topic usually being the location of the major treatment of the material.

Many aetiological studies are site orientated (what is the cause of oral cancer?), rather than the converse (what are the cancers caused by exposure to ionizing irradiation?). Both types of study occur, but an important point about the former is that they are the usual approach when there is no definite evidence of a specific carcinogen involved, and also they are required when there is conflicting evidence about the importance of a number of different agents in causing a specific malignancy (such as the wealth of data on a wide range of occupational causes of lung cancer, and some dispute as to the role of synergism or interaction with cigarette smoking). Also, presentation of the material site by site forms a convenient way in which to consider the extent of present knowledge, the suggestive but unproven leads, and the gaps in our knowledge (and thus consideration of the steps required in the future to further unravel the causes of cancer).

However, the main positive leads for primary prevention are then collated in the final subsection, with a table listing the known causes by site of malignancy (see p. 66 and Table 3.5).

Carcinogenesis: general considerations

When discussing the epidemiological approaches to the identification of human carcinogens, Alderson (1980a) deliberately contrasted the present knowledge on nitrosamines and arsenic. For the former, there is a wealth of laboratory information on the carcinogenic properties of a wide range of compounds but no adequate human data to indicate (let alone confirm) risk of cancer to those exposed to or producing nitrosamines. The opposite applies to arsenic; case reports from medical use, and studies of those drinking arsenic-contaminated water or exposed by occupation, document the risk of cancer—with no matching laboratory evidence of adequate standard.

Other examples could be chosen; laboratory tests have cast doubt about the safety of phenobarbitone but prospective studies of patients regularly consuming this drug over many years have not indicated an enhanced cancer mortality (see for example Clemmesen et al., 1974; Jancar, 1980). The converse is true of the epidemiological data of occupational risk from benzene exposure (see leukaemia, p. 46) which are inadequately supported by laboratory studies.

Another puzzle relates to isoniazid, which has been associated with excess tumours at various sites in mice; again, prospective studies on patients treated with this drug have failed to demonstrate a clear risk of malignancy (see Stott et al., 1976; Howe et al., 1979).

It must be accepted that some leads from the laboratory have been confirmed; for example, mutagenicity tests on ethylene oxide gave positive results, though two small animal studies were negative (IARC, 1976). Hogstedt et al. (1979) have now reported excess cancer on follow-up of a small group of exposed workers, involving leukaemia, alimentary tract and urogenital malignancy; the specific chemical associated with this could not be identified, though ethylene oxide and ethylene dichloride were suspect.

Occasionally a useful substance has been withdrawn when short-term tests of mutagenicity have been positive. For example, the main flame retardant used in children's polyester pyjamas was found to be a potent mutagen (Blum and Ames, 1977); after further laboratory studies, but with no human data relevant to assessing carcinogenicity, its use was banned in the United States. As a contrast, a recent study on 1551 deaths amongst veterinarians in the US demonstrates the limited direct contribution from some epidemiological work. This showed an excess of deaths from leukaemia, Hodgkin's disease, and cancers of the brain and skin (Blair and Hayes, 1980). Such a study cannot do more than indicate topics for detailed investigation; other work had suggested that pesticides, anaesthetics, radiation, or zoonotic viruses might influence their risk of cancer. Interesting as these findings and suggestions are, they require a range of further studies of daunting complexity to unravel the possible aetiological factors responsible. It has been suggested (Alderson, 1980d) that it is not necessary to determine the carcinogenic mechanisms involved in order to institute preventive measures; the identification of the specific factor and its portal of entry to the human body are of prime importance. Consideration of the numbers of individuals exposed, their levels of exposure, and the additional number of cancers generated is then relevant to the consideration of methods of prevention.

One of the most crucial aspects of identifying previously unsuspected carcinogens is the source of the initial lead. Alderson (1977) has briefly discussed the generation of hunches in general; leads in the cancer field have come from observation of astute clinicians (from scrotal cancer in chimney sweeps—Potts, 1775), from laboratory work (e.g. on nitrogen mustard), from serendipity in epidemiological studies (e.g. nasal cancer in boot and shoe workers—Acheson *et al.*, 1970). In many fields, advances have come not from clearly delineated research programmes but from the follow-up of the unexpected. Thus hunches, however they are derived (and if not biologically plausible), may require cross-checking; the selection of promising leads then being a matter for flair and judgement. Mixed exposure to a range of environmental agents is an accompaniment of life; case reports of an unusual association between a factor and a few patients with cancer may be the only evidence from human study of an aetiological agent.

The details of screening chemicals for carcinogenicity have been reviewed by Purchase (1980), whilst the approaches to mathematical extrapolation from animal results to man have been discussed by Gaylor and Shapiro (1979) and Albert *et al.* (1979); some of the major pitfalls have been delineated by Paddle (1980). However, these reviews do not offer an adequate blueprint for dealing with future (contentious) issues. The steps in the process are:

(i) independent scientific assessment of the validity of results from short-term animal and human studies;

(ii) extrapolation from laboratory to man, in the absence of hard data from human exposure on dose and response;

(iii) judgement of whether a chemical is a human carcinogen;

(iv) decision as to the appropriate method(s) of prevention for declared carcinogens.

Clemmesen (1977), in discussing the controversy over anticonvulsants, has hinted at the dismay of an epidemiologist when relevant human data are ignored and animal studies given emphasis. The present work is not the appropriate forum for expanding on this topic; the following sections deal with human data (particularly from epidemiological studies, but also relevant case reports). This is not to emphasize the contribution from such studies and denigrate laboratory work on carcinogenesis; it is merely a reflection of the contributor's field of work and, to a lesser extent, an acknowledgement of the wealth of literature that already exists on the assessment of carcinogenesis from other fields of work (for example, the admirable series of monographs published by the International Agency for Research in Cancer). The aim of the following sections is to cover the main literature on cause of cancer site by site, distinguishing confirmed from suggested carcinogens. One reason for concentrating upon human data is that, in the absence of definitive evidence of a specific causative factor, the material may clearly indicate variation in risk in different sub-groups of the population; this may be of value when planning early detection programmes. Despite a wealth of studies and literature that is voluminous, the confirmed hazards only account for a relatively small proportion of cancers—particularly in women. Circumstantial evidence may point to aspects of environment (including personal behaviour, or 'lifestyle'); this is of limited value for primary prevention. The injunction 'change your lifestyle' is not a feasible or acceptable approach—ignoring the important issue raised by Mill over 100 years ago in his book *On Liberty* (Mill, 1859), questioning the right of government or society to influence the behaviour of an individual.

Validity of data

Before reviewing information relevant to the consideration of the causes of cancer, it is essential to consider the validity of such material. The general comments which follow must be read and borne in mind when considering any of the evidence that then follows; it is impossible to deal in a relatively short contribution with a detailed appraisal of the validity of each separate item of information that is presented. Use has to be made of these general comments to help guide the interpretation of the remaining material.

In considering the value of routine mortality or morbidity data, attention must be paid to the denominator used in producing the rates; this is especially so for the more detailed statistics that relate to sub-groups of the population such as statistics by race, religion, urban/rural residence, or migrants by country of origin. A comparable issue is the suitability of the data that are used in collation studies (e.g. relating mortality rates for a specific malignancy to estimates of the per capita intake of certain nutrients); there are the two rather different problems of the validity of the population data and the appropriateness of this as a measure of genuine differences in populations' risks of exposure to specific carcinogens.

The other aspect of the routine mortality and morbidity data is the validity of the diagnostic information. For mortality, has the cause of death been correctly identified, and if so, is this incorporated in the statistics (is the certification, coding and processing correct)? For morbidity, the issues are similar, but begin with the concern that there may be variation in the completeness of registration (are all recognized cancers appropriately documented so that details about them are incorporated in the statistics?). Again, there is concern that the recognition of different sites of malignancy may vary from one sub-group in the population to another, or from one period of time to another.

An important point about all these considerations is that the chief use of such statistics is to identify variation in the rate of incidence or mortality from cancer, and then seek for (environmental) explanations for such variation. Obviously variation in the quality of the statistics can generate false degrees of variation, and lead to major problems of interpretation.

Alderson (1981) has discussed at some length the validity of such statistics; in summary, comparisons over time within one country and between countries for the same time period can be readily distorted by variation in the accuracy of the basic statistics. The causes of bias and error in the data must be carefully considered before trying to interpret such data. Sub-groups of the population may have very different health care facilities, with quite different degrees of diagnostic precision or certification efficiency. Change over time may also be due to system effects, rather than to genuine differences in exposure to environmental carcinogens. In particular, care must be taken with collation studies, which may utilize very imprecise data on estimates of population exposure to various agents. In addition, the tendency to examine many different causes of death and a wide range of 'environmental' factors can result in a very large number of statistical comparisons being made; it then becomes difficult to distinguish the false positive (chance) correlations that may be found from those that genuinely reflect the biological relationships underlying the cause of disease.

As far as aetiological studies are concerned, routine mortality and morbidity statistics are really only a starting point, either in stimulating ideas about possible aetiology, or to help in sifting leads derived from other sources. They are not really appropriate for specific hypothesis testing which requires the use of purpose collected data from case-control or prospective studies. Such studies may require careful consideration of the specific design being used, as well as the innate validity of the type of data collected, before they can be adequately interpreted. Alderson (1977) reviewed some general points concerned with the validity of data derived from self-completion questionnaires, interview, examination, or investigation. It must be remembered that many studies are launched without adequate investigation being carried out to test rigorously the validity of the data collection system. It is often assumed that material collected in various forms of special study is of adequate quality.

Quite different is the need to consider the study design in some detail. As with mortality data, the crucial issue is whether there has been any (hidden) bias in the selection of subjects or in the validity of the data collected from cases and controls, or the other sub-groups in the study population. One general aspect of this is the response rate amongst the individuals invited to participate.

Case-control studies

As far as the design of the studies is concerned, the following points need to be borne in mind.

1. Has the source of cases and controls introduced bias in the likelihood of exposure to various factors, irrespective of whether they are aetiologically important?

2. Has the response rate been different in these groups, and are the responders a biased sub-group of the total population?

3. Has any characteristic of the cases or controls affected the validity of the data collected from them, independent of the relationship of the item to the cause of the malignancy being studied?

Prospective studies

In general, these involve selecting 'healthy' subjects, collecting exposure data from each of the respondents, following the subjects up to an agreed end point, and then analysing the dose response. Obviously, this is over-simplification of the complexity that can be involved in prospective studies; there are many variations from the basic study design.

In considering the interpretation of data, the following points need to be borne in mind.

1. Was the study population biased in any way that would affect either the validity of the initial data collection or the subsequent incidence/mortality of the cancer being studied?

2. Was the response rate from the subjects adequate?

3. Was valid data collected from each of the subjects? (This may be estimated by replicate interviewing, cross-interviewing of different individuals knowing the respondent, checking supporting evidence for any information obtained, reviewing pathology etc. where appropriate, comparison of the distribution of results obtained from the respondents with other sets of statistics, validating the overall data collection system on a small sample by detailed study.)

4. Has involvement in a prospective study and the 'observation' of the respondents resulted in any change in their behaviour—either a change in degree of exposure to an aetiological agent, or change that would alter the efficiency with which the subsequent incidence or mortality from cancer is identified?

5. Has the drop-out rate of individuals during the follow-up been such that the results are distorted?

6. Have an adequate number of 'events' (either incidence or mortality) occurred?

7. Was the length of follow-up adequate for cancers to develop with the anticipated latent interval?

In considering the interpretation of any study, the method of analysis needs to be considered; the basic method may be to examine the incidence or mortality in exposed and non-exposed individuals. Where appropriate data are available, the dose–response relationship may be investigated. It is important to consider whether there are other confounding or intervening factors that influence the likelihood of the various respondents developing the cancer being studied. In certain circumstances (particularly with historical prospective studies which will be discussed in the following section), the observed events are compared with calculated 'expected' events. These expected figures may either be based on the survey data or derived from application of national or other 'external' rates which are not derived from the study population.

The ultimate point being whether the prospective study leads to support of an inference of causality, it has been suggested that Mill's canons apply. These indicate that the following should be considered: the method of difference (for example, variation in exposure being followed by variation in risk of development of the cancer), the method of agreement (with replication of the study producing similar results), the method of concomitant variation (various sub-groups, for instance different age, sex and racial groups, all showing the same overall relationship between exposure and risk of disease), or the method of residues (for example, studying lung cancer risk in urban and rural areas in non-smokers). The absolute number of subjects followed may not be as important in such studies as the duration of follow-up. However, where there has been lengthy follow-up, it may mean that the subjects developing the disease may have been exposed to conditions many years ago which no longer now apply. When considering such findings, caution has to be observed to see that the data are still relevant to the present day or the future.

Historical prospective study

Particularly in the occupational field, prospective studies may be carried out by retrieving data which identify individuals exposed in the past to a particular environment, and then so organizing the study that the subsequent incidence or mortality from malignant disease in the subjects is obtained. The following points require consideration.

1. How accurate are the old records, particularly in identifying all the individuals, and the quality of the documented 'exposure'?

2. Has adequate follow-up been permitted by the use of such records in order to generate reliable data on the numbers developing or dying from malignancy?

3. Is the calculated expected figure (often based on national mortality or

incidence data after adjusting for age, sex and calendar period) appropriate to the study population?

Investigation of exposed/unexposed individuals

Such a study is not particularly suitable for cancer, but is more often used when searching for the development of a chronic disease which is likely to have a relatively high prevalence in the exposed individuals. It may be suitable in the malignant disease field where a search can be made for either in-situ and pre-cancerous lesions or other change, such as the development of chromosome abnormality in the exposed individuals. Analysis should permit comparison of the prevalence of such measures in sub-groups with different levels of exposure to some suspect agent.

Was the study designed as descriptive or hypothesis testing?

Many papers reporting a positive association between particular exposure and development of cancer do not clearly indicate on what basis the study was designed, or whether the observed 'significant results' were deliberately sought in testing a hypothesis. The important point here is that, where an extensive survey has been designed as a descriptive or exploratory study, it may be possible to carry out a large number of internal comparisons of the data. Whatever level of significance is chosen to indicate findings unlikely to be due to chance, with a very large number of comparisons authors can report 'positive' findings that are no more than would have been anticipated due to the repeated probing of the data. If some adjustment for such a procedure has not been carried out, the cautious approach is to require replication of the study in some other locality (perhaps using a slightly different technique) and await confirmatory results from such a further study.

Cancer of different sites

Digestive organs

Cancers of the alimentary tract as an entity are a major cause of mortality, though the overall extent is usually 'hidden' by presenting data separately for individual sites of malignancy (as in Table 2.1, and Figs. 2.7 and 2.8). For males in England and Wales in 1978, the sites oral cavity, oesophagus, stomach, large intestine, rectum, liver, gall bladder and pancreas together were responsible for 20 907 deaths—a figure only exceeded by that for lung cancer.

Over the present century the trend in England and Wales has been one of declining mortality for six of the sites concerned; the exception is the fairly steady rise for pancreas for the whole period. The rate of decline appears to be slowing at the present time for some of the other sites, whilst liver and oesophagus appear to have a rising mortality for the recent years. This suggests that 'environmental' changes in the beginning of the century may have been beneficial, except for some additional hazard for pancreatic cancer; in addition, more recent changes have added again to the risk of oesophageal and liver cancer. The extent to which improved diagnosis is responsible for change in these statistics is difficult to quantify.

Oral cavity

This is a site with major inter- and intranational variation (Sanghvi *et al.*, 1955; Blot and Fraumeni, 1977). Evidence strongly suggests that smoking, chewing tobacco, oral snuff usage, and alcoholic beverages were aetiological factors (Sanghvi *et al.*, 1955; Wynder and Bross, 1957; Brown *et al.*, 1965; Larsson *et al.*, 1975; Graham *et al.*, 1977). Chewing tobacco includes the use of betel-nut and betel leaf and lime in some communities.

Variation in occupational groups has been reported but no specific process has been adequately demonstrated as being involved. Moss and Lee (1974) indicated that textile workers had a higher mortality from this cancer, but a case-control study in two main textile regions in England failed to confirm that any specific process was associated with increased risk (Whitaker *et al.*, 1979).

Nasopharynx

This is another infrequent site for cancer amongst Whites in Europe and America; the Chinese constitute a unique high-risk group in the Orient. The standardized mortality ratio (SMR) is lower in second than first generation Chinese migrants in the US (King and Haenszel, 1973).

There appears to be a genetic component to this condition, with an increased frequency of HLA-2 in patients. It has been suggested that this may be linked to the ability to metabolize a potential carcinogen (Henderson *et al.*, 1976).

The main aetiological agent identified is the increased prevalence of Epstein–Barr infection (identified in cells from the tumours or in patients' sera). Hospital studies showed an increased prevalence of infection in staff nursing these cancer patients, which increased in relation to the proximity of patient and staff (Ho, Kwan *et al.*, 1978). A case-control study investigated a number of carcinogens known to induce nasal or lung cancer; these showed no association with nasopharyngeal cancer (Ho, Huang and Fong, 1978). However, such patients were found to be more likely to eat traditional foods, such as salted fish. The significance of this was not clear.

Oesophagus

Many authors have delineated a high-risk zone involving parts of East Africa, the Middle East through Northern Iran, southern portions of the USSR, Afghanistan into China (Day, E. and Munoz, N., personal communication). Evidence suggests that there is a number of different aetiological agents, not all of which are present in each high-risk zone.

Work in the UK and Iran suggests that there is a genetic component which can influence risk of the disease. It is only likely to be responsible for a small proportion of the total cases (Howell-Evans *et al.*, 1958; Pour and Ghadirian, 1974). Alcohol undoubtedly plays a part, for example in Northern France (where distilled apple spirits are drunk), and an independent effect of smoking has been noted. Analysis of data on both factors indicates there is a multiplicative effect in persons smoking and drinking (Tuyns *et al.*, 1977). Extensive studies in Northern Iran and China have not yet identified specific causal factors—though alcohol is certainly not responsible. There is a strong suggestion that dietary deficiency is associated with high risk (Cook-Mozaffari *et al.*, 1979), whilst one paper has incriminated a particular usage of opium (Hewer *et al.*, 1978). Elsewhere, dietary deficiency (in the form of Plummer–Vinson syndrome) had also been identified as a risk factor (Wynder *et al.*, 1957).

Though no specific dietary carcinogen has been identified, consumption of food at high temperatures appears to increase the risk of this cancer (de Jong *et al.*, 1974). A specific but rare aetiological factor was lye burns (Imre and Kopp, 1972). Occupational studies have suggested increased risk in those exposed to asbestos; this is not one of the major risks associated with asbestos (Selikoff and Hammond, 1975). Comparison of the occupational mortality supplements for England and Wales for 1959–63 and 1970–72 showed farming as the only consistently increased SMR, and the increase was less than twofold (Registrar General, 1971; 1978).

Stomach

The decrease in mortality in Western countries and the international variation have not clearly pointed to aetiological factors. The importance of the environment is emphasized by the decreasing risk of stomach cancer in Japanese migrants to Hawaii and the US; there is a lowered risk in second generation individuals, whilst there is an even lower risk amongst US native Whites (Haenszel and Kurihara, 1968).

Genetic studies, despite their limitations, do suggest that gastric cancer is concentrated in some families (Graham and Lilienfeld, 1958). There is also increased incidence in persons with blood group A (Aird *et al.*, 1954), ABH non-secretors (Doll *et al.*, 1961), Blacks compared with Whites in the US (Wynder *et al.*, 1963), and those with pernicious anaemia (Mosbech and Videbaek, 1950)— though it was not clear whether this was due to changes resulting simply from the presence of the pernicious anaemia or some common aetiological factor.

Collation and case-control studies suggest that deficiency of fresh fruit, vegetables and salads is associated with increased risk; no specific carcinogen in the diet has been identified (Saxen, 1961; Dungal and Sigurjonsson, 1967; Haenszel *et al.*, 1976). Endogenous and exogenous nitrosamines have been proposed as relevant on somewhat tenuous evidence (Alderson, 1980a).

Other work indicates that cigarette smoking (Hammond and Horn, 1958), atmospheric pollution (Stocks, 1960), and work in dusty jobs such as coal-mining (Registrar General, 1978) may all be associated with increased incidence or mortality from stomach cancer. In contrast to the US study, there was no association with smoking in the UK doctors (Doll and Peto, 1976; Doll *et al.*, 1980). Specific studies have also incriminated poor dental hygiene or oral sepsis (Herbert and Bruske, 1936), and use of liquid paraffin as a purgative (Boyd and Doll, 1954); these findings have not been confirmed in other studies. Conflicting views also exist on whether the subsequent risk of stomach cancer following peptic ulcer is different from that in the general population (Hirohata, 1968; Stalsberg and Taksdal, 1971; Nicholls, 1974).

Colorectal cancer

Cancers of the colon and rectum show comparable mortality trends this century in England and Wales, with a decrease and then more recent suggestion of rise at the same ages in both males and females. Though the rates roughly parallel the trends of stomach cancer, this is not reflected in the international variation in mortality rates; countries with high rates of stomach cancer tend to have low colorectal cancer mortality rates and vice versa. Persons living in rural areas tend to have low rates (Clemmesen, 1977). Mormons have a lower rate of these cancers than the general population (Enstrom, 1978), whilst a recent study suggests this is also so for Seventh Day Adventists (Phillips, 1975). There appears to be no clear social class trend for colon cancer, but higher mortality for rectal cancer in Social Class III manual, IV and V (Registrar General, 1978). Migrant studies show low rates for Japanese living in Japan, which rise in first and then second generation migrants into the US (Haenszel and Kurihara, 1968). There are other examples of rates rising on migration, and this change may occur within relatively few years of migration (Haenszel and Dawson, 1965). Collation of national statistics has suggested that increased risk of colorectal cancer is associated with: increased average temperature (McVay, 1968); diets containing excess fat and animal protein (Gregor et al., 1969; Shrauzer, 1976), and those that are deficient in fibre, particularly the pentose fraction (Bingham et al., 1979); excess beer consumption (Knox, 1977; Enstrom, 1977; McMichael, 1979).

A definite genetic component exists, though this is only directly responsible for a small proportion of the cancers that develop. In addition to familial polyposis coli (Bussey, 1975), there is increased incidence in (1) other syndromes with multiple colonic adenoma—such as Garner's and Turcot's syndromes, and (2) other hereditary large bowel disease—such as coeliac disease, Crohn's disease, and ulcerative colitis (Wennstrom et al., 1974). Quite apart from such hereditary disease it has been suggested that bowel cancers are more likely to follow appendicectomy (Hyams and Wynder, 1968; Hornbak and Amtrup, 1970), schistosomiasis (Ch'en et al., 1965), and uretero-sigmoidostomy (Haney and McGarity, 1971).

The international data on diet have stimulated a search for an association with specific nutrients in case-control studies. There are very limited positive results; one study suggested that excess meat intake was a factor to consider (Haenszel et al., 1973), whilst a small case-control study suggested that the cases had a diet that combined high saturated fat food with low fibre-containing foods (Dales et al., 1979). Many other studies were negative for both fat and meat intake— perhaps a reflection of the great difficulty of such studies (Stocks, 1957; Pernu, 1960; Higginson, 1966; Wynder and Shigematsu, 1967; Wynder et al., 1969; Bjelke, 1971; Bjelke, 1974; IARC, 1977; Graham et al., 1978). International comparisons had suggested that the bacterial flora and faecal bile acids were different in high- and low-risk populations; the hypothesis was advanced that diet influenced the flora and hence the production of carcinogenic metabolites (Aries et al., 1969; Hill et al., 1971). It was of great interest when support for this was obtained from a small case-control study of in-patients (Hill et al., 1975). However, subsequent findings from this research team's work have generated some unexplained results (Bone et al., 1975; IARC, 1977); and a number of other groups carrying out comparable projects in metabolic epidemiology failed to confirm the work (Finegold et al., 1974; Mower et al., 1979).

The international data suggested beer consumption might be a risk factor. Excess large bowel adenoma were reported in one study of alcoholics (Diamond,

1952). The confusing results from case-control studies are discussed in the section on alcohol (p. 47). Three historical prospective studies have explored the subsequent incidence or mortality from colorectal cancer in those thought to consume about average quantities of alcohol (particularly beer) (Hakulinen *et al.*, 1974; Dean *et al.*, 1979; Jensen, 1979). Only one of these (Dean *et al.*, 1979) showed an appreciable excess of large bowel cancer (that was significant for rectum, but not for colon).

Other factors highlighted by one or more case-control studies have been constipation and the use of laxatives (Boyd and Doll, 1954), prior irradiation (Brinkley and Haybittle, 1969; Smith and Doll, 1976), and a raised risk in women having higher parity than control subjects (Bjelke, 1971; 1974). Occupational studies confirm an increased risk in those exposed to asbestos (McDonald *et al.*, 1971); there is a suggestion of higher mortality in chemists (Li *et al.*, 1969; Olin, 1976) and in workers at refineries (Hanis *et al.*, 1979; Rushton and Alderson, 1980). No specific associations with particular processes or chemicals have been reported.

Liver

This section is chiefly concerned with primary hepatocellular cancer of the liver; some comments are also made about angiosarcoma of the liver.

There are clusters of high mortality of liver cancer in (1) Eastern South Asia, (2) south of the Sahara, and (3) in South and East Europe (Aoki, 1978). Many of the populations so involved are not covered by adequate incidence or mortality statistics; where mortality statistics are available the distinction between primary and secondary cancers may vary in precision.

Glycogen-storage disorders and haemachromatosis, which have a genetic aetiology, are associated with an increased risk of such cancers (Mulvihill, 1975).

Studies in Africa, Asia, Australia, Greece, UK and the US have shown more frequent evidence of present or past infection with hepatitis B in cases compared with controls (Vogel *et al.*, 1970; Anthony *et al.*, 1972; Maupas *et al.*, 1975; Larouze *et al.*, 1976; Tabor *et al.*, 1977; Turbitt *et al.*, 1977; McCaugham *et al.*, 1979). That this was not so for patients with liver metastases suggests that it is not the presence of the cancer in the liver that is leading to the evidence of infection (Trichopoulos *et al.*, 1978). There is indication that prior infection with typhoid (Welton *et al.*, 1979) is more likely to be followed by liver cancer; this is only thought to be relevant to a small proportion of cases.

In Africa surveys have indicated an association between high incidence of the cancer in populations and the degree to which they eat aflatoxin-contaminated foods (Peers and Linsell, 1973). There is some suggestion that prior infection with hepatitis or dietary deficiency may be an added risk factor in such populations (Shank, 1977).

The evidence on cirrhosis and alcohol is somewhat confusing. Patients with cancer of the liver have a higher prevalence of cirrhosis than controls (Mori, 1967). A case-control study of liver cancer found an association with alcohol intake (Williams and Horn, 1977). However, a number of prospective studies of individuals consuming an excess of alcohol have failed to find a raised mortality from liver cancer (Schmidt and de Lindt, 1972; Pell and D'Alonzo, 1973; Nicholls *et al.*, 1974; Monson and Lyon, 1975; Robinette *et al.*, 1979); others have suggested an excess (Hakulinen *et al.*, 1974), one report without observed and expected deaths (Rubin and Lieber, 1975).

A limited role has been suggested for various drug usage, such as anabolic steroids (Johnson *et al.*, 1972), immunosuppression (Kinlen *et al.*, 1979), and oral contraceptives (Baum *et al.*, 1973; Klatskin, 1977). The latter risk is thought to be very low in the UK (Vessey *et al.*, 1977).

It must be emphasized that angiosarcoma of the liver is a much less frequent tumour that is still predominantly of unexplained aetiology. However, increased risk occurs in individuals exposed to arsenic, anabolic steroids, thorotrast, and vinyl chloride monomer (Falk *et al.*, 1979).

Gall bladder and biliary tract

Biliary tract cancer is much less common than primary liver cancer. In a US study, patients with cancer of the gall bladder had a significantly higher prevalence of gall-stones than would be expected from the population incidence of this condition (Maram *et al.*, 1979).

Autopsy studies in the Far East have shown that biliary tract cancer may be associated with parasite infestations, such as *Clonorchis sinensis* (Hou, 1956) or opisthorchiasis (Bhamarapravati and Viranuvatti, 1966; Sonakul *et al.*, 1978).

Pancreas

This site provides the predominant exception to trend data for digestive organ cancers; the mortality from pancreatic cancer shows an appreciable rise during the century, with high rates in developed countries. Two studies in the US showed particularly high rates amongst Blacks (Krain, 1971; Mancuso and Sterling, 1974), whilst English data showed no social class gradient (Registrar General, 1978).

Japanese migrants to the US appear to have higher mortality from pancreas cancer than Japanese in Japan or Whites in the US (Haenszel and Kurihara, 1968), whilst rates rise for migrants from a number of European countries going to the US (Haenszel, 1961).

Collation studies have shown associations with consumption of coffee (Stocks, 1970), sugar or sweets (Shenn and Bishop, 1974), alcohol (Breslow and Enstrom, 1974), egg and animal protein (Armstrong and Doll, 1975). Dietary studies of patients have not confirmed any of these suggestions.

Case-control studies of alcohol consumption have given conflicting results (Burch and Ansari, 1968; Wynder *et al.*, 1973), whilst follow-up of those known to take excess alcohol show virtually the same observed and expected deaths when pooling six studies (Pell and D'Alonzo, 1973; Hakulinen *et al.*, 1974; Monson and Lyon, 1975; Dean *et al.*, 1979; Jensen, 1979; Robinette *et al.*, 1979).

Three case-control studies showed an excess of diabetics (Clark and Mitchell, 1961; Karmody and Kyle, 1969; Wynder *et al.*, 1973), whilst follow-up of a large cohort of diabetics confirmed that a significant excess developed pancreatic cancer (Kessler, 1970). There have also been case reports (Bartholomew *et al.*, 1958; Gambill, 1971) and case-control studies indicating an association with pancreatitis (Wynder *et al.*, 1973), but it is not clear if this is due to confounding with alcohol consumption. One case-control study showed an association with prior cholecystectomy (Wynder *et al.*, 1973).

Case-control studies (Wynder *et al.*, 1973) and prospective studies (e.g. Doll and Peto, 1976) have clearly shown an increased risk with cigarette smoking, which is compatible with the trends in mortality for this cancer.

Limited evidence indicates an association of increased mortality with work involving chemicals (Li *et al.*, 1969); the only specific lead is from exposure to β-naphthylamine (Mancuso and El-Attar, 1967).

Nasal cancer

This is a very rare form of cancer; less than 0.1 per cent of deaths from cancers in males were due to this neoplasm in England and Wales in 1978. All the accepted aetiological leads point to a range of occupational factors. Evidence suggests the following work potentiates the risk: (1) boot and shoe manufacture (Acheson *et al.*, 1970; Cecchi *et al.*, 1980)—the dusty parts of the plant appear to be at highest risk, but the agent involved is not yet identified; (2) isopropyl alcohol manufacture (Weil *et al.*, 1952; Alderson and Rattan, 1980)—again the chemical that is responsible has yet to be confirmed, though there is evidence that it may be an alkyl sulphate (Lynch *et al.*, 1979); (3) nickel refinery workers have an increased risk of nasal cancer in addition to lung cancer (Doll *et al.*, 1977; see p. 34); (4) wood workers, particularly those exposed to the dust from hard woods, have a greatly increased risk of nasal cancer (Acheson *et al.*, 1967)—the specific agent has not been confirmed.

Larynx

Mortality rates in England and Wales increased in the early part of this century and then declined; this decline has now ceased and at some ages the mortality is again increasing. Collation studies have suggested an association with the chemical industry (Hoover and Fraumeni, 1975), low economic status (Blot *et al.*, 1978), and alcohol and cigarette consumption (McMichael, 1978a and 1978b).

This is not a site for which an appreciable genetic component is usually suggested, but Trell *et al.* (1976) have found that an excess proportion of male patients possess the appropriate enzymes for aryl hydrocarbon hydroxylase inducibility.

Smoking and alcohol consumption have both been indicated as associated with increased risk of the disease, in case-control (Wynder *et al.*, 1956; Hinds *et al.*, 1979) and prospective studies (Jensen, 1979; Robinette *et al.*, 1979). There was also a suggestion from a Swedish case-control study that sideropenic dysphagia was more frequent in the cases with extrinsic cancer (Wynder *et al.*, 1956); this was not found in the associated American study.

Irradiation, which has clearly been shown to cause cancer at other sites, has been noted in one larynx study as associated with the cases—especially more frequent dental x-ray (Hinds *et al.*, 1979).

A number of occupations appear to carry an enhanced risk of laryngeal cancer, though the specific factor has not always been identified: asbestos workers (Stell and McGill, 1973); nickel refining (Pederson *et al.*, 1973); exposure to leather and wood dust (Viadana *et al.*, 1976; Wynder *et al.*, 1976).

Lung

This site shows the greatest relative and absolute rise in mortality rate; the male rates rose earlier than those for females and there is now a halt in this for males but not females. A similar picture exists for many other western countries, though the extent of the rise and the level attained differs between countries (the UK having one of the highest). There is a higher rate in urban areas (OPCS, 1979); Jewish males show a lower rate than Catholics or Protestants (MacMahon, 1960; Haenszel, 1971), whilst Seventh Day Adventists (Lemon et al., 1964) and Mormons (Enstrom, 1978) have very low rates. Migrants to the US from Japan (Haenszel and Kurihara, 1968) and China (King and Haenszel, 1973) show a steep rise in first but not second generation; migrants from most European countries show rates intermediate between those in their countries of origin and the US (Haenszel, 1961).

Familial clustering had been reported (Tokuhata and Lilienfeld, 1963); a possible explanation was the genetically transmitted ability to induce aryl hydrocarbon hydroxylase (Kellermann et al., 1973). The early work was not confirmed by other groups until recently (Emery et al., 1978).

Smoking has been indicted as the main causal agent; this is on the basis of collation (Waller, 1967), case-control (e.g. Doll and Hill, 1950), and prospective studies (e.g. Doll and Peto, 1976; Doll et al., 1980). A powerful point in the argument is the lower risk of cancer in those who give up smoking compared with those who continue; this has been indicated in broad sub-groups of the population and confirmed in prospective studies. Various aspects of smoking are associated with increased risk of lung cancer: cigarette compared with pipe or cigar (Doll and Peto, 1976); early age of starting to smoke (Hammond, 1966); inhaling (Royal College of Physicians, 1977); increased puff frequency (Graham, 1968); retaining the burning cigarette in the mouth (Brett and Benjamin, 1968); extinguishing and relighting the cigarette (Dark et al., 1963); leaving a short butt length (Doll et al., 1959); use of plain rather than filter cigarettes (Bross and Gibson, 1968; Dean et al., 1977). All these may be directly or indirectly linked to the degree of exposure of the bronchial tree to the products of combustion. Some authors have questioned the causal relationships, suggesting that genetic liability to lung cancer might be associated with a desire for smoking. Some of the arguments against the generally accepted hypothesis have been set out by Burch (1980).

Atmospheric pollution has been associated with increased risk of lung cancer (Gardner et al., 1969); in a number of countries there is evidence that persons living in towns smoke more than rural dwellers. There appears to be about a twofold increase in lung cancer after adjusting for this (Wicken, 1966). Both smoking and air pollution increase the incidence of chronic bronchitis; it is thus not straightforward to determine whether the presence of chronic bronchitis per se adds to the risk of lung cancer developing, but several studies suggest this is so (Finke, 1956; Rimington, 1968 and 1971).

Recent work has indicated that persons with an adequate intake of vitamin A are at reduced risk of developing cancer in general and lung cancer in particular (Bjelke, 1975; Wald et al., 1980).

In addition to the major hazard from smoking, there is evidence of a wide range of occupations associated with increased risk of lung cancer. These are now listed in alphabetical order (rather than increment in risk or numbers of workers involved): arsenic exposure (Hill *et al.*, 1948; Pinto *et al.*, 1977) particularly from smelting; asbestos workers (see p. 50); cadmium smelting (Lemen *et al.*, 1976); chloromethyl ether plants (Weiss and Figueroa, 1976); chloroprene plants (Lloyd, 1976); chromate manufacture (Machle and Gregorius, 1948; Bidstrup, 1951); coke ovens (Kennaway and Kennaway, 1947; Doll *et al.*, 1972); foundry workers (McLaughlin and Harding, 1956; Decoufle and Wood, 1979); herbicide usage (Axelson and Sundell, 1974); mining involving atmospheric contamination with radon and its daughter products (Lorenz, 1944; Archer *et al.*, 1976) though this was not shown definitely to be the factor in ferrite miners in the UK (Boyd *et al.*, 1970); mustard gas manufacture (Case and Lea, 1955; Beebe, 1960); nickel refining (Doll *et al.*, 1977; Pedersen *et al.*, 1973); oil mist exposure (Waterhouse, 1971); printing workers (Ask-Upmark, 1955; Moss *et al.*, 1972); talc miners and millers (Kleinfeld *et al.*, 1967 and 1974)—though a deficiency of lung cancer was found in an Italian study (Rubino *et al.*, 1976).

Bone

This is a relatively uncommon cancer, with 395 male deaths in England and Wales in 1978—0.5 per cent of all deaths from neoplasms. Unlike many tumours, there is a double rise in incidence; there is a peak incidence in adolescence and also in the elderly.

There is a genetic component to one variety of bone neoplasm; patients with retinoblastoma, or their relatives, are at increased risk of bone sarcoma (Sagerman *et al.*, 1969; Matsunaga, 1980).

Rather different is the definite association between Paget's disease and oesteogenic sarcoma occurring in the deformed bones (Price, 1962).

Women in the luminous dial industry were exposed to radium which has a lengthy half-life and became deposited in bone. Early on, blood disorders occurred in these workers (Martland *et al.*, 1925); the relation of dose and latent interval to subsequent bone cancer has now been quantified (Polednak *et al.*, 1978; Rowland *et al.*, 1978).

Melanoma

This is a relatively uncommon tumour that has increased in incidence and mortality in many countries in the recent past (Lee and Carter, 1970; Swerdlow, 1979). In England and Wales this rise in mortality from melanoma has been accompanied by a fall in skin cancer; the former increasing from rates of about 1/3 that of other skin cancer to being the commonest form of skin cancer within a 25-year period.

There are major racial differences, with much higher rates in Whites than in Blacks when living at the same latitude (Lancet, 1968). A familial tendency has been reported (Wallace *et al.*, 1971); in addition, a rare pigmented skin lesion that is genetically determined is a precursor for melanoma (Reimer *et al.*, 1978). There is also an increased risk of melanoma in subjects with xeroderma pigmentosa (Frichot *et al.*, 1977).

Collation studies indicate an association between latitude, or sunshine, and mortality rates for melanoma (Elwood *et al.*, 1974; Swerdlow, 1979). Migrants to

Israel had increasing risk of melanoma the longer they had stayed in the country (Movshovitz and Modan, 1973). Case-control studies indicate a relationship with light complexions and sensitivity to sunlight (Lancaster and Nelson, 1957; Klepp and Magnus, 1979). Less clearly defined are possible associations with: oestrogen consumption or parity (Sadoff *et al.*, 1973; Rampen and Mulder, 1980); alcohol intake (Williams, 1976); and trauma (Lea, 1965). The latter is difficult to quantify, whilst the alcohol findings have been disputed (Lyon *et al.*, 1976).

Routine occupational mortality (Registrar General, 1978) and case-control studies suggest professional workers are at higher risk of this cancer (Williams and Horn, 1977). A 'fishing' analysis in the US had identified an excess of blacksmiths, excavators, labourers handling paper, mill wrights, and roofers (Bross *et al.*, 1978). Another study showed a cluster of cases in men exposed to polychlorinated biphenyls (Bahn *et al.*, 1976). There is also some indication of excess deaths from melanoma in oil refinery workers (Rushton and Alderson, 1980). These associations have yet to be confirmed.

Skin—other than melanoma

Now the cause of approximately the same number of deaths as melanoma, skin cancer has shown a very different time trend, with steady decrease throughout the century. However, the same international variation exists.

A racial difference exists, with Whites having higher rates than Blacks living at the same latitude (Schreek, 1944). There is an association with xeroderma and a number of other rare genetic skin disorders (Schimke, 1978).

Scrotal cancer in chimney-sweeps was the first occupational cancer to be recognized (Pott, 1775); over the past 100 years a number of other jobs involving pitch, tar or oil exposure have been confirmed as involving excess skin cancer risk (Bell, 1876; Whitaker *et al.*, 1979).

The geographical variation accords with study of populations and patients indicating that increased ultraviolet radiation from sunlight is an aetiological factor (Jablon, 1975). Accepted but less frequent causes are: chronic bacterial infection (Davies, 1975); presence of scars (Templeton, 1975); irradiation (Ingram and Comaish, 1967); exposure to arsenic from occupation or medicinal use (Hutchinson, 1888; Hill *et al.*, 1948); treatment with immunosuppressive drugs (Kinlen *et al.*, 1979).

Breast

This is the commonest cancer in women, with an incidence that has a plateau around the age of the menopause—instead of rising steadily with advancing age. There is appreciable international variation, with very low rates in Japan, and increasing mortality from East Europe across to West Europe with highest rates in North America (Segi and Kurihara, 1972). Recent trends suggest a rising mortality, especially in the young.

Catholics in the US have lower rates than Jews or Protestants (MacMahon, 1960), whilst both Japanese and Polish migrants show rising mortality in second generation women in the US (Haenszel and Kurihara, 1968). International collation studies have shown an association with fat, oil and meat consumption (Armstrong and Doll, 1975; Howell, 1976; Shrauzer, 1976; Knox, 1977); alcohol consumption was associated with mortality within the US (Breslow and Enstrom, 1974). Time trends for Canada, England and Wales, and the US show a negative association with estimates of fertility (Armstrong, 1976; Wigle, 1977a).

There is a wealth of case reports indicating a familial association (e.g. Teasdale et al., 1976); the genetic (rather than environmental) basis of this has been suggested by work showing very high risks in daughters where mothers and sisters have bilateral premenopausal cancer (Anderson, 1974). A Danish twin study estimated hereditability at about 0.3–0.40 (Holm et al., 1980). Considerable epidemiological research has been focused on breast cancer; though 'risk factors' have been identified, no clear leads emerge from much of this work for primary prevention. Parity and marital status had been associated with variation in risk (e.g. Fraumeni et al., 1969); a seven-country study showed that the age at first pregnancy was the relevant factor, with risk rising with older childbearing (Mac-Mahon, Cole et al., 1970; MacMahon, Lin et al., 1970). Prospective studies have indicated that women with benign breast disease have an increased likelihood of subsequent cancer (Donnelly et al., 1975; Hutchinson et al., 1980); this has been disputed, partly on the basis of missed cancer in the original diagnosis and the validity of the calculated expected values (Levene, 1976). Artificial (early) menopause (Feinleib, 1968), thyroid disease (Mittra and Hayward, 1974), excess fat intake (Hill et al., 1971; Miller et al., 1978), use prior to first pregnancy of combination oral contraception in young women (WHO, 1978), and hormone replacement therapy (Hoover et al., 1976) have all been suggested as risk factors. This is aligned with evidence of hormonal imbalance in subjects who develop breast cancer (Bulbrook and Hayward, 1967; Adams and Wong, 1968) and the hypothesis that these various aspects may be particularly linked to the hazard of anovulatory menstrual cycle with unopposed oestrogens (Korenman, 1980).

Disputed evidence has been reported on the influence of: alcohol consumption (Lyon et al., 1976; Williams, 1976), treatment with Rauwolfia (Boston Collaborative Drug Surveillance Program, 1974a; Christopher et al., 1977), use of hair dyes (Kinlen et al., 1977; Nasca et al., 1980), or virus infection (Fraumeni and Miller, 1971; Henderson et al., 1974). The negative evidence presently seems persuasive. Quite different is the acknowledged impact that irradiation from thorotrast, fluoroscopy, therapy for mastitis, and nuclear weapons can have upon subsequent risk of breast cancer (Brody and Cullen, 1957; MacKenzie, 1965; Mettler et al., 1969; Jablon and Kato, 1972; Boice and Monson, 1977). Though an accepted aetiological agent, irradiation only accounts for a very small proportion of these cancers. There is thought to be a near-linear relationship with dose, which is important for considerations of prevention.

Cervix

Unlike many other cancers, the incidence rises until about the age of 50 and then hardly alters. There has been some fluctuation in incidence and mortality in England and Wales and other countries but no clear time trend (Higgins, 1971; Hakama and Pukkala, 1977). Examination of cohort data for England and Wales suggested there may have been an increase in mortality in women who were young adults in 1940 (Hill and Adelstein, 1967). The incidence is lower in rural areas (OPCS, 1979), high in the divorced (Leck et al., 1978) and very low in Jews (MacMahon, 1960). Japanese women have a lower rate of mortality if they migrate to the US compared to those who remain in their own country, which is even lower in the second generation migrants (Haenszel and Kurihara, 1968).

Many epidemiological studies have been reported, which deal with 'risk factors' rather than explicit aetiological agents. There is a close inverse relationship of risk to age at first intercourse (Wynder et al., 1954; Moghissi et al., 1968); there is an interrelationship of this to virginity (Gagnon, 1950), marital status (Leck et al., 1978), parity (Boyd and Doll, 1964), number of marriages (Rotkin, 1967) and numbers of consorts (Stephenson and Grace, 1954).

Collation studies show a parallel trend in venereally transmitted infection (Beral, 1974); case-control studies have reported increased risk in prostitutes (Rojel, 1953) and persons having had a venereal infection such as syphilis, gonorrhoea, or trichomonas infection (Levin et al., 1942; Terris and Oalmann, 1960). A prospective study showed cervical cancer was more likely to develop in women with antibodies to herpes simplex type 2 (Choi et al., 1977). This is more persuasive evidence than differences in prevalence of such infections in cases compared with controls (Punnonen et al., 1974). Other lines of work have indicated the malignant potential of vulval warts (Zur Hausen, 1976) and the greatly increased frequency of cellular abnormalities associated with such lesions in cervical smears with mild dysplasia (Reid et al., 1980).

Minor support for the role of infection is the suggestion that women are at lower risk of cervical cancer if their husbands use an obstructive method of contraception (Stern and Dixon, 1961; Aitken-Swan and Baird, 1965).

Choriocarcinoma

Hydatidiform mole occurs in about 1:2500 pregnancies in Europe and North America, but is thought to be ten times as common in Asia. The incidence of choriocarcinoma is also believed to be much higher in Asia than in Europe and America. Childbearing in late menstrual life increases the risk of molar pregnancies and may partly account for the geographical variation (Bagshawe, 1967).

Uterus—body

There has been a modest decline in mortality from uterine cancer in many countries (Adelstein et al., 1971; Kinlen and Doll, 1973; Weiss, 1978). The data for England and Wales suggest that all age groups were equally affected at the same period of time. Mortality is high in rural areas (OPCS, 1979), amongst the single (Fraumeni et al., 1969), and in Jews compared with Catholics (Newill, 1961; Seidman, 1970). Collation studies suggest an association with fat or meat intake (Armstrong and Doll, 1975).

Case-control studies indicate higher risk in the nulliparous, those marrying late, first having intercourse at an 'older age', or having a 'late' menopause (Stewart et al., 1966; Elwood et al., 1977). The cancer is associated with obesity, diabetes, hypertension and arthritis (Elwood et al., 1977); a syndrome exists with increased incidence of breast, ovary and uterine cancer in the same patients or in families (Thiessen, 1974).

All the above items relate to general indicators of risk. Quite different is an extensive series of studies that have explored the relationship to use of hormone replacement therapy. Nine studies noted a positive association, though there were queries about the selection of controls, the reason for therapy and the variation in case ascertainment. It was concluded that there was a genuine relationship because (i) the higher the dose of oestrogen, the higher the risk of endometrial cancer, (ii) the risk increased with increasing duration of use, and (iii) decreased after hormone therapy ceased (see review: Lancet, 1979).

A WHO study group concluded that there was some evidence of an increased risk of endometrial cancer among women using sequential oral contraceptives, which have now been withdrawn in a number of countries (WHO, 1978).

Ovary

This is the fifth commonest cause of death from neoplasms in England and Wales; this prominence has been reached by a steady fourfold rise in rate throughout the century. Internationally the variation between countries is relatively slight, developed countries showing higher rates; these have risen as in England (Lingeman, 1974). Studies in the US have shown relatively minor variation in mortality between Blacks, Chinese, Hispano and Japanese living in the same locality (Weiss and Peterson, 1978). The rates are low in Japan; migrants from there to Hawaii show increased mortality from ovarian cancer (Haenszel and Kurihara, 1968).

Case-control studies (Stewart et al., 1966; Newhouse et al., 1977; Casagrande et al., 1979) have indicated an increased risk in women first having intercourse, pregnancy or marrying after the age of 20; having few children; having an early menopause; making limited use of oral contraceptives. These points can be aggregated into estimated 'total anovular time' which is indirectly related to risk of the cancer (Casagrande et al., 1979). This agrees with collation data which indicated an indirect association between ovarian cancer mortality and average family size for eighteen countries (Beral et al., 1978). The increase in mortality this century in England and Wales could be 'accounted for' by the decrease in completed family size.

A minimal contribution is postulated for genetic factors, though family clusters have been reported (Lewis and Davison, 1969; Li et al., 1970) and a tenuous association of specific histological types with blood group A (Osborne and de George, 1963).

Two specific factors have been investigated. There is some suggestion of an increased risk in women who have been on hormone replacement therapy (Hoover et al., 1977), though the analysis was disputed (Annegers et al., 1977). In a limited study it was suggested that talc particles occurred more frequently in ovaries involved in cancer than normal ovaries (Henderson et al., 1971). These tentative findings were criticized on publication (Lancet, 1977a) and no definitive support for the hypothesis has since appeared (Roe, 1979).

There has been an indication of higher frequency of obesity and gall bladder disease in ovarian cancer patients (West, 1966; Casagrande et al., 1979). Limited support for this comes from international collation studies which showed a high correlation between total fat intake and mortality from ovarian cancer (Armstrong and Doll, 1975).

Vagina

A very rare, clear cell adenocarcinoma was reported in seven adolescent girls (Herbst and Scully, 1970). The following year this was associated with prior consumption of diethylstilboestrol during pregnancy (Herbst *et al.*, 1971). This therapy had been widely used in the US in 1948–70 for threatened miscarriage and an increasing number of affected patients has been reported (Herbst *et al.*, 1972). Less extensive use had been made of this in England and Wales (Kinlen *et al.*, 1974), but cases have now been identified (Monaghan and Sirisena, 1978; Shepherd *et al.*, 1979).

Prostate

This is the third commonest cause of male deaths from neoplasm in England and Wales; there has been about a twofold rise in mortality rate during this century, though some of this may be diagnostic. There is appreciable international variation (Tulinius, 1977), with more marked increase in mortality in Blacks than Whites in the US (Henschke *et al.*, 1973); a genuine cohort effect appeared likely rather than altered precision of the data (Ernster *et al.*, 1978)—this is a site with widely varying estimates of the prevalence of in-situ cancer (see Breslow *et al.*, 1977).

Family clusters have been reported (Lynch *et al.*, 1966) and an increased risk in blood group A subjects (Bourke and Griffin, 1962). However, the genetic influence is thought to be minor (Wynder *et al.*, 1971).

Case-control studies have reported differences in sexual habits (Wynder *et al.*, 1971; Rotkin, 1977; Schumann *et al.*, 1977); though the items examined have varied, there appears to be consistency in the reported excess risk with aspects of sexual drive: early age at first intercourse, number of consorts, coital frequency, age at marriage, number of children, prior venereal disease. Two rather different hypotheses have been suggested; one associates dietary differences to altered hormone profile and thus sexual behaviour and risk of prostate cancer. Collation studies had indicated a broad association with fat intake (Armstrong and Doll, 1975; Shrauzer, 1976; Blair and Fraumeni, 1978); though no detailed dietary studies have been reported, one case-control study did find an indication of high lipid/cholesterol intake (Rotkin, 1977). Another hypothesis suggests that the behaviour affects the risk of sexually transmitted infection (Zeigel *et al.*, 1977); there is some limited information on variation in prevalence of virus antibodies in cases and controls (Schumann *et al.*, 1977).

Conflicting findings from two prospective studies on patients with benign prostatic hypertrophy suggest no increased risk (Greenwald *et al.*, 1974) and about a fourfold increase (Armenian *et al.*, 1974). This discrepancy has not been resolved.

A number of studies have reported differences in occupational histories, but no jobs were consistently identified from 'fishing' studies (Henry *et al.*, 1931; Rotkin, 1977; Ernster *et al.*, 1979). A report, based on very small numbers, suggested that workers exposed to cadmium were at increased risk of prostate cancer (Potts, 1965). Three other studies also observed a relationship with cadmium exposure (Kipling and Waterhouse, 1967; Lemen *et al.*, 1976; Kolonel and Winkelstein, 1977), whilst a fourth did not (Ross *et al.*, 1979). The positive results were all based on small numbers and two were not significant; if a specific hazard exists, it can only affect a small group of workers and the relative risk cannot be greatly raised.

A number of studies have commented on the excess of patients who have been circumcised (Gibson, 1954). Prostate cancer is uncommon in Jews (Ravich and Ravich, 1951; Seidman, 1970); no report has been able to confirm whether the practice of circumcision or another aspect of behaviour is the key factor.

Testis

This is another rare tumour, 22nd in the list of sites (see Table 2.1) and accounting for only about 0.3 per cent of deaths from neoplasms. During this century there have been different trends at different ages, with an increase in mortality rates in the young but stable or decreasing rates in the older adults; this was apparent in Denmark (Clemmesen, 1968), England and Wales (Petersen and Lee, 1972), and US (Li and Fraumeni, 1972). There are four quite different histological tumours: embryonal carcinoma occurring in the youngest subjects, teratoma, seminoma, and carcinoma in the oldest (Grumet and MacMahon, 1958). Inadequate attention has been paid to examining the different aetiologies of each of these forms of tumour.

The urban/rural variation shows anomalies, with higher incidence in large cities in Denmark (Clemmesen, 1968), but low mortality in urban areas in England and Wales (Lipworth and Dayan, 1969).

There is an extensive literature on the relationship of cryptorchism to risk of testicular cancer, with considerable inconsistency in the findings (Gilbert and Hamilton, 1940; Campbell, 1959; Morrison, 1976). This may be partly due to the difficulty in obtaining either a valid history from the cancer patients or of determining the prevalence in the general population. The weight of evidence supports an association between the two conditions.

Antecedent orchitis has also been suggested as an aetiological factor, but two major studies were negative (Gilbert, 1944; Ehrengut and Schwartau, 1977).

Other case-control studies have noted differences between cases and controls, but with no consistency to clearly identify risk factors or causal agents. There was an indication of association with professional occupations (Graham and Gibson, 1972; Mustacchi and Millimore, 1976) and of trauma (Mustacchi and Millimore, 1976), though the latter is very difficult to document in an unbiased way.

Penis

This is a rare malignancy, accounting for only 95 deaths in England and Wales out of a total of nearly 69 000 (i.e. about 0.1 per cent). There is appreciable variation from country to country, which is not thought to be due solely to chance fluctuation from small numbers (Paymaster and Gangadharan, 1967).

Studies in East Africa and India have both shown the 'incidence' of the condition varies in relation to circumcision practice, being rare in those communities practising this (Dodge and Linsell, 1963; Paymaster and Gangadharan, 1967).

A number of years ago there was a suggestion of excess cervical cancer in wives of men with penile cancer (Martinez, 1969). Two prospective studies of wives of such men have confirmed this (Graham et al., 1979; Smith et al., 1980); this association only involved a very small proportion of cervical cancer patients. Neither study was appropriate to determine the mechanism, but it was thought to be compatible with a common virological aetiology for both cancers.

Bladder

There has been about a fourfold rise in bladder cancer mortality this century in England and Wales (depending on the specific age and sex group examined). Rates are highest in the UK and most of the countries in Western Europe; intermediate rates occur in North America, Australasia, Scandinavia and Southern Europe (Staszewski, 1980). These data suggest that some of the changes of modern society (either of way of life or of occupation) may be associated with increased risk of this cancer; however, Davies (1980) has pointed out that this still leaves a hard core of cancers unexplained, as the mortality was appreciable at the beginning of this century.

A number of studies have indicated a relative risk of 2.0 to 4.0 for smokers (see Morrison and Cole, 1976, for a review). Because of the prevalence of smoking, this makes an appreciable contribution to the overall toll from this site.

It has been known for many years that workers in the dyestuff industry were exposed to a hazard of bladder cancer; research in a number of countries confirmed the risk (e.g. Case et al., 1954). The hazard involved the manufacture of β-naphthylamine, benzidene, auramine, and magenta (Case, 1966). Similar chemicals were used in the curing of rubber, and rubber was used in cable manufacture; workers in these industries had increased risk of bladder cancer (Case and Hosker, 1954; Davies, 1965). Doll et al. (1965) demonstrated a risk in gas workers producing coal-gas; they were also exposed to aromatic amines in the work environment. It was suggested that hairdressers were at increased risk, but this did not show on follow-up in England and Wales (Alderson, 1980b). A number of other occupations have been associated with a raised risk of bladder cancer, though the reasons have not been identified: shoe and leather workers (Wynder et al., 1963); sailors, tin- and coppersmiths (Dunham et al., 1968); tailors, textile workers, and health service staff (Anthony and Thomas, 1970).

Coffee drinking has been suggested as increasing the risk of bladder cancer (Simon et al., 1975). Other studies have tentatively implicated alcohol, artificial sweeteners, Coca-Cola, and opium (Morgan and Jain, 1974; Miller, 1977; Sadeghi and Behmard, 1978). These suggestions have not been substantiated.

It was postulated that nitrosamines might be formed in an infected bladder and support came from studies on Egyptian and English patients (Hicks et al., 1977). However, more recent studies of bladder cancer patients and controls showed no significant difference in levels of various nitrosamine compounds (IARC, 1978).

Egypt has a considerably higher bladder cancer mortality than other countries. This is thought to be due to the endemic schistosomiasis. Patients with this infection have an appreciably raised risk of bladder cancer (Hashem, 1961; Dunham et al., 1973).

Kidney

English data show steadily rising mortality this century; the original level was higher in males than in females and the rise has been steeper for them, with about a threefold excess in the present rates for males compared with females. Jews showed higher mortality rates than Catholics and Protestants (MacMahon, 1960), whilst Mormons had lower rates than the US population (Enstrom, 1978). Migrants from Europe and America had higher and those from Asia and Africa lower mortality than the native born in Israel (Halevi *et al.*, 1971). Collation studies have shown associations with beer (Breslow and Enstrom, 1974), coffee drinking (Armstrong and Doll, 1975), and lead levels in water (Berg and Burbank, 1972).

Children developing Wilm's tumour are more likely to have a range of other congenital abnormalities, whilst adult renal tumours occur in excess in the rare congenital tuberous sclerosis (Mulvihill, 1975).

Three quite different genito-urinary conditions are associated with increased frequency of renal tumours: Balkan nephropathy (Petkovic *et al.*, 1966), phenacetin abuse (Johansson *et al.*, 1974), and renal stone (MacLean and Fowler, 1965). These are relatively rare or restricted conditions and together they can only account for a small proportion of all renal tumours. It is not clear whether the cause of each of the three conditions directly affects the risk of renal tumours, or indirectly via the long-standing changes that occur in the kidney.

An American study 'fishing' for occupational relationships had suggested that metal workers, masons and roofing workers had an excess of renal cancer (Houten *et al.*, 1977). The only specific occupational study to show an excess was on coke-oven workers (Redmond *et al.*, 1972).

Smoking has been suggested as relevant, but the large British prospective study showed no indication of this (Doll and Peto, 1976).

Central nervous system

Brain tumours were the tenth commonest cause of deaths from neoplasm in males in England and Wales in 1978; the other sites in the central nervous system are considerably less frequently involved. During this century there has been a steady increase, fourfold for men and threefold for women; the extent of improved diagnosis is not clear. There is only limited international variation (Segi and Kurihara, 1972), and no clear urban–rural trend (OPCS, 1979); this is a site affecting the professional classes to a greater extent in the US (Buell *et al.*, 1960). Collation studies show an association with fat intake, for which no adequate explanation exists (Armstrong and Doll, 1975).

Case reports have indicated the occasional family clusters of brain tumours; better data exist for a number of rare syndromes, such as tuberose sclerosis in which there is an increased risk of central nervous system tumours (Mulvihill, 1975). A study of children with brain tumours showed that their siblings and mothers were more likely to have suffered from seizures, epilepsy or stroke (Gold *et al.*, 1979). It is accepted that exposure to ionizing radiation can increase the risk of brain tumours (Jablon *et al.*, 1971; Preston-Martin *et al.*, 1980).

Trauma has been reported prior to development of brain tumours, but there is great difficulty in assessing the validity of such a history. A case-control study suggested a history was associated with double the risk of brain tumours (Preston-Martin *et al.*, 1980).

Occupational mortality statistics for England and Wales indicate a significantly raised SMR for farmers, farm managers and market gardeners (Registrar General, 1978). This has also been noted in other studies of patients; one case-control study found a significant excess of children with brain tumours had had contact with either farm animals or pets who had been sick (Gold *et al.*, 1979).

There have recently been suggestions that certain occupational groups have an increased risk of brain tumours: vinyl chloride workers (Monson *et al.*, 1974); professional chemists (Olin and Ahlbom, 1980); workers in petrochemical plants (Theriault and Goulet, 1979; Thomas *et al.*, 1980). For the latter group there is no consistency in the findings, nor indication of any particular agent (Alderson and Rushton, 1980).

Thyroid

This is a relatively rare cancer and one of the few cancers with higher incidence in females; it was ranked twenty-second in the sites causing deaths in England and Wales in 1978. There has been little trend in mortality this century in England, though incidence data for New York showed a cohort increase in those aged under 55 in the period 1941–62 (Carroll *et al.*, 1964). In general, there is limited variation in the mortality in different countries, despite the major concern about the validity of the data; thyroid cancer can occur in occult form, and variation in case-finding may appreciably affect the statistics (Saxen *et al.*, 1969; Maruchi *et al.*, 1971).

It is accepted that there is a rare familial medullary thyroid cancer (Hillyard *et al.*, 1978). Also thyroid cancer can occur as one of the manifestations of the rare familial syndrome of multiple endocrine adenoma (Schimke, 1976).

There is evidence that some patients have an enhanced likelihood of tumours of the breast and thyroid (Schottenfeld and Berg, 1971), though the mechanism of this remains obscure. Somewhat more controversial is whether individuals who have suffered goitre are at increased risk of cancer of the thyroid. Some population statistics suggest an association (Wegelin, 1928), though this has been disputed (Saxen and Saxen, 1954). Histology reports of the prevalence of thyroid abnormalities in patients with cancer are compatible with a common aetiology (Wahner *et al.*, 1966), rather than a direct sequence of benign lesions later becoming malignant.

A well-defined aetiological agent is ionizing radiation; this has been shown in several countries for children given treatment for 'enlarged thymus' in infancy, scalp ringworm, or other disease of the head and neck (Duffy and Fitzgerald, 1950; Hempelmann *et al.*, 1975; Modan *et al.*, 1977). Therapeutic irradiation of adults has also been followed by cancer of the thyroid, but has not been numerically such a problem (Goolden, 1958). There is no evidence from large-scale prospective studies that ^{131}I has been associated with increased risk of cancer when used for diagnostic or therapeutic purposes (Pochin, 1960; Dobyns *et al.*, 1974).

Occupational mortality statistics for England and Wales give no clear indication of a particular hazard for this site and no studies in industry have indicated a risk (Registrar General, 1978). One laboratory generated hypothesis, that ethylene thiourea might induce thyroid cancer, was not substantiated in a study of exposed workers (Smith, 1976).

A more extensive review of the epidemiology has been published (Alderson, 1980c).

Hodgkin's disease

This is a relatively rare condition, accounting for about 0.5 per cent of all deaths from neoplasms in males and females. The age distribution is atypical, with a peak in childhood and also early adult life; though referred to as one disease, there are a variety of histological sub-types each with differing age distribution (Newell *et al.*, 1970). There has been about a twofold increase in mortality this century in England and Wales. There is appreciable variation between different countries (MacMahon, 1966), or from one area of a country to another (Cole *et al.*, 1968); the trends in various countries have been different (MacMahon, 1966). There is evidence that the disease is more common in the professional classes; in the latest data for England and Wales (Registrar-General, 1978) Social Class I had the highest SMR of 113 and the gradient across the classes was slight. In the US the mortality in adults is higher in Whites than non-Whites (Fraumeni and Li, 1969), and in Jews than Catholics or Protestants (MacMahon, 1960).

There are studies indicating an excess of patients in families; this is more commonly around the same period rather than when members achieve the same age, suggesting an environmental factor (Razis *et al.*, 1959).

Circumstantial evidence suggested an infective origin to the disease; formal mathematical tests for clustering have been negative (Fraumeni and Li, 1969; Alderson and Nayak, 1971). An episode in New York suggested that the family and friends of an original group of patients had a raised incidence of the disease (Vianna *et al.*, 1971); interpretation of such observational data is extremely difficult. A more vigorous examination of school pupils suggested an association between affected pupils or schools with cases and subsequent development of Hodgkin's disease (Vianna and Polan, 1973). An examination of the network of contacts in patients and controls in Oxford failed to identify any difference (Smith *et al.*, 1973). It was suggested that New York doctors had an increased incidence of Hodgkin's (Vianna *et al.*, 1974), but this was not found in other American (Matanoski *et al.*, 1975) or English doctors (Smith *et al.*, 1974). Very different to these studies is the follow-up of large numbers of patients with infectious mononucleosis; a small but significant excess of Hodgkin's disease has been observed (Rosdahl *et al.*, 1974; Kvale *et al.*, 1979). A number of studies have suggested that children or young adults with Hodgkin's are more likely to have had tonsillectomy than their siblings (Vianna *et al.*, 1971; Gutensohn *et al.*, 1975). There is some evidence that woodworkers have a higher incidence than expected (Spiers, 1969; Petersen and Milham, 1974), but this has not been universally observed nor the reasons for the original observations demonstrated. Other studies have suggested an increased mortality from lymphoma in chemists (Li *et al.*, 1969; Olin, 1978).

A case-control study suggested excess consumption of amphetamines (Newell *et al.*, 1973), but this was not confirmed in other work (Boston Collaborative Drug Surveillance Program, 1974b). Follow-up of college students indicated that those who were obese or drank and smoked more than others were at increased risk of developing Hodgkin's (Paffenbarger *et al.*, 1977); it is possible that this reflects confounding with affluence.

Lymphoma

This condition is the main component of the entry 'other neoplasms of lymphoid tissue' in Tables 2.1 and 2.2 and Figs. 2.17 and 2.18. It ccounts for just under 1 per cent of deaths from neoplasms in males and females, and the mortality rate has risen sharply over the past twenty years (though how much of this is diagnostic is not clear). There is major variation throughout the world, with very high mortality in some Arab countries and in Israel (Haghighi *et al.*, 1979; Aghai *et al.*, 1974); this so-called Mediterranean lymphoma is particularly common in children and especially involving the alimentary tract.

Limited evidence indicates a possible familial association (Freedlander *et al.*, 1978). The disease also occurs in excess in patients with coeliac disease—in itself a familial condition (Gough *et al.*, 1962; Whorwell *et al.*, 1976).

Follow-up of patients treated with immunosuppressive drugs shows a significant excess of lymphoma (Kinlen *et al.*, 1979; 1980), some occurring a relatively short while after initial treatment associated with renal transplant. Increase in lymphoma has been reported in patients with rheumatoid arthritis (Isomaki *et al.*, 1979); this observation has not been confirmed, nor has it been indicated whether this is thought to be a reflection of the cause of the arthritis, the presence of the arthritis, or the treatment given.

A collation study in the US showed an association with counties in which food packing occurred; it was not clear if this was a reflection of other associated industry in these counties (Cantor and Fraumeni, 1980). Studies in Sweden (Olin, 1978; Olin and Ahlbom, 1980), the UK (Searle, 1978) and US (Li *et al.*, 1969) indicated an excess of lymphoma in professional chemists. No specific reasons for this have been advanced, but other work in Scandinavia has shown an excess of patients with lymphoma report exposure to chlorophenols (Hardell, 1979). Other associations have been noted with residence near a solvent-refining plant (Capurro and Eldridge, 1978), work in petroleum refineries (Tabershaw, 1974), exposure to benzene (Vianna and Polan, 1979), rubber tyre production (Monson and Fine, 1978), and work in medical laboratories (Harrington and Shannon, 1975).

Very different is the lymphoma in children described by Burkitt (1959). This occurs in restricted localities in Africa, shows space–time clustering (Williams *et al.*, 1978) and marked seasonal variation (Williams *et al.*, 1974). A prospective study of a large number of children in Uganda, who had sera collected on entry to the study, showed higher titres of viral capsid antigen than matched controls (de Thé *et al.*, 1978). The disease only occurs in areas where malaria is endemic (apart from very rare cases of rather different nature in developed countries). It has been suggested that neonatal infection with Epstein–Barr virus may initiate the malignancy, which is then promoted by major immunological stress such as from malaria (de Thé, 1977).

Leukaemia

For all ages, leukaemia accounts for about 2.5 per cent of the deaths from malignancy; there is relatively high incidence and mortality in children. There has been a rise in mortality throughout this century, affecting the young and the elderly; the trends by cell type vary at different ages. There is relatively little variation in international rates, especially at ages 20–44 years, and the trends are comparable to those in England. The age and cytology differences in trends suggest that improved diagnosis plays only a minor part (see Alderson (1980d) for extensive review of leukaemia epidemiology).

If one child develops leukaemia, the likelihood of a second child so doing in the sibship is twice that of the population risk (Draper *et al.*, 1977). Patients with Down's syndrome have a chromosomal abnormality and are at greatly increased risk of leukaemia (Stewart *et al.*, 1958). No adequate-sized twin study is available to permit familial and genetic factors to be distinguished (Cederlöf *et al.*, 1977).

Ionizing radiation from various sources has been shown to be leukaemogenic. Diagnostic investigation in early pregnancy (Stewart *et al.*, 1958; MacMahon, 1962), therapeutic irradiation for malignant (Li *et al.*, 1975) or benign disease (Brinkley and Haybittle, 1969; Smith *et al.*, 1977), occupational exposure (March, 1950; Polednak *et al.*, 1978) are all confirmed hazards—though some work on low-level radiation has been discounted (Reissland, 1978). Diagnostic x-ray other than of the fetus (Gibson *et al.*, 1972) or use of ^{131}I (Pochin, 1967) has not been shown to constitute a hazard in controlled use. There is no evidence that background irradiation ever reaches an adequate level for a measurable leukaemogenic risk (Court Brown *et al.*, 1960).

Leukaemia is associated with certain immunological deficiencies (Kersey *et al.*, 1973) and other rare syndromes (Mulvihill, 1975). Excess mortality has been recorded in subjects with rheumatoid arthritis (Lea, 1964) and pernicious anaemia (Blackburn *et al.*, 1968) but this is as yet unexplained.

Medical treatment with immunosuppressive drugs (Sieber and Adamson, 1976; Stutman, 1976), cytotoxic drugs for chronic disease (Sieber and Adamson, 1976), or chemotherapy for other malignant disease (Canellos *et al.*, 1975) have been shown to increase the risk of leukaemia. A similar hazard has been suggested from butazolidine and chloramphenicol (Fraumeni, 1967) but this is not confirmed.

Apart from irradiation, occupational exposure to benzene has been followed by increased rate of mortality from leukaemia (Tyroler *et al.*, 1976).

The most confusing area has been the search for an infective agent. There is some indication that virus infections in pregnancy increase the risk of the child developing leukaemia (Stewart *et al.*, 1958; Fedrick and Alberman, 1972; Hakulinen *et al.*, 1973); other studies have produced negative results (Leck and Steward, 1972; McCrea Curnen *et al.*, 1974). Patients have reported excess contact with hospitals (Timonen and Ilvonen, 1978), farm animals (Fasel *et al.*, 1967; Milham, 1971), and sick pets (Bross *et al.*, 1972) compared with controls; there is little consistency in these studies (Schneider and Riggs, 1973; Linos *et al.*, 1980). Many studies of mathematical clustering in space and time of incident cases in populations have failed to confirm the original suggestive findings from the north-east of England (Knox, 1964; Gunz and Spears, 1968; Glass and Mantel, 1969). This may be due partly to the inappropriateness of the mathematical approach; alternative examination of networks of contacts of cases and controls has also been substantially negative (Schimpff *et al.*, 1976; Zack *et al.*, 1977). Laboratory studies have produced results that as yet fail to demonstrate an infective aetiology (Karpas *et al.*, 1978).

Specific aetiological factors

The following subsections discuss the main specific aetiological factors that have been identified. These will have already been mentioned in the preceding section on cancer by site; cross-reference should be made to this earlier material, as some studies mentioned there are not also covered in the following material. The intention in the following subsections is to identify some of the general issues raised by research on these agents, such as assessment of the weight of evidence, conflict from studies of different types or research carried out in different countries, and the issue of multiplicative effect between different agents.

The final subsection attempts to provide a brief synopsis of the present knowledge about the aetiology of cancer.

Alcoholic beverages

This topic may be studied in a variety of different ways, each with major problems of interpretation.

Collation studies have attempted to look at the relationships between national (or regional) per capita intake of alcoholic beverage and age-adjusted cancer mortality in these populations. Apart from concern about the validity of the data, and the number of multiple comparisons that can be readily generated, there is the difficulty that some authors only present a subsection of their findings and it is not possible to tell whether absence of a result indicates a low correlation was found or the correlation was not actually calculated (it is more likely to be the former in these papers and this distorts the balance of the published results). Table 3.1 presents the results from three of these publications; due to the incompleteness

Table 3.1 Correlation coefficients (r) derived from three collated studies between per capita intake of three alcoholic beverages and age-adjusted mortality for various sites of malignancy

Site	Knox (1977)		Breslow and Enstrom (1974)			Schrauzer (1976)		
	Beer	Wine	Beer	Wine	Spirits	Beer	Wine	Spirits
Mouth		0.70	0.45	0.59	0.44	0.79	—	—
Nasopharynx			—		0.46			
Oesophagus		0.51	0.67	0.60	0.68	0.74	—	—
Stomach			0.62	—	—			
Colon	0.85		0.73	0.45	0.60	0.69	—	—
Rectum	0.66		0.78	0.52	0.54	0.65	—	—
Liver						—	0.53	—
Pancreas			—	0.42	0.42			
Larynx		0.84	0.45	0.62	0.48	0.89	—	—
Lung			—	0.58	0.53			
Skin						0.52	—	—
Prostate			0.15	—	−0.25			
Kidney			0.75	—	0.49			
Bladder			0.73	0.64	0.59			
r for p = 0.01	0.73	0.66	0.39	0.39	0.39	0.61	0.61	0.61

Where a non-significant value was reported the above table uses —; a blank indicates no value was provided.

of the tabulated results, it is suggested that a correlation with a probability of < 0.01 should be merely used as an indication of sites worth reviewing and for which further studies of a different nature could be considered.

A number of prospective studies have followed groups known or thought to have increased alcohol intake and have analysed subsequent cancer incidence or mortality. Obviously a cohort of known high alcohol intake may be a very 'atypical' group of individuals in whom variation in mortality patterns from that of the general population may reflect other aspects of their 'way-of-life'. The results from nine of these studies are presented in Table 3.2; for any given site of malignancy the data have been pooled from published results. Again there is the

Table 3.2 Observed (O) and expected (E) deaths and ratio for various sites of malignancy, derived from nine prospective studies

Site*	O	E	O:E	χ^2	P
Mouth 1, 2, 5, 7, 8	47	25.39	1.85	18.4	<0.001
Oesophagus 1, 2, 4, 5, 6, 7, 8	177	107.48	1.65	45.0	<0.001
Stomach 1, 4, 5, 6, 7, 8, 9	184	199.24	0.92	1.2	<0.3
Colon 1, 4, 5, 6, 7, 8	202	201.57	1.00	—	
Rectum 2, 5, 6, 7, 8	105	81.47	1.29	6.8	<0.01
Liver 4, 5, 6, 7	121	82.95	1.46	17.4	<0.001
Pancreas 2, 4, 5, 6, 7, 8	74	66.50	1.11	0.8	<0.4
Larynx 1, 2, 4, 5, 6, 7, 8	55	21.2	2.60	54.1	<0.0001
Lung 1, 2, 4, 5, 7, 8, 9	656	461.63	1.42	81.8	<0.0001
Prostate 1, 2, 4, 5, 8	15	17.1	0.88	0.2	<0.7
All cancers	1528	1331.89	1.15	28.9	<0.001

* Results pooled from the following studies:

1. Schmidt and de Lint (1972)
2. Pell and D'Alonzo (1973)
3. Nicholls et al. (1974)
4. Hakulinen et al. (1974)
5. Monson and Lyon (1975)
6. Dean et al. (1979)
7. Jensen (1979)
8. Robinette et al. (1979)
9. Thorarinsson (1979)

problem that not all results are included in published papers, and it is quite possible that some have excluded data when no excess of observed deaths occurred. Another point is that the method of the study varies; the majority provided estimated person-years-at-risk and enabled expected deaths to be calculated from national age/sex/calendar period mortality rates. Pell and D'Alonzo (1973) compared deaths occurring in a comparison population in their industrial study, whilst Robinette et al. (1979) followed a comparison group of war veterans to obtain control mortality; Monson and Lyon (1975) calculated expected deaths from proportional mortality as they did not have complete ascertainment of their subjects on follow-up. The numbers of subjects involved in the different reports vary markedly and thus the pooled data are heavily weighted by the results from the larger studies. It must also be noted that this pooling of results is a relatively crude process, particularly if the mortality rates in the different countries (and thus the basic cancer deaths 'expected') vary to any extent. Again, it is suggested that this material is used as a background to consideration of more specific studies.

Case-control studies have examined the relative risk of high alcoholic consumption in patients with various head and neck cancers (mouth, pharynx, larynx, other miscellaneous sites), oesophagus, colon, rectum, liver, pancreas and lung cancers.

There have been two rather different kinds of exploration, either concentrating upon alcohol as the focus of enquiry or studies of a range of aetiological agents including questioning about alcohol consumption. References to these studies appear in the site-specific subsections; the weight of evidence suggests that consumption of alcoholic beverage is associated with an increased risk of the head and neck sites, oesophagus and liver. The position is not so clear for either large bowel or pancreas.

Out of the 13 case-control studies on colorectal cancer, 3 identified an association with beer consumption (Stocks, 1957; Wynder and Shigematsu, 1967; IARC, 1977); 4 observed no appreciable effect from alcohol consumption (Pernu, 1960; Higginson, 1966; Wynder *et al.*, 1969; Bjelke, 1971); 2 found a negative association (Schwartz *et al.*, 1962; Modan *et al.*, 1975); 4 do not comment about this topic (Haenszel *et al.*, 1973; Bjelke, 1974; Graham *et al.*, 1978; Dales *et al.*, 1979). The results from the collation and prospective studies on high alcohol consumers are thus difficult to explain. There is no indication whether there is confounding between alcohol intake and other environmental factors that have generated these positive results. It is suggested that more detailed study of 'healthy' populations who have been investigated in some detail and followed up may be required. Laboratory studies of bile acids, flora and other identifiable carcinogens or mutagens in the stools of subjects on different diets may also shed light on the controversy.

Evidence from case-control studies in which smoking and alcohol have been assessed indicate that these two aetiological factors combine in exposed subjects.

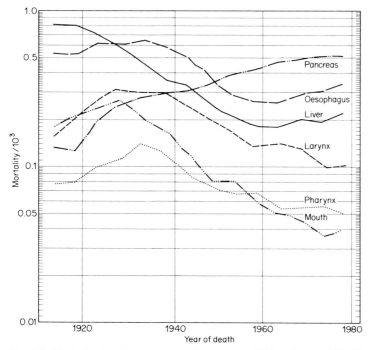

Fig. 3.1 Alcohol-related cancers: mortality rates per 1000 males aged 65–69 years in England and Wales, 1911–78.

For example, Tuyns *et al.* (1977) demonstrate the multiplicative effect, with very high risk suffered by those who both drink and smoke heavily. It has been suggested that this interaction of these two powerful factors results in 90 per cent of the risk of oesophageal cancer in North America and Western Europe being due to alcohol or tobacco usage (Day and Munoz, personal communication).

Tuyns and Griciute (1980) discussed the carcinogenic substances in alcoholic beverages; though this has yet to be resolved from laboratory studies, there is epidemiological evidence that the risk is a function of the amount of ethanol consumed.

Figure 3.1 shows the trend in mortality rates for males aged 65–69 years in England and Wales in 1911–78 for six 'alcohol-related' sites. The remarks above suggest the evidence is least defined for pancreas, which is the one site showing a very different trend (and one that is consistent with the major impact of smoking on this malignancy). Alcohol consumption decreased in the first half of the twentieth century in England and Wales, and has then increased in the past twenty-five years; this shows a closer relationship with the trends for oesophagus and liver. This suggests that there are other important factors associated with the risk of mouth, pharynx and laryngeal cancer.

Asbestos

The first reports of an association between asbestos exposure and malignancy indicated an increased risk of lung cancer; by 1955 sixty-one such cases had been reported (Doll, 1955). In the late 1950s a series of pleural tumours was referred for treatment in South Africa from the north-western Cape Province; investigation showed that all but one of thirty-three patients with pleural mesothelioma had exposure to asbestos (Wagner *et al.*, 1960). Investigation of asbestos patients having coroner's autopsies in the east of London showed that ten had primary mesothelioma of the peritoneum (Enticknap and Smither, 1964). Follow-up of various categories of exposed workers has also indicated an excess risk of alimentary tract cancers (see review by Miller, 1978).

Studies of various occupational groups have demonstrated a risk from exposure in miners (e.g. Wagner *et al.*, 1960; Liddell and McDonald, 1977), asbestos-factory workers (Peto *et al.*, 1977), insulation workers (Selikoff *et al.*, 1964), and dockyard workers (Lumley, 1976). In addition, increased risk was demonstrated for households with members working with asbestos and also those living in the vicinity of a factory (Newhouse and Thompson, 1965). In a recent case-control study of malignant mesothelioma in North America occupational exposure to asbestos was found in 50 per cent of the males but only 5 per cent of the female cases; there was no evidence of an increased risk in those exposed at work to man-made mineral fibres, living near zeolite deposits, or who smoked (McDonald and McDonald, 1980). Follow-up studies of insulation workers had shown the risk of lung cancer was greatly increased in those who smoked (Selikoff *et al.*, 1968). A further study on amosite asbestos factory workers showed an eighty-fold excess risk of lung cancer in those who smoked (Selikoff *et al.*, 1980).

In a necropsy series in east London, after excluding subjects with asbestosis, mesothelioma, or known occupational exposure to asbestos, the prevalence of asbestos bodies in the lungs was studied. These were identified in 42 per cent of 216 males and 30 per cent of 178 females, though in much lower numbers than found in subjects with asbestosis; the numbers were increased in men with stomach cancer and women with breast cancer, though no explanation for this could be found.

Though there is a significant increase in gastrointestinal cancer in workers exposed to asbestos, there is no evidence that the minute quantities of fibres present in the natural water supply pose a hazard (Wigle, 1977b; Harrington *et al.*, 1978).

Diet

This section includes many of the points already made under the site-specific sections, though dealing with the material from the opposite aspect. (The references for these are not repeated, but may be found in the earlier sections.) Various nutrients, beverages (other than alcohol), contaminants and additives are covered; specific mention is then made of the role of vitamin A, nitrosamines and blood lipids.

Information on possible associations between diet and cancer has come from collation studies of national (or regional) mortality or incidence statistics and estimates of per capita intake of different nutrients. Such studies can only provide suggestions for further study; unfortunately, due to the complexity of studying diet in either retrospective or prospective studies, the data from hypothesis-testing studies are relatively limited.

It has been observed that there is an association between increased intake of fat and risk of cancer of the colon and rectum, breast, uterus body, ovary, prostate and kidney. Apart from the large bowel and kidney there are neoplasms associated with hormonal balance and it has been suggested that variation in the intake of fat may be linked to alteration in hormone balance. A similar list of sites has been linked to intake of excess protein: colorectal, pancreatic, breast, uterus body and renal cancer. There is a difficulty as far as the collation studies are concerned in that the intake of fat and protein are interrelated, but multivariate analysis suggests that independent effects exist. Low fibre intake (especially the pentose fraction) has been associated with increased risk of large bowel cancer. High coffee intake is associated with increased risk of pancreatic, bladder and kidney cancer. These are three sites which are related to smoking and it is known that coffee consumption is higher in smokers than non-smokers; though adjustment for smoking has been made in some of the studies, it is not clear whether this completely removes any confounding effect.

Population studies in East Africa have demonstrated a relationship between the degree to which diet is contaminated with aflatoxin and the incidence of liver cancer.

Much laboratory work is devoted to the testing of food additives for carcinogenicity. One class of additives identified as potentially hazardous is artificial sweeteners; case-control studies have produced some conflicting results, but the balance of evidence is that such agents cannot have contributed an appreciable risk of cancer.

Epidemiological studies of varying kinds (use of retrievable data, case-control and prospective) have suggested that reduced vitamin A intake may increase the risk of cancer, particularly of bladder and lung (Bjelke, 1975; Wald *et al.*, 1980). Men attending a medical screening centre in London had a sample of their serum stored; follow-up of about 16 000 men from 1975-78 identified 86 who developed or died from cancer. Their sera and control samples had the retinol levels assayed; low retinol levels were associated with an increased risk of cancer that was not accounted for by variation in age, smoking or initial serum cholesterol levels. The relationship was most marked for lung cancer (Wald et al., 1980). An intervention study has been planned for a randomized controlled trial in about 25 000 subjects (British Medical Journal, 1980).

Laboratory studies have identified over ninety nitrosamine compounds that are carcinogens in many species of animals. In addition to the nitrosamines taken in to the body, these compounds may be found in the stomach and bladder in man as a result of the intake of nitrates or nitrites; the compounds can be metabolized by the human liver to produce carcinogenic metabolites. However, the present epidemiological evidence is extremely tenuous, whether derived from collation studies or case-control studies (see review: Alderson, 1980a). It is not clear whether this is due to the great difficulty in mounting an adequate study to test the hypothesis in man, or due to some unrecognized species difference that makes man resistant to these potent animal carcinogens.

A puzzle comes from some recent studies on blood lipids (initially designed in relationship to ischaemic heart disease). One of the five follow-up studies using dietary control of blood lipids showed an increase in cancer incidence and mortality (see Ederer et al., 1971; Pearce and Dayton, 1971). A WHO trial to lower serum cholesterol by drugs identified a significant excess of gastrointestinal cancers (Committee of Principal Investigators, 1978); a further report on this study confirmed an increase in deaths from cancer in the treated group, though no site was particularly involved (Committee of Principal Investigators, 1980). There has now been published evidence that individuals with low cholesterol at initial examination have an increased risk of subsequently developing malignant disease (Rose et al., 1974). It had been suggested that this might be a reflection of incipient disease (Rose and Shipley, 1980), but a recent report showed the increased risk remained for individuals followed for seven to thirteen years (Kark et al., 1980). No explanation has been yet accepted for these findings.

Drugs

This section relates to various substances that are or have been prescribed as part of medical treatment; only 'chemical' treatments are included, as diagnostic and therapeutic irradiation is covered in the general section on irradiation. The majority of the substances require prescriptions, though use of oral contraceptives, phenacetin and purgatives is also included. Most of the substances have already been referred to in the preceding site-specific sections, but review here enables the text to be ordered alphabetically by drug, noting those which appear to influence risk of cancer at several sites. A few drugs are included where there has been a suggestion, from laboratory or human studies, of a carcinogenic hazard which has as yet not been confirmed. It should also be remembered that the availability of drugs varies from country to country and some of those mentioned below will have been withdrawn from use.

Alkylating agents
These powerful chemicals may be used to treat certain chronic diseases which are responding poorly to other forms of therapy (Sieber and Adamson, 1976), or they

can be given as treatment for malignant disease. Only with improved survival of such patients have there arisen a number of patients followed over several years who have developed a second malignancy (Canellos *et al.*, 1975). In the majority of reported cases this has been the development of leukaemia (for example, following treatment of Hodgkin's disease).

Amphetamines
Limited data suggested an increased risk of Hodgkin's disease (Newell *et al.*, 1973); these findings have not been confirmed, despite the widespread use of this drug (Boston Collaborative Drug Surveillance Program, 1974b).

Anticonvulsants
Laboratory studies suggested that phenobarbitone was a carcinogen. Examination of data for a hospital in Denmark where epilepsy had been controlled for many years suggested there was no increase in malignancy (Clemmesen *et al.*, 1974). Other studies support this negative finding (Jancar, 1980).

Arsenic
Long-continued use of arsenic increases the risk of skin cancer and possibly angiosarcoma of the liver (Hutchinson, 1888; Falk *et al.*, 1979).

Butazolidine
There is limited evidence that this increases the risk of leukaemia (Woodliff and Dougan, 1964).

Chloramphenicol
There is limited evidence that this increases the risk of leukaemia (Fraumeni, 1967).

Chlornaphazine
A review (IARC, 1974) referred to eleven cases of bladder cancer reported after use of this drug and accepted that it was carcinogenic.

Hormones
Many studies have investigated the effects of various contraceptive pills; the widespread use of such drugs makes it important to assess their long-term effects. Present results indicate that certain combined oral contraceptives may increase the risk of breast cancer (WHO, 1978), sequential oral contraceptives may increase the risk of cancer of the body of the uterus (WHO, 1978), whilst the more commonly used pill results in a low but significant level of benign and malignant liver neoplasms (Baum *et al.*, 1973).

Hormone replacement therapy in menopausal women has been associated with added risk of cancer of the breast (Hoover *et al.*, 1976), body of uterus (Lancet, 1979), and ovary (Hoover *et al.*, 1977). These findings have not yet been confirmed let alone quantified in terms of type of preparation used, dose and duration of use, or latent interval.

Anabolic steroids increase the risk of both primary hepatocellular cancer (Johnson *et al.*, 1972) and angiosarcoma of the liver (Falk *et al.*, 1979).

Use of diethylstilboestrol in pregnancy has been followed by a rare form of neoplasm in girls born from such pregnancies—clear cell adenocarcinoma of the vagina (Herbst *et al.*, 1972).

Immunosuppression

Drugs used for this purpose have been used in high dosage for patients having renal (and other) transplants. Relatively shortly after such treatment there is increased risk of non-Hodgkin's lymphoma, and also liver cancer and leukaemia (Kinlen *et al.*, 1979).

Isoniazid

This is another drug which laboratory studies suggested was carcinogenic. Studies of patients treated for tuberculosis and followed up have failed to confirm an increased risk of cancer (Stott *et al.*, 1976; Howe *et al.*, 1979).

Phenacetin abuse

Persistent consumption of high doses of phenacetin can lead to an abnormality in the renal pelvis (with papillary necrosis). Studies of women in Scandinavia, where this abuse seems to have been particularly prevalent, have indicated the increased risk of renal neoplasms (Johansson *et al.*, 1974).

Purgatives

One case-control study of the use of purgatives in patients with alimentary tract cancer has indicated an increased risk with regular use of purgatives (Boyd and Doll, 1954). This finding has not been adequately investigated in other studies to determine whether the original report was a chance finding, a causal relationship or confounding of use in those at high risk of such cancers.

Rauwolfia

Examination of material in a file established to monitor adverse drug reactions suggested there was increased use of this drug in women who developed breast cancer (Boston Collaborative Drug Surveillance Program, 1974a). Though this was supported by further case-control studies, subsequent studies have failed to confirm a significant excess of women have taken such a drug (see Christopher *et al.*, 1977). The original findings and subsequent non-significant excess use of this drug reported by women with breast cancer have not been adequately explained. Rather than dismissing the original findings as chance, it seems more likely that there is a 'weak' aetiological relationship, or confounding with high-risk women more likely to have had treatment with Rauwolfia due to some other characteristic of such women.

Environment

For many years the product of combustion of fossil fuels has led to pollution of the atmosphere, particularly over towns. Initially coal smoke was the predominant pollutant, though industry and the motor vehicle have added other substances of proven or potential toxicity. The mixture of chemicals present in polluted air is often complex, but for many years the only data in the UK related to deposited matter (i.e. soot), smoke and sulphur dioxide levels.

The main health stimulus to environmental control has been the relationship to chest disease (particularly chronic bronchitis and other chronic respiratory disorder); this has been associated with general consideration of damage to buildings. Lawther (1974) reviewed the health hazards from air pollution, and did not mention malignant disease as a specific risk (apart from the suggested relationship to diesel fumes, which were shown not to be a carcinogen).

A number of studies have shown some association between atmospheric pollution and variation in the incidence or mortality from malignant disease; there is a twofold gradient in England and Wales for lung cancer from urban to rural areas. A case-control study in Northern Ireland demonstrated a threefold increase in risk from residence in rural areas to central Belfast; this was contrasted with a twentyfold increase from a non-smoker to someone smoking twenty cigarettes a day (Wicken, 1966).

A review of this topic concluded that some element of the British urban environment produced, in those sufficiently exposed, an increased liability to lung cancer. The exact role of air pollution had not been clarified (Royal College of Physicians, 1970).

A much more specific problem can exist in the vicinity of industrial complexes, in the absence of modern operating systems and devices to prevent pollution. This has already been referred to in the section on asbestos, and will be referred to also in the section on irradiation.

Genes

This section briefly indicates the various categories of familial or genetic contribution in influencing cancer risk; it relies heavily upon two recent books (Mulvihill *et al.*, 1977; Schimke, 1978).

Rare recessive syndromes

The following rare autosomal recessive syndromes have been identified as bearing an increased risk of malignancy: ataxia telangiectasia (leukaemia, lymphoma, gastric, ovarian, brain tumours); Bloom syndrome (leukaemia); Chediak–Higashi syndrome (lymphoma and Hodgkin's); Fanconi's panmyelopathy (leukaemia, oesophagus, skin, liver); Werner syndrome (sarcomas, breast, thyroid, liver, leukaemia); xeroderma pigmentosa (skin including melanoma, tongue, leukaemia).

The risk of malignancy varies and has not always been fully evaluated due to the rarity of the syndromes and shortened life expectancy of those affected.

Premalignant conditions

Polyposis coli occurs as a dominant condition in families and is associated with a greatly increased risk of colon cancer in affected individuals. The cancers are often multiple and occur at a younger age than in other patients. Screening of asymptomatic blood relatives demonstrated the presence of malignancies in 14 per cent.

Bolande (1977) drew attention to work on childhood malignancies, which had indicated that 41 per cent of the affected children had evidence of congenital malformations, with only 13 per cent in controls. He suggested that developmentally anomalous tissue was particularly at risk. Apart from the rare syndromes already referred to, increased risk of malignancy occurs with: aniridia (Wilms); genito-urinary malformations (Wilms); glycogen storage disorders (liver);

hemihypertrophy (Wilms, liver, adrenal cortex); mongolism (leukaemia, retino-blastoma); nevoid basal cell carcinoma syndrome (basal cell cancer, medullo-blastoma, rhabdomyosarcoma); Poland syndrome (leukaemia); 13q-syndrome (retinoblastoma).

Cancer families
The literature documents an appreciable number of families where there appears to be a markedly increased risk of cancer. This may involve a constellation of sites in different members of the families, whilst individual members may have an increased risk of cancer at two or more sites. There is great difficulty in interpreting such reports because: (i) members may share common environments and patterns of behaviour, in addition to genes; (ii) reporting aggregations of cases that are recognized cannot readily be subject to statistical evaluation (unlike the planned search for such groups in cancer registry data). Schimke (1978) suggests there are two types of family syndrome: (a) adenocarcinoma of the breast, ovary, endo-metrium, prostate and colon (plus less frequent involvement of other sites); (b) breast cancer with soft tissue sarcoma and embryonal tumours. Lynch *et al.* (1977) suggested that of all patients with cancer 7 per cent have cancer in three or more first-degree relatives, and this is the group which contributes to the cancer family syndrome. Obviously such a statistic will depend on the size of sibships and the age to which members of the nuclear family are traced.

Genetically determined increase in risk of a specific cancer
Breast cancer is an example where there is a small, but accepted, increase in risk of other cases in sisters or daughters. This is not thought to be due to shared environment (or a breast cancer virus). There is evidence for a slight increase in risk in relatives of patients with cancer of the oesophagus, stomach, colon, rectum, lung, prostate, testis, ovary and leukaemia. There is overlap between the concept of 'cancer families' with increased risk of a range of malignancies and familial risk of a specific cancer; because of the relative frequency of the different cancers and the fact that many of the reports have not been obtained from incidence in completely documented families, it is not straightforward to set out the absolute increment in risk (let alone partition the contribution from common patterns of behaviour or environment).

Genetically determined cancers
Retinoblastomas develop in about 1 in 18 000 live-born children; at least 30 per cent are due to hereditary transmission of an autosomal dominant. About 30 per cent of gene carriers have unilateral disease, whilst the remainder have bilateral or multifocal disease.

Sipple (1961) reported the occurrence of phaeochromocytoma in patients with thyroid cancer. The cancer was subsequently shown to be a medullary tumour derived from C cells (unlike the usual follicular cancer); the tumour secretes large quantities of calcitonin, which may be detected by radio-immunoassay of plasma.

Certain neuroblastoma with multiple tumours may represent a hereditable form of the disease, possibly an autosomal dominant with incomplete penetrance.

Irradiation

The sections on malignancy by site had suggested that irradiation is associated with increased risk of neoplasms of colon and rectum, liver, larynx, bone, skin, breast, brain, thyroid and leukaemia. This section discusses the various sources of irradiation, their relative contribution to additional malignancies, dose-response, and the influence of age at exposure.

Ionizing irradiation can come from therapeutic and diagnostic use of x-rays; therapeutic and diagnostic use of radioactive chemicals; occupation; nuclear warfare; background radiation. Each of these is briefly discussed in turn.

Therapeutic x-rays have been used for non-malignant and malignant conditions. Though there is only limited use of x-rays to treat non-malignant conditions at present, this has been used in the past to treat appreciable numbers of (i) infants with minor upper respiratory symptoms and suggestions of 'enlarged thymus' (Hempelmann et al., 1975), (ii) children with tinea capitis (Modan et al., 1977), (iii) adults with ankylosing spondylitis (Court Brown and Doll, 1965), (iv) women with menorrhagia (Smith and Doll, 1976). X-ray of the head and head and neck in childhood has been followed by raised incidence of thyroid tumours. The treatment of adults is more closely linked to leukaemia. As survival from malignant disease improves, the long-term increment in leukaemia becomes more readily apparent (for example in adolescents treated for Hodgkin's disease), though other forms of therapy may also be leukaemogenic (Li et al., 1975).

Diagnostic x-rays, by virtue of their much lower dose than required for therapy, pose much less hazard. However, there is direct evidence of increased breast cancer in women who have had repeat fluoroscopy (MacKenzie, 1965). The influence of much lower dosage than this is discussed later, in commenting on the dose–response relationship.

A very special category of risk is that of the fetus exposed to x-rays taken (usually) for some diagnostic process during pregnancy. Stewart and her colleagues (1956, 1958) demonstrated that an excess of mothers whose children died from leukaemia reported antenatal x-ray more frequently than control mothers. Using a quite different approach MacMahon (1962) replicated these findings and pointed out that the published studies on this topic were all compatible with about a twofold increase in risk of leukaemia. Mole (1974) demonstrated that the results were not due to selection of high leukaemia-risk subjects for x-ray. The contribution of prenatal x-ray to leukaemia in childhood has decreased since the initial findings, probably due to lower dose per film and fewer films being taken (Bithell and Stewart, 1975).

Considerable care has been taken to assemble data on groups of patients receiving radioactive isotopes for diagnostic or therapeutic purposes. Thorotrast is an exception, in that case reports and subsequently carefully conducted follow-up studies showed an increase in risk of liver angiosarcoma and leukaemia (Horta et al., 1965). There is no evidence that ^{131}I, which has been used on large numbers of patients for diagnostic and therapeutic purposes, increases the risk of malignant disease (see Pochin, 1967), though it has been pointed out that longer follow-up may be required to identify carcinogenicity with a lengthy latent interval (Hoffman and Lundin, 1978).

Occupational exposure occurs in three categories of workers: staff involved in medical care and laboratory research; workers in the construction industry testing the viability of metal welds; workers in the nuclear power industry. The pioneer radiologists and radiographers, working without clear guidance on safe levels of radiation, developed skin changes (telangiectasis, pigmentation, atrophy) that were followed by multiple skin cancers often leading to tragic deaths (Ingram and Comaish, 1967). However, such complications do not occur below a total lifetime exposure of 1000 rads—well above the levels that should occur with present-day safety measures. There has also been a suggestion that the 'early' radiologists had an increased risk of mortality from leukaemia (March, 1950).

Work in America has suggested that workers exposed in the past thirty years to low levels of ionizing radiation had an excess of malignancies such as myeloma (Mancuso et al., 1977) or leukaemia (Najarian and Colton, 1978). Both these studies have provoked debate and criticism and their findings are not generally accepted (see Reissland, 1978). There is no accepted evidence demonstrating an increase in any malignancy amongst workers in the nuclear power industry.

Very different to the above has been the clearly defined hazard of bone cancer and leukaemia in luminizers or radium dial workers (see Polednak et al., 1978). Another category is men working in mines where the air is contaminated by radon and other radioactive particles (Wagoner et al., 1965). Other jobs have been suggested as hazardous, such as the use of artificial radionuclides in activation analysis, oil-well drilling, and tracer chemistry, or astronauts exposed to cosmic rays (Archer, 1977). No epidemiological data have demonstrated the risks in such workers.

One of the medium- to long-term hazards from nuclear warfare is the question of excess malignancies at a number of sites; this has been documented in a series of papers based on detailed follow-up of persons surviving the atomic bomb explosions at Hiroshima and Nagasaki (BEIR Committee, 1980; Morgan, 1980). More recent experience stems from the further testing of nuclear weapons, such as the generation of thyroid cancer in those exposed to radioactive iodine fall-out in the Pacific (Conard et al., 1970). Much more controversial has been the suggestion of an increased risk of leukaemia in US military involved in manœuvres after a nuclear explosion (Bond and Hamilton, 1980; Caldwell et al., 1980).

Compared with the points raised above, the natural background radiation, which varies within and between countries, is of low magnitude and shows no clear relationship to risk of malignancy (Court Brown et al., 1960; Pincet and Massé, 1975).

In considering prevention of risk from irradiation it is important that an indication of the dose–response relationship can be provided, at the level of exposure postulated as 'safe' (Gloag, 1980). The carcinogenic process is thought to be initiated by an effect on the cell nucleus; the probability of this event decreases with the reduction in dose and very large numbers of individuals must have their exposure measured and then be followed up to determine the relationship. A linear relationship has been suggested for the commonly occurring types of radiation (β-particles, γ-rays or x-rays); there is inadequate evidence on this point and it has been argued that this may under- or overestimate the actual hazard at very low levels (BEIR report, 1980).

There is evidence that age influences the radiosensitivity and this may affect the likelihood of cancer in different organs at different ages. Breast cancer seems most likely to be generated by exposure at age 10–19 years (Land, 1980); the thyroid seems more sensitive in childhood, though reappraisal did not confirm this (Dolphin, 1980); leukaemia has been shown to have a linear relationship with increasing age at exposure in UK data (Doll, 1972), though this was not so for Japanese atomic bomb survivors under the age of 20 (Doll, 1977).

Occupation

This section includes both specific clearly defined carcinogens present in occupational environments and the more general leads that have come from studies on groups of workers. For example, woodworkers have been identified as at particularly high risk of nasal cancer, though there is no indication of the carcinogen involved other than a relationship between risk and degree of dust exposure. In many occupational studies the individual workers will have been potentially exposed to a wide range of specific chemicals at work (irrespective of variation in non-occupational carcinogens). No further mention is made of asbestos or irradiation, which have already been covered; some occupations may directly or indirectly affect the consumption of alcohol or tobacco and again this is not dealt with in the following comments.

The following occupations are dealt with in alphabetical order, either of the specific agent involved or the job involved.

Arsenic
Many years ago it was recognized that exposure to arsenic in a smelter or use of pesticides containing arsenic could increase the risk of skin cancer (Hill *et al.*, 1948). Subsequently a hazard of liver and lung cancer was demonstrated (Pinto *et al.*, 1977).

Benzene
Initially, case reports identified the hazard of blood dyscrasias (Delore and Borgamano, 1928). Subsequent studies of workers using benzene as a solvent, for example in shoe making or rubber production, demonstrated an excess of leukaemia (Aksoy *et al.*, 1974; Tyroler *et al.*, 1976). There is less well documented evidence of an increase in lymphoma (Vianna and Polan, 1979).

Cadmium
An excess of deaths from prostate cancer was found amongst a small group of workers (Potts, 1965). Three out of four further studies indicated a relationship, but only one of these results was significant (Kipling and Waterhouse, 1967; Lemen *et al.*, 1976; Kolonel and Winkelstein, 1977; Ross *et al.*, 1979).

Chemists
A number of studies have indicated that professional chemists have an increased risk of a variety of malignant disease: colon and rectum; pancreas; brain tumours; Hodgkin's disease; lymphoma (Li *et al.*, 1969; Olin, 1978; Olin and Ahlbom, 1980).

Chloromethyl ether, chloroprene; chromates
Workers exposed to these chemicals have an increased risk of lung cancer (Bidstrup, 1951; Lloyd, 1976; Weiss and Figueroa, 1976). The numbers of workers involved are relatively small and the risk is not greatly raised.

Dusts—inorganic

A number of studies have suggested that coal-miners have an increased risk of stomach cancer (Matolo *et al.*, 1972; Registrar General, 1978) and one prospective study has shown that this is related to levels of dust exposure (Jacobson, 1976). There is some indication of increase in lung cancer in talc miners and millers (Kleinfeld *et al.*, 1974). The 1970-72 occupational mortality statistics for England and Wales suggested a more general association of stomach cancer with a number of 'dusty' jobs (Registrar General, 1978).

Dusts—organic

Nasal cancer has been associated with exposure to dust of hard woods and from leather in shoe manufacture (Acheson *et al.*, 1967; 1970). Less clear cut are the suggestions of increased risk of laryngeal cancer and Hodgkin's disease in wood-workers (Petersen and Milham, 1974; Bross *et al.*, 1978).

Dyestuffs

As a result of case reports, studies were mounted and demonstrated an increased risk of bladder cancer in workers exposed to β-naphthylamine, auramine, benzidene and magenta (Case *et al.*, 1954; Case, 1966). It was subsequently shown that β-naphthylamine had been used as a curing agent in producing rubber; workers manufacturing rubber and producing cable coated with rubber were also shown to be at increased risk of bladder cancer (Case and Hosker, 1954; Davies, 1965). Gas retort workers who were exposed to aromatic amines were found to have an increased risk of bladder cancer (Doll *et al.*, 1965). It has also been suggested that β-naphthylamine increases the risk of pancreatic cancer.

Foundry workers

An increased risk of lung cancer has been recorded, but a specific carcinogen has not been demonstrated (Decoufle and Wood, 1979).

Isopropyl alcohol

Limited studies on small groups of workers involved in manufacture of isopropyl alcohol have been shown to indicate an increased risk of nasal cancer (Alderson and Rattan, 1980). This is thought to be associated with the alkyl sulphates that were involved in the process (Lynch *et al.*, 1979).

Mustard gas

Manufacture of this is associated with an increased risk of lung cancer (Beebe, 1960).

Nickel refining

Workers have an increased risk of nasal, laryngeal and lung cancer (Pederson *et al.*, 1973; Doll *et al.*, 1977).

Polycyclic hydrocarbons

Over 250 years ago it was reported that chimney-sweeps, who were exposed to soot, had an increased risk of scrotal cancer. In the present century, oil, pitch and tar exposure has been shown to increase the risk of skin cancer. This class of compounds may also be the agent responsible for the increased lung cancer that occurs in coke-oven workers (Doll *et al.*, 1972), and those exposed to oil mists (Waterhouse, 1971).

Petroleum refinery workers
A number of studies have reported the patterns of mortality of refinery workers and though there is not consistency in all the findings—let alone identification of any aetiological agents—there have been indications of an increased risk of colorectal cancer, melanoma and brain tumours in some of the studies (Hanis *et al.*, 1979; Rushton and Alderson, 1980; Thomas *et al.*, 1980).

Vinyl chloride
Case reports identified a few deaths from the very rare angiosarcoma of the liver in men who had been heavily exposed to vinyl chloride monomer in the US. Subsequent studies confirmed the hazard in workers on vinyl chloride plants in a number of countries (Falk *et al.*, 1979). Relatively few workers were involved and though the risk of angiosarcoma was greatly raised, it still remained an uncommon hazard in the occupation. There has been evidence of increased risk of other neoplasms, particularly tumours of the brain (Monson *et al.*, 1974).

It is not a simple matter to extend the above comments to quantification of the proportion of cancers that are due to occupation. It has been suggested that most cancers are attributable to environmental factors (WHO, 1964; Clayson, 1967; Boyland, 1967; Lancet, 1977b). This is agreed particularly on the basis of international variation in incidence site by site, with the lowest rate for any country giving an indication of the genetic contribution to cancer. By considering the number of workers exposed to various carcinogens and the relative risks involved, it has been suggested that perhaps 1–5 per cent of cancers are due to occupation (Higginson and Muir, 1976; Doll, 1977b; Wynder and Gori, 1977); another estimate was 10–15 per cent (Cole, 1977). A report from the US has suggested that 23–38 per cent of total cancer mortality in future decades might be occupationally related (Bridbord *et al.*, 1978); this report, which received wide publicity, has been criticized as being out of line with present evidence and incorporating ill-founded extrapolations (e.g. Lancet, 1978; Peto, 1980).

Smoking

The site-specific sections mentioned a relationship with smoking for mouth (p. 27), oesophagus (p. 27), pancreas (p. 31), larynx (p. 32), lung (p. 33), and bladder (p. 41). Figure 3.2 presents the trends in mortality for males aged 65–69 years for these six eites. This shows a very marked rise in lung cancer (note a log scale is used on the vertical axis). The trends for the other sites are quite different, indicating that the component of the disease associated with smoking is in a very different proportion in these sites. This section is devoted to some general issues, though it particularly overlaps with the items covered in the lung section on the debate over causality. An important issue is the interaction between smoking and other environmental agents; this has already been briefly dealt with in the section on alcohol (p. 47).

Smoking is a prevalent habit in many societies, including populations in all developed and many developing countries (this aspect is dealt with further in a later chapter—see Figs. 5.1 to 5.5). It is an example of a health hazard that

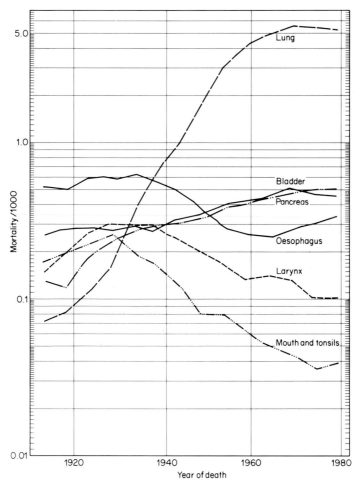

Fig. 3.2 Smoking-related cancers: mortality rates per 1000 males aged 65–69 years in England and Wales, 1911–78.

influences the risk of many diseases, affecting different organs, a wide age range, and chronic diseases as well as malignant conditions. The extent of the general public health problem is beyond the scope of this book, but an indication of this is warranted as it is a crucial background to the consideration of priority for action. Restricting consideration to the development of fatal disease in the middle aged and elderly, there is firm evidence that the 'all-cause' mortality rates of smokers are double that of non-smokers in males under 70 years, and increased by 50 per cent for those over the age of 70 (Doll and Peto, 1976). Table 3.3 presents data derived from follow-up of a large number of male British doctors for twenty years; death rates (adjusted for age) are given for four causes for non-smokers and heavy smokers, i.e. those smoking more than twenty-four cigarettes daily. These data are then converted into a ratio of the rates and the attributable death rate (i.e. the increment in the death rate if the heavy smoking was a causal

Table 3.3 Age-adjusted death rates from four diseases in non-smokers and those smoking more than 24 cigarettes daily, with rate ratio and attributable rate. (Based on data from Doll and Peto, 1976.)

Cause	Non-smokers	Heavy smokers	Rate ratio	Attributable rate
Lung cancer	10	251	25.1	241
Chronic bronchitis and emphysema	3	114	38.0	111
Ischaemic heart disease	413	792	1.9	379
Cerebral thrombosis	86	137	1.6	51
All causes	1317	2843	2.2	1526

agent). Comparison of the magnitude of the rate ratios and the attributable rate shows quite marked differences; this presents these conditions in different perspectives. The rate ratio is a measure of the chance of an individual dying from a given disease if he smokes heavily (taking into account the mortality from that condition in the non-smoker). The attributable rate shows the additional burden of mortality in the population from the influence of heavy smoking. The risk of lung cancer is greatly raised in the heavy smoker, whilst the population burden comes predominantly from the extra deaths from ischaemic heart disease. Such data can be further manipulated to provide estimates of the impact upon such diseases of the cessation of smoking in the population (by calculating the percentage of deaths in the community that are attributable to present/past smoking). This interesting aspect is again beyond the scope of this limited contribution. Comparable data are shown in Table 3.4 for four other sites of malignancy; again the two indices give varying estimates of the importance of smoking as far as individual risks and population effects are concerned.

Table 3.4 Age-adjusted death rates from four sites in non-smokers and those smoking more than 24 cigarettes daily, with rate ratio and attributable rate. (Based on data from Doll and Peto, 1976.)

Site	Non-smokers	Heavy smokers	Rate ratio	Attributable rate
'Other respiratory'*	1	33	33	32
Oesophagus	3	21	7	18
Pancreas	14	29	2	15
Bladder	9	13	1.4	4

* Combination of lip, tongue, mouth, pharynx except nasopharynx, larynx, and trachea.

The evidence for causality, rather than mere association between smoking and certain diseases, stems from a variety of aspects of past work. The range of studies, involving different methods, different countries, different time periods, provides a very convincing body of evidence. The strength of the associations is a major point against bias being the reason for the findings. As far as lung cancer is concerned, there is evidence that many aspects of smoking are associated with variations in risk and all are likely 'markers' of the degree of exposure of the bronchial tree to the products of cigarette combustion (see p. 33). Examination of histological specimens in Norway showed a major change in type of lung cancer: that type which had increased in prevalence was associated with smoking (Kreyberg, 1956). Follow-up of groups with known smoking habits has demonstrated

Table 3.5 Accepted causes of cancer, showing source and site affected

Cause	Source	Pharynx	GI tract	Liver	Nose	Larynx	Lung	Meso-thelioma	Bone	Skin	Breast	Female genital	Prostate	Bladder	Kidney	Brain	Haematopoietic
Acrilonitrile	Manufacture		+				+										
Aflatoxin	Diet		+	+													
Alcohol	Diet	+		+		+											
Alkylating agents	Therapy													+			+
4-Aminodiphenyl	Manufacture													+			
Arsenic	Occupation; therapy			+			+			+							+
Asbestos	Occupation		+			+	+	+									
Benzene	Occupation								+								+
Beryllium	Occupation						+										
Butazolidine	Therapy																+
Cadmium	Occupation						+						+				
Chloramphenicol	Therapy																+
Chlornaphazine	Occupation													+			
Chloromethyl ether	Occupation						+										
Chloroprene	Manufacture						+										
Chromates	Occupation	+			+		+										
Dust: inorganic	Occupation		+														
Dust: organic	Occupation		+		+												
Dyestuffs	Occupation													+			
Ethylene oxide	Occupation		+														
Foundry workers	Occupation						+										
Haematite	Mining						+										+

Cause	Source	Pharynx	GI tract	Liver	Nose	Larynx	Lung	Meso-thelioma	Bone	Skin	Breast	Female genital	Prostate	Bladder	Kidney	Brain	Haemato poietic
Hormones:																	
androgens	Therapy			+													
diethylstilboestrol	Therapy										+	+					
oestrogens	Therapy			+								+					
oral contraception												+					
Immunosuppression	Therapy	+	+														+
Irradiation	Medical care, occupation, warfare, background			+		+			+	+	+	+				+	+
Isopropyl alcohol	Manufacture	+			+	+											
Mustard gas	Manufacture				+	+	+										
Nickel	Refining				+		+										
Phenacetin	Therapy													+	+		
Polycyclic aromatic hydrocarbons	Environment, occupation		+			+	+			+				+			
Smoking		+	+			+	+							+			
Vinyl chloride	Manufacture		+	+			+									+	+
u.v. light	Sunlight									+							

a relative decrease in risk of lung cancer in those who gave up smoking compared with those who continue. Despite such evidence, it has still been suggested that smoking may be a reflection of genetically determined patterns of behaviour, and that risk of lung cancer was also genetically high in those destined to smoke. The major Swedish twin study does not indicate that this is an adequate explanation of the situation (Cederlöf *et al.*, 1977).

Follow-up of over 6000 British women doctors for twenty-two years (Doll *et al.*, 1980) was still only able to provide an early warning of the possible hazards from smoking in women. This was because of the relatively low prevalence of the habit in women born before 1915 and the low numbers of deaths by smoking category and cause from which to calculate rates. It was shown that there was a significant association for ischaemic heart disease, lung cancer and chronic obstructive airways disease. An indication of the potential hazard was not only the increased prevalence of smoking in the younger generation, but the increase in number of cigarettes smoked and the proportion inhaling. The latter was reported as an ill-omen, though earlier work had shown some anomalous results in relation to the males' inhaling (Doll and Peto, 1976).

Detailed analysis of the data from the British doctors (Doll and Peto, 1978) indicates the relationship between cigarette consumption per day and duration of smoking against incidence of lung cancer. The best fit was found for those who started smoking aged 16–25 years, using a second-order polynomial, i.e. 0.26 $(\text{dose}+6)^2$ and raising the age to a power between 4 and 5. This indicates a powerful effect from duration of smoking, and that smoking is likely to affect more than one stage in the genesis of cancers.

Overview of cancer aetiology

In order to provide a concise basis for the subsequent chapters on prevention, Table 3.5 is provided. This indicates those causes that are accepted at present, the source of exposure and the sites affected. Much of the information condensed into this table has been discussed in preceding sections of this chapter.

A major review of the chemicals and industrial processes associated with cancer in humans dealt with sixty chemicals for which there were published case reports or epidemiological data (International Agency for Research in Cancer, 1979). This was the core of substances for which human data existed, following detailed review of 442 substances in the first twenty volumes of the IARC monographs on evaluation of carcinogenic risk of chemicals to humans. Others have produced comparable tables, though the classification and layout vary (e.g. Doll, 1980).

References

Acheson, E. D., Cowdell, R. H. and Jolles, B. (1970). *British Medical Journal* **1**, 385.
Acheson, E. D., Hadfield, E. H. and MacBeth, R. G. (1967). *Lancet* **i**, 311.
Adams, J. B. and Wong, M. S. F. (1968). *Lancet* **ii**, 1163.
Adelstein, A. M., Hill, G. B. and Maung, L. (1971). *British Journal of Preventive and Social Medicine* **25**, 186.
Aghai, E., Hulu, N., Virag, I., Kende, G. and Ramot, B. (1974). *Cancer* **33**, 1411.
Aird, I., Bentall, H. H., Mehigan, J. A. and Roberts, J. A. F. (1954). *British Medical Journal* **2**, 315.
Aitken-Swan, J. and Baird, D. (1965). *British Journal of Cancer* **19**, 217.
Aksoy, M., Erdem, S. and Guncag, D. (1974). *Blood* **44**, 837.

Albert, R. E., Burns, F. J. and Altshuler, B. (1979). In *New Concepts in Safety Evaluation*, pp. 89–95. Ed. by M. A. Mehlman, R. E. Shapiro and H. Blumenthal. Hemisphere Publishing, New York.

Alderson, M. R. (1977). *An Introduction to Epidemiology*. Macmillan, London.

Alderson, M. R. (1980a). In *Human Health and Environmental Toxicants*, pp. 107–125. Ed. by L. Wood. Academic Press and Royal Society of Medicine, London.

Alderson, M. R. (1980b). *Journal of Epidemiology and Community Health* **34**, 182.

Alderson, M. R. (1980c). In *Recent Results in Cancer Research*, Vol. 73, pp. 1–22. Ed. by W. D. Duncan. Springer, Berlin.

Alderson, M. R. (1980d). *Advances in Cancer Research* **31**, 2.

Alderson, M. R. (1981). *International Mortality Statistics*. Macmillan, London.

Alderson, M. R. and Nayak, R. (1971). *British Journal of Preventive and Social Medicine* **25**, 168.

Alderson, M. R. and Rattan, N. (1980). *British Journal of Industrial Medicine* **37**, 85.

Alderson, M. R. and Rushton, L. (1980). *An Epidemiological Survey of Eight Oil Refineries in the UK—Final Report*. Institute of Petroleum, London.

Anderson, D. E. (1974). *Cancer* **34**, 1090.

Annegers, J. F., O'Fallon, W. and Kurland, L. T. (1977). *Lancet* **ii**, 869.

Anthony, H. M. and Thomas, G. M. (1970). *Journal of the National Cancer Institute* **45**, 879.

Anthony, P. P., Vogel, C. L., Sadikali, F., Barker, L. F. and Peterson, M. R. (1972). *British Medical Journal* **1**, 403.

Aoki, K. (1978). *World Health Statistics Quarterly* **31**, 28.

Archer, E. (1977). *Cancer* **39**, 1802.

Archer, V. E., Gillam, J. D. and Wagoner, J. K. (1976). *Annals of the New York Academy of Science* **271**, 280.

Aries, V., Crowther, J. S., Drasar, B. S., Hill, M. J. and Williams, R. E. O. (1969). *Gut* **10**, 334.

Armenian, H. K., Lilienfeld, A. M., Diamond, E. L. and Bross, I. D. J. (1974). *Lancet* **ii**, 115.

Armstrong, B. (1976). *International Journal of Cancer* **17**, 204.

Armstrong, B. and Doll, R. (1975). *International Journal of Cancer* **15**, 617.

Ask-Upmark, E. (1955). *Diseases of the Chest* **27**, 427.

Axelson, O. and Sundell, L. (1974). *Work–Environmental Health* **11**, 21.

Bagshawe, K. D. (1967). In *The Prevention of Cancer*, pp. 276–80. Ed. by R. W. Raven and F. J. C. Roe. Butterworths, London.

Bahn, A. K., Rosenwaike, I., Herrmann, N., Grover, P., Stellman, J. and O'Leary, K. (1976). *New England Journal of Medicine* **295**, 450.

Bartholomew, L. G., Gross, J. B. and Comfort, M. W. (1958). *Gastroenterology* **35**, 473.

Baum, J. K., Holtz, F., Bookstein, J. J. and Klein, E. W. (1973). *Lancet* **ii**, 926.

Beebe, G. W. (1960). *Journal of the National Cancer Institute* **25**, 1231.

BEIR Committee (1980). National Academy of Science, 3rd report.

Bell, J. (1876). *Edinburgh Medical Journal* **22**, 135.

Beral, V. (1974). *Lancet* **i**, 1037.

Beral, V., Fraser, P. and Chilvers, C. (1978). *Lancet* **i**, 1083.

Berg, J. W. and Burbank, F. (1972). *Annals of the New York Academy of Sciences* **199**, 249.

Bhamarapravati, N. and Viranuvatti, V. (1966). *American Journal of Gastroenterology* **45**, 267.

Bidstrup, P. L. (1951). *British Journal of Industrial Medicine* **8**, 302.

Bingham, S., Williams, D. R. R., Cole, J. J. and James, W. P. T. (1979). *British Journal of Cancer* **40**, 456.

Bithell, J. F. and Stewart, A. (1975). *British Journal of Cancer* **31**, 271.

Bjelke, E. (1971). In *Oncology Vol. 5: Proc. 10th International Cancer Congress*, pp. 320–34. Ed. by R. L. Clarke, R. C. Cumley, J. E. McCoy and M. M. Copeland. Year Book Medical, Chicago.

Bjelke, E. (1974). *Scandinavian Journal of Gastroenterology* **9**, Suppl. 31, 1.

Bjelke, E. (1975). *International Journal of Cancer* **15**, 561.

Blackburn, E. K., Callender, S. T., Dacie, J. V., Doll, R., Girdwood, R. H., Mollin, D. L., Saracci, R., Stafford, J. L., Thompson, R. B., Varadi, S. and Wetherley-Mein, G. (1968). *International Journal of Cancer* **3**, 163.

Blair, A. and Fraumeni, J. F. (1978). *Journal of the National Cancer Institute* **61**, 1379.

Blair, A. and Hayes, H. M. (1980). *International Journal of Cancer* **25**, 118.

Blot, W. J. and Fraumeni, J. F. (1977). *Journal of Chronic Diseases* **30**, 745.

Blot, W. J., Fraumeni, J. F. and Morris, L. E. (1978). *Lancet* **ii**, 674.

Blum, A. and Ames, B. N. (1977). *Science* **195**, 17.
Boice, J. D. and Monson, R. A. (1977). *Journal of the National Cancer Institute* **59**, 823.
Bolande, R. P. (1977). In *Genetics of Human Cancer*, pp. 43–75. Ed. by J. J. Muluihill, R. W. Miller and J. F. Fraumeni. Raven Press, New York.
Bond, V. P. and Hamilton, L. D. (1980). *Journal of the American Medical Association* **244**, 1610.
Bone, E., Drasar, B. S. and Hill, M. J. (1975). *Lancet* **i**, 1117.
Boston Collaborative Drug Surveillance Program (1974a). *Lancet* **ii**, 669.
Boston Collaborative Drug Surveillance Program (1974b). *Journal of the American Medical Association* **229**, 1462.
Bourke, J. B. and Griffin, J. P. (1962). *Lancet* **ii**, 1279.
Boyd, J. T. and Doll, R. (1954). *British Journal of Cancer* **8**, 231.
Boyd, J. T. and Doll, R. (1964). *British Journal of Cancer* **18**, 419.
Boyd, J. T., Doll, R., Faulds, J. S. and Leiper, J. (1970). *British Journal of Industrial Medicine* **27**, 97.
Boyland, E. (1967). *Practitioner* **199**, 277.
Breslow, N., Chan, C. W., Dhom, G., Drury, R. A. B., Franks, L. M., Gellei, B., Lee, Y. S., Lundberg, S., Sparke, B., Sternby, N. H. and Tulinius, H. (1977). *International Journal of Cancer* **20**, 680.
Breslow, N. E. and Enstrom, J. E. (1974). *Journal of the National Cancer Institute* **53**, 631.
Brett, G. Z. and Benjamin, B. (1968). *British Medical Journal* **3**, 82.
Bridbord, K., Decoufle, P., Fraumeni, J. F., Hoel, O. G., Hoover, R. N., Rall, D. P., Saffioti, W., Schneiderman, M. A. and Upton, A. C. (1978). *Estimates of the fraction of cancer in the United States related to occupational factors*. National Institutes of Health, Washington.
Brinkley, D. and Haybittle, J. L. (1969). *British Journal of Radiology* **42**, 519.
British Medical Journal (1980). *British Medical Journal* **281**, 957.
Brody, H. and Cullen, M. (1957). *Surgery* **42**, 600.
Bross, I. D. J., Berteu, R. and Gibson, R. (1972). *American Journal of Public Health* **62**, 1520.
Bross, I. D. J. and Gibson, R. (1968). *American Journal of Public Health* **58**, 1396.
Bross, I. D. J., Viadana, E. and Houten, L. (1978). *Archives of Environmental Health* **33**, 300.
Brown, R. L., Suh, J. M. and Scarborough, J. E. (1965). *Cancer* **18**, 2.
Buell, P. (1973). *Journal of the National Cancer Institute* **51**, 1479.
Buell, P., Dunn, J. E. and Breslow, L. (1960). *Journal of Chronic Disease* **12**, 600.
Bulbrook, R. D. and Hayward, J. L. (1967). *Lancet* **i**, 519.
Burch, G. E. and Ansari, A. (1968). *Archives of Internal Medicine* **122**, 273.
Burch, P. R. J. (1980). *Journal of Chronic Diseases* **33**, 221.
Burkitt, D. (1959). *British Journal of Surgery* **46**, 218.
Bussey, H. J. R. (1975). *Familial Polyposis Coli*. Johns Hopkins University, Baltimore.
Caldwell, G. G., Kelley, D. B. and Heath, C. W. (1980). *Journal of the American Medical Association* **244**, 1575.
Campbell, H. E. (1959). *Journal of Urology* **81**, 663.
Canellos, G. P., DeVita, V. T., Arsenaan, J. L., Whang-Peng, J. and Johnson, R. E. C. (1975). *Lancet* **i**, 947.
Cantor, K. P. and Fraumeni, J. F. (1980). *Cancer Research* **40**, 2645.
Capurro, P. U. and Eldridge, J. E. (1978). *Lancet* **i**, 942.
Carroll, R. E., Haddon, W., Handy, V. H. and Wieben, E. E. (1964). *Journal of the National Cancer Institute* **33**, 277.
Casagrande, J. T., Pike, M. C., Ross, R. K., Louie, E. W., Roy, S. and Henderson, B. E. (1979). *Lancet* **ii**, 170.
Case, R. A. M. (1966). *Annals of the Royal College of Surgeons of England* **39**, 223.
Case, R. A. M. and Hosker, M. E. (1954). *British Journal of Preventive and Social Medicine* **8**, 39.
Case, R. A. M., Hosker, M. E., McDonald, D. B. and Pearson, J. T. (1954). *British Journal of Industrial Medicine* **11**, 75.
Case, R. A. M. and Lea, A. J. (1955). *British Journal of Preventive and Social Medicine* **9**, 62.
Cecchi, F., Buatti, E., Kriebel, O., Nastasi, L. and Santucci, M. (1980). *British Journal of Industrial Medicine* **37**, 222.
Cederlöf, R., Friberg, L. and Lundman, T. (1977). *Acta Medica Scandinavica Supplement* **612**.
Ch'en, M-C., Hu, J-C., Chang, P'Y., Chuang, C-Y., Ts'ao, P. F., Chang, S-H., Wang, F. P., Chen, T. L. and Choo, S. C. (1965). *Chinese Medical Journal* **84**, 513.

Choi, N. W., Shettigara, P. T., Abu-Zeid, H. A. H. and Nelson, N. A. (1977). *International Journal of Cancer* **19,** 167.

Christopher, L. J., Crooks, J., Moir, D. and Weir, R. D. (1977). *Lancet* **i,** 140.

Clark, C. G. and Mitchell, P. E. G. (1961). *British Medical Journal* **2,** 1259.

Clayson, D. B. (1967). *European Journal of Cancer* **3,** 405.

Clemmesen, J. (1968). *Acta Pathologica et Microbiologica Scandinavica* **72,** 348.

Clemmesen, J. (1977). *Statistical Studies in Malignant Neoplasms*, Vol. V. Munksgaard, Copenhagen.

Clemmesen, J., Fuglsang-Frederiksen, V. and Plum, C. M. (1974). *Lancet* **i,** 705.

Cole, P. (1977). *Cancer* **39,** 1788.

Cole, P., MacMahon, B. and Aisenberg, A. (1968). *Lancet* **ii,** 1371.

Committee of Principal Investigators (1978). *British Heart Journal* **40,** 1069.

Committee of Principal Investigators (1980). *Lancet* **ii,** 379.

Conard, R. A., Dobyns, B. M. and Sutow, W. W. (1970). *Journal of the American Medical Association* **214,** 316.

Cook-Mozaffari, P. J., Axordegan, F., Day, N. E., Ressicaud, A., Sabai, C. and Aramesh, B. (1979). *British Journal of Cancer* **39,** 293.

Court Brown, W. M. and Doll, R. (1965). *British Medical Journal* **2,** 1327.

Court Brown, W. M., Doll, R., Spiers, F. W. and Duffy, R. J. (1960). *British Medical Journal* **1,** 1753.

Dales, L. G., Friedman, G. D., Ury, H. K., Grossman, S. and Williams, S. R. (1979). *American Journal of Epidemiology* **109,** 132.

Dark, J., O'Connor, M., Pemberton, M. and Russell, M. H. (1963). *British Medical Journal* **2,** 1164.

Davies, J. M. (1965). *Lancet* **ii,** 143.

Davies, J. M. (1982). The epidemiology of bladder cancer. In *Scientific Foundations of Urology*, 2nd edn. Ed. by D. Innes Williams and G. D. Chisholm. Heinemann Medical, London. In press.

Davies, J. N. P. (1975). In *Persons at High Risk of Cancer*, pp. 373–81. Ed. by J. F. Fraumeni. Academic Press, New York.

Dean, G., Lee, P. N., Todd, G. F. and Wicken, A. J. (1977). *Report on a Second Retrospective Mortality Study in North East England, Part I*. Tobacco Research Council, London.

Dean, G., MacLennan, R., McLoughlin, H. and Shelley, E. (1979). *British Journal of Cancer* **40,** 581.

Decoufle, P. and Wood, D. J. (1979). *American Journal of Epidemiology* **109,** 667.

Delore, P. and Borgamano, C. (1928). *Journal de Médecine, Lyon* **9,** 227.

Diamond, M. (1952). *American Journal of Digestive Diseases* **19,** 47.

Dobyns, B. M., Sheline, G. E., Workman, J. B., Tomkins, E. A., McConahey, W. M. and Becker, D. V. (1974). *Journal of Clinical Endocrinology and Metabolism* **38,** 976.

Dodge, O. G. and Linsell, C. A. (1963). *Cancer* **16,** 1255.

Doll, R. (1955). *British Journal of Industrial Medicine* **12,** 81.

Doll, R. (1972). *The Epidemiology of Leukaemia*. Leukaemic Research Fund, London.

Doll, R. (1977a). Personal Communication.

Doll, R. (1977b). *Journal of the Royal College of Physicians* **11,** 125.

Doll, R. (1980). *Cancer* **45,** 2475.

Doll, R., Drane, H. and Newell, A. C. (1961). *Gut* **2,** 352.

Doll, R., Fisher, R. E. W., Gammon, E. J., Gunn, W., Hughes, G. O., Tyrer, F. H. and Wilson, W. (1965). *British Journal of Industrial Medicine* **22,** 1.

Doll, R., Gray, R., Hafner, B. and Peto, R. (1980). *British Medical Journal* **280,** 967.

Doll, R. and Hill, A. B. (1950). *British Medical Journal* **2,** 739.

Doll, R., Hill, A. B., Gray, P. G. and Parr, E. A. (1959). *British Medical Journal* **i,** 322.

Doll, R., Mathews, J. D. and Morgan, L. G. (1977). *British Journal of Industrial Medicine* **34,** 102.

Doll, R. and Peto, R. (1976). *British Medical Journal* **1,** 1525.

Doll, R. and Peto, R. (1978). *Journal of Epidemiology and Community Health* **32,** 303.

Doll, R., Vessey, M. P., Beasley, R. W. R., Buckley, A. R., Fears, E. C., Fisher, R. E. W., Gammon, E. J., Gunn, W., Hughes, G. O., Lee, K. and Norman-Smith, B. (1972). *British Journal of Industrial Medicine* **29,** 394.

Dolphin, G. W. (1980). In *Thyroid Cancer*, pp. 23–30. Ed. by W. D. Duncan. Springer Verlag, Berlin.

Donnelly, P. K., Baker, K. W., Carney, J. A. and O'Fallon, W. M. (1975). *Mayo Clinic Proceedings* **50, 650**.

Draper, G. J., Heaf, M. M. and Kinnier Wilson, L. M. (1977). *Journal of Medical Genetics* **14**, 81.

Duffy, B. J. and Fitzgerald, P. J. (1950). *Journal of Clinical Endocrinology* **10**, 1296.

Dungal, N. and Sigurjonsson, J. (1967). *British Journal of Cancer* **21**, 270.

Dunham, L., Bailar, J. C. and Lacquer, G. L. (1973). *Journal of the National Cancer Institute* **50**, 1119.

Dunham, L. J., Rabson, A. S., Stewart, H. L., Frank, A. S. and Young, J. L. (1968). *Journal of the National Cancer Institute* **41**, 683.

Ederer, F., Lerem, P., Turpeinen, O. and Frantz, I. D. (1971). *Lancet* **ii**, 203.

Ehrengut, W. and Schwartau, M. (1977). *British Medical Journal* **2**, 191.

Elwood, J. M., Cole, P., Rothman, K. J. and Kaplan, S. D. (1977). *Journal of the National Cancer Institute* **59**, 1055.

Elwood, J. M., Lee, J. A. H., Walter, S. D., Mo, T. and Green, A. E. S. (1974). *International Journal of Epidemiology* **3**, 325.

Emery, A. E. H., Anand, R., Danford, N., Duncan, W. and Paton, L. (1978). *Lancet* **i**, 470.

Enstrom, J. E. (1977). *British Journal of Cancer* **35**, 674.

Enstrom, J. E. (1978). *Cancer* **42**, 1943.

Enticknap, J. B. and Smither, W. J. (1964). *British Journal of Industrial Medicine* **21**, 20.

Ernster, V. L., Selvin, S., Brown, S. M., Sacks, S. T., Winkelstein, W. and Austin, D. F. (1979). *Journal of Occupational Medicine* **21**, 175.

Ernster, V. L., Selvin, S. and Winkelstein, W. (1978). *Science* **200**, 1165.

Falk, H., Thomas, L. B., Popper, H. and Ishak, K. G. (1979). *Lancet* **ii**, 1120.

Fasal, E., Jackson, E. W. and Klauber, M. R. (1967). *American Journal of Epidemiology* **87**, 267.

Fedrick, J. and Alberman, E. (1972). *British Medical Journal* **2**, 485.

Feinleib, M. (1968). *Journal of the National Cancer Institute* **41**, 315.

Finegold, S. M., Attebery, H. R. and Sutter, V. L. (1974). *American Journal of Clinical Nutrition* **27**, 1456.

Finke, W. (1956). *International Record of Medicine* **169**, 61.

Fraumeni, J. F. (1967). *Journal of the American Medical Association* **201**, 828.

Fraumeni, J. F. and Li, F. P. (1969). *Journal of the National Cancer Institute* **42**, 681.

Fraumeni, J. F., Lloyd, J. W., Smith, E. M. and Wagoner, M. S. (1969). *Journal of the National Cancer Institute* **42**, 455.

Fraumeni, J. F. and Miller, R. W. (1971). *Lancet* **ii**, 1196.

Freedlander, E., Kissen, L. H. and McVie, J. G. (1978). *British Medical Journal* **1**, 80.

Frichot, B. C., Lynch, H. T., Guirgis, H. A., Harris, R. E. and Lynch, J. F. (1977). *Lancet* **i**, 864.

Gagnon, F. (1950). *American Journal of Obstetrics and Gynecology* **60**, 516.

Gambill, E. E. (1971). *Mayo Clinic Proceedings* **46**, 174.

Gardner, M. J., Crawford, M. D. and Morris, J. N. (1969). *British Journal of Preventive and Social Medicine* **23**, 133.

Gaylor, D. W. and Shapiro, R. E. (1979). In *New Concepts in Safety Evaluation*, pp. 65–87. Ed. by M. A. Mehlman and R. E. Shapiro. Blumenthal H. Hemisphere Publishing, Washington.

Gibson, E. C. (1954). *British Journal of Urology* **26**, 227.

Gibson, R., Graham, S., Lilienfeld, A., Schuman, L., Dowd, J. E. and Levin, M. L. (1972). *Journal of the National Cancer Institute* **48**, 301.

Gilbert, J. B. (1944). *Journal of Urology* **51**, 296.

Gilbert, J. B. and Hamilton, J. B. (1940). *Surgery, Gynecology and Obstetrics* **71**, 731.

Glass, A. G. and Mantel, N. (1969). *Cancer Research* **29**, 1995.

Gloag, D. (1980). *British Medical Journal* **281**, 1479.

Gold, E., Gordis, L., Tonascia, J. and Szklo, M. (1979). *American Journal of Epidemiology* **109**, 309.

Goolden, A. W. G. (1958). *British Medical Journal* **2**, 954.

Gough, K. R., Read, A. E. and Nash, J. M. (1962). *Gut* **3**, 232.

Graham, S. (1968). *Cancer* **21**, 523.

Graham, S., Dayal, H., Rohrer, T., Swanson, M., Sultz, H., Shedd, D. and Fischman, S. (1977). *Journal of the National Cancer Institute* **59**, 1611.

Graham, S., Dayal, H., Swanson, M., Mittelman, A. and Wilkinson, G. (1978). *Journal of the National Cancer Institute* **61**, 709.

Graham, S. and Gibson, R. W. (1972). *Cancer* **29**, 1242.

Graham, S. and Lilienfeld, A. M. (1958). *Cancer* **11**, 945.

Graham, S., Priore, R., Graham, M., Browne, R., Burnett, W. and West, D. (1979). *Cancer* **44**, 1870.

Greenwald, P., Kirmss, V., Polan, A. K. and Dick, V. S. (1974). *Journal of the National Cancer Institute* **53**, 335.

Gregor, O., Toman, R. and Prusova, F. (1969). *Gut* **10**, 1031.

Grumet, R. F. and MacMahon, B. (1958). *Cancer* **11**, 790.

Gunz, F. W. and Spears, G. F. S. (1968). *British Medical Journal* **4**, 604.

Gutensohn, N., Li, F. P., Johnson, R. E. and Cole, P. (1975). *New England Journal of Medicine* **292**, 22.

Haenszel, W. (1961). *Journal of the National Cancer Institute* **26**, 37.

Haenszel, W. (1971). *Israel Journal of Medical Sciences* **7**, 1437.

Haenszel, W., Berg, J. W., Segi, M., Kurihara, M. and Locke, F. B. (1973). *Journal of the National Cancer Institute* **51**, 1765.

Haenszel, W. and Dawson, E. (1965). *Cancer* **18**, 265.

Haenszel, W. and Kurihara, M. (1968). *Journal of the National Cancer Institute* **40**, 43.

Haenszel, W., Kurihara, M., Locke, F. B., Shimuzu, K. and Segi, M. (1976). *Journal of the National Cancer Institute* **56**, 265.

Haghighi, P., Mostafavi, N., Dezhbakhsh, F., Ariazad, M., Ghassemi, H., Cook, A., Salmassi, S., Nabizadeh, I. and Asvadi, S. (1979). *Cancer* **44**, 254.

Hakama, M. and Pukkala, E. (1977). *British Journal of Preventive and Social Medicine* **31**, 238.

Hakulinen, T., Hovi, L., Karkinen-Jaaskelainen, M., Penttinen, K. and Saxen, L. (1973). *British Medical Journal* **4**, 265.

Hakulinen, T., Lehtimaki, L., Lehtonen, M. and Teppo, L. (1974). *Journal of the National Cancer Institute* **52**, 1711.

Halevi, H. S., Dreyfuss, F., Peritz, E. and Schmelz, W. O. (1971). *Israel Journal of Medical Sciences* **7**, 1386.

Hammond, E. C. (1966). *National Cancer Institute Monographs* **19**, 127.

Hammond, E. C. and Horn, D. (1958). *Journal of the American Medical Association* **166**, 1294.

Haney, M. J. and McGarity, W. C. (1971). *Archives of Surgery* **103**, 69.

Hanis, N. M., Stavraky, K. M. and Fowler, J. L. (1979). *Journal of Occupational Medicine* **21**, 167.

Hardell, L. (1979). *Lancet* **i**, 55.

Harrington, J. M., Craun, G. F., Meigs, J. W., Landrigan, P. J., Flannery, J. T. and Woodhull, R. S. (1978). *American Journal of Epidemiology* **107**, 96.

Harrington, J. M. and Shannon, H. S. (1975). *British Medical Journal* **4**, 329.

Hashem, M. (1961). *Journal of the Egyptian Medical Association* **44**, 857.

Hempelmann, L. H., Hall, W. J., Philips, M., Cooper, R. A. and Ames, W. R. (1975). *Journal of the National Cancer Institute* **55**, 519.

Henderson, B. E., Louie, E., Jing, J. S., Buell, P. and Gardner, M. B. (1976). *New England Journal of Medicine* **295**, 1101.

Henderson, B. E., Powell, D., Rosario, I., Keys, C., Hanisch, R., Young, M., Casagrande, J., Gerkins, V. and Pike, M. C. (1974). *Journal of the National Cancer Institute* **53**, 609.

Henderson, W. J., Joslin, C. A. F., Turnbull, A. C. and Griffiths, K. (1971). *Journal of Obstetrics and Gynaecology of the British Commonwealth* **78**, 266.

Henry, S. A., Kennaway, N. M. and Kennaway, E. L. (1931). *Journal of Hygiene* **30**, 125.

Henschke, U. K., Lasalle, D. L., Mason, C. H., Reinhold, A. W., Schneider, R. L. and White, J. E. (1973). *Cancer* **31**, 763.

Herbert, W. E. and Bruske, J. S. (1936). *Guy's Hospital Reports* **86**, 301.

Herbst, A. L., Ijfelder, J. and Poskanzer, D. C. (1971). *New England Journal of Medicine* **284**, 878.

Herbst, A. L., Kurman, R. J., Scully, R. E. and Poskanzer, D. C. (1972). *New England Journal of Medicine* **287**, 1259.

Herbst, A. L. and Scully, R. E. (1970). *Cancer* **25**, 745.

Hewer, T., Rose, E., Ghadirian, P., Castegnaro, M., Malavelle, C., Bartsch, H. and Day, N. (1978). *Lancet* **ii**, 494.

Hicks, R. M., Walters, C. L., Elsebai, I., El Aasser, A-B., Merzebani, M. and Gough, T. (1977). *Proceedings of the Royal Society of Medicine* **70**, 413.

Higgins, I. T. T. (1971). *Lancet* **ii**, 1141.

Higginson, J. (1966). *Journal of the National Cancer Institute* **37**, 527.
Higginson, J. and Muir, L. S. (1976). *Cancer Detection and Prevention* **1**, 79.
Hill, A. B., Faning, E. L., Perry, K., Bowler, R. G., Buckell, H. M., Druett, H. A. and Schilling, R. S. F. (1948). *British Journal of Industrial Medicine* **5**, 1.
Hill, G. B. and Adelstein, A. M. (1967). *Lancet* **ii**, 605.
Hill, M. J., Crowther, J. S., Drasar, B. S., Hawksworth, G., Aries, V. and Williams, R. E. O. (1971). *Lancet* **i**, 95.
Hill, M. J., Drasar, B. S., Williams, R. E. O., Meade, T. W., Cox, A. G., Simpson, J. E. P. and Morson, B. C. (1975). *Lancet* **i**, 535.
Hillyard, C. J., Evans, I. M. A. and Hill, P. A. (1978). *Lancet* **i**, 1009.
Hinds, M. W., Thomas, D. B. and O'Reilly, H. P. (1979). *Cancer* **44**, 1114.
Hirohata, T. (1968). *Journal of the National Cancer Institute* **41**, 895.
Ho, H. C., Kwan, H. C., Poon, Y. F., Tse, K. C. and Ng, M. H. (1978). *Lancet* **i**, 710.
Ho, J. H. C., Huang, D. P. and Fong, Y. Y. (1978). *Lancet* **ii**, 626.
Hoffman, A. and Lundin, F. E. (1978). *New England Journal of Medicine* **299**, 662.
Hogstedt, C., Rohlen, O., Berndtsson, B. S., Axelson, O. and Ehrenberg, L. (1979). *British Journal of Industrial Medicine* **36**, 276.
Holm, L. E., Lundell, G. and Wallinder, G. (1980). *Journal of the National Cancer Institute* **64**, 1055.
Hoover, R. and Fraumeni, J. F. (1975). *Environmental Research* **9**, 196.
Hoover, R., Gray, L. A., Cole, P. and MacMahon, B. (1976). *New England Journal of Medicine* **295**, 401.
Hoover, R., Gray, L. A. and Fraumeni, J. F. (1977). *Lancet* **ii**, 533.
Hornbak, J. and Amtrup, F. (1970). *Acta Pathologica et Microbiologica Scandinavica Suppl.* **212**, 158.
Horta, J. da S., Abbatt, J. D., Motta, L. C. and Roriz, M. L. (1965). *Lancet* **i**, 201.
Hou, P. C. (1956). *Journal of Pathology and Bacteriology* **LXXII**, 239.
Houten, L., Bross, I. D. J., Viadana, E. and Sonnesso, G. (1977). *Advances in Experimental Medicine and Biology* **91**, 93.
Howe, G. R., Lindsay, J., Coppock, E. and Miller, A. B. (1979). *International Journal of Epidemiology* **8**, 305.
Howell, M. A. (1976). *Journal of Chronic Diseases* **29**, 243.
Howell-Evans, W., McConnell, R. B., Clarke, C. A. and Sheppard, P. M. (1958). *Quarterly Journal of Medicine* **27**, 413.
Hutchinson, J. (1888). *Transactions of the Pathological Society, London* **39**, 352.
Hutchinson, W. B., Thomas, D. B., Hamlin, W. B., Roth, G. J., Peterson, A. V. and Williams, B. (1980). *Journal of the National Cancer Institute* **65**, 13.
Hyams, L. and Wynder, E. L. (1968). *Journal of Chronic Diseases* **21**, 391.
Imre, J. and Kopp, M. (1972). *Thorax* **27**, 594.
Ingram, J. T. and Comaish, S. (1967). In *The Prevention of Cancer*, pp. 212–15. Ed. by R. W. Raven and F. J. C. Roe. Butterworth, London.
International Agency for Research in Cancer (1974). *IARC Monograph* **4.**
International Agency for Research in Cancer (1976). *IARC Monograph* **11**, 161.
International Agency for Research in Cancer–Intestinal Microecology Group (1977). *Lancet* **ii**, 207.
International Agency for Research in Cancer (1978). Annual Report, p. 58.
International Agency for Research in Cancer (1979). *IARC Monograph Supplement* **1.**
Isomaki, H., Hakulinen, T. and Joutsenlahti, U. (1979). *Lancet* **i**, 392.
Jablon, S. (1975). In *Persons at High Risk of Cancer*, pp. 151–65. Ed. by J. F. Fraumeni. Academic Press, New York.
Jablon, S. and Kato, H. (1972). *Radiation Research* **50**, 649.
Jablon, S., Tachikawa, K., Belsky, J. L. and Steer, A. (1971). *Lancet* **i**, 927.
Jacobson, M. (1976). PhD Thesis. Edinburgh University.
Jancar, J. (1980). *Lancet* **i**, 484.
Jensen, O. M. (1979). *International Journal of Cancer* **23**, 454.
Johansson, S., Angervall, L., Bengtsson, U. and Wahlqvist, L. (1974). *Cancer* **33**, 743.
Johnson, F. L., Feagler, J. R., Lerner, K. G., Majerus, P. W., Siegel, M., Hartmann, J. R. and Thomas, E. D. (1972). *Lancet* **ii**, 1273.
Jong, U. W. de, Breslow, N., Goh Ewe Hong, J., Sridharan, M. and Shanmugarathnam, K. (1974). *International Journal of Cancer* **13**, 291.

Kark, J. D., Smith, A. H. and Hames, C. G. (1980). *Journal of Chronic Diseases* **33**, 311.

Karmody, A. J. and Kyle, J. (1969). *British Journal of Surgery* **56**, 362.

Karpas, A., Wreghitt, T. G. and Nagington, J. (1978). *Lancet* ii, 1016.

Kellermann, G., Shaw, C. R. and Luyten-Kellerman, M. (1973). *New England Journal of Medicine* **289**, 934.

Kennaway, E. L. and Kennaway, N. M. (1947). *British Journal of Cancer* **1**, 260.

Kersey, J., Spector, B. and Good, R. A. (1973). *International Journal of Cancer* **12**, 333.

Kessler, I. I. (1970). *Journal of the National Cancer Institute* **44**, 673.

King, H. and Haenszel, W. (1973). *Journal of Chronic Diseases* **26**, 623.

Kinlen, L. J., Badaracco, M. A., Moffett, J. and Vessey, M. P. (1974). *Journal of Obstetrics and Gynaecology, British Empire* **81**, 849.

Kinlen, L. J. and Doll, R. (1973). *British Journal of Preventive and Social Medicine* **27**, 146.

Kinlen, L. J., Eastwood, J. B., Keer, D. N. S., Moorhead, J. F., Oliver, D. O., Robinson, B. H. B., de Wardener, H. E. and Wing, A. J. (1980). *British Medical Journal* **280**, 1401.

Kinlen, L. J., Harris, R., Garrod, A. and Rodriguez, K. (1977). *British Medical Journal* **2**, 366.

Kinlen, L. J., Sheil, A. G. R., Peto, J. and Doll, R. (1979). *British Medical Journal* **2**, 1461.

Kipling, M. D. and Waterhouse, J. A. H. (1967). *Lancet* i, 730.

Klatskin, G. (1977). *Gastroenterology* **73**, 386.

Kleinfeld, M., Messite, J. and Kooyman, O. (1967). *Archives of Environmental Health* **15**, 177.

Kleinfeld, M., Messite, J. and Zaki, M. H. (1974). *Journal of Occupational Medicine* **15**, 345.

Klepp, O. and Magnus, K. (1979). *International Journal of Cancer* **23**, 482.

Knox, E. G. (1964). *British Journal of Preventive and Social Medicine* **18**, 17.

Knox, E. G. (1977). *British Journal of Preventive and Social Medicine* **31**, 71.

Kolonel, L. and Winkelstein, W. (1977). *Lancet* ii, 566.

Korenman, S. G. (1980). *Lancet* i, 700.

Krain, L. S. (1971). *Journal of Chronic Diseases* **23**, 685.

Kreyberg, L. (1956). *British Journal of Preventive and Social Medicine* **10**, 145.

Kvale, G., Hiby, E. A. and Pedersen, E. (1979). *International Journal of Cancer* **23**, 593.

Lancaster, H. O. and Nelson, J. (1957). *Medical Journal of Australia* **44**, 452.

Lancet (1968). *Lancet* i, 76.

Lancet (1977a). *Lancet* i, 1348.

Lancet (1977b). *Lancet* i, 685.

Lancet (1978). *Lancet* ii, 1238.

Lancet (1979). *Lancet* i, 1121.

Land, E. (1980). *Cancer* **46**, 868.

Larouze, B., London, W. T., Saimot, G., Werner, B. G., Lustbader, E. D., Payet, M. and Blumberg, B. S. (1976). *Lancet* ii, 534.

Larsson, L., Sandstrom, A. and Westling, P. (1975). *Cancer Research* **35**, 3308.

Lawther, P. J. (1974). In *Occupational Health*, pp. 221-4. Ed. by S. Gauvain. Heinemann, London.

Lea, A. J. (1964). *Annals of the Rheumatic Diseases* **23**, 480.

Lea, A. J. (1965). *Annals of the Royal College of Surgery* **37**, 169.

Leck, I., Sibary, K. and Wakefield, J. (1978). *Journal of Epidemiology and Community Health* **32**, 108.

Leck, I. and Steward, J. K. (1972). *British Medical Journal* **4**, 631.

Lee, J. A. H. and Carter, A. R. (1970). *Journal of the National Cancer Institute* **45**, 91.

Lemen, R. A., Lee, J. S., Wagoner, J. K. and Blejer, H. P. (1976). *Annals of the New York Academy of Sciences* **271**, 273.

Lemon, F. R., Walden, R. T. and Woods, R. H. (1964). *Cancer* **17**, 486.

Levene, A. (1976). *Lancet* ii, 475.

Levin, M. L., Kress, L. C. and Goldstein, H. (1942). *New York State Journal of Medicine* **42**, 1737.

Lewis, A. C. W. and Davison, B. C. C. (1969). *Lancet* ii, 235.

Li, F. P., Cassady, J. R. and Jaffe, N. (1975). *Cancer* **35**, 1230.

Li, F. P. and Fraumeni, J. F. (1972). *Journal of the National Cancer Institute* **48**, 1575.

Li, F. P., Fraumeni, J. F., Mantel, N. and Miller, R. W. (1969). *Journal of the National Cancer Institute* **43**, 1159.

Li, F. P., Rapoport, A. H., Fraumeni, J. F. and Jensen, R. D. (1970). *Journal of the American Medical Association* **214**, 1559.

Liddell, F. D. K., McDonald, J. C. and Thomas, D. C. (1977). *Journal of the Royal Statistical Society, Series A* **140**, 469.

Lingeman, C. H. (1974). *Journal of the National Cancer Institute* **53**, 1603.

Linos, A., Kyle, R. A., O'Fallon, W. M. and Kurland, L. T. (1980). *International Journal of Epidemiology* **9**, 131.

Lipworth, L. and Dayan, A. D. (1969). *Cancer* **23**, 1119.

Lloyd, J. W. (1976). *Annals of the New York Academy of Sciences* **271**, 91.

Lorenz, E. (1944). *Journal of the National Cancer Institute* **5**, 1.

Lumley, K. P. S. (1976). *British Journal of Industrial Medicine* **33**, 108.

Lynch, H. T., Larsen, A. L., Magnuson, C. W. and Krush, A. J. (1966). *Cancer* **19**, 1891.

Lynch, H. T., Lynch, J. and Lynch, P. (1977). In *Genetics of Human Cancer*, pp. 235–53. Ed. by J. J. Mulvihill, R. W. Miller and J. F. Fraumeni. Raven Press, New York.

Lynch, J., Hanis, N. M., Bird, M. G., Murray, J. M. and Walsh, J. P. (1979). *Journal of Occupational Medicine* **21**, 333.

Lyon, J. L., Klauber, M. R., Gardner, J. W. and Smart, C. R. (1976). *New England Journal of Medicine* **294**, 129.

McCaugham, G., Parsons, C. and Gallagher, N. D. (1979). *Medical Journal of Australia* **1**, 304.

McCrea Curnen, M. G., Varma, A. A. O., Christine, B. W. and Turgeon, L. R. (1974). *Journal of the National Cancer Institute* **53**, 943.

McDonald, A. D. and McDonald, J. C. (1980). *Cancer* **46**, 1650.

McDonald, J. C., McDonald, A. D., Gibbs, G. W., Siemiatyki, J. and Rossiter, C. E. (1971). *Archives of Environmental Health* **22**, 677.

MacKenzie, I. (1965). *British Journal of Cancer* **XIX**, 1.

McLaughlin, A. I. G. and Harding, H. E. (1956). *AMA Archives of Industrial Health* **14**, 350.

MacLean, J. T. and Fowler, V. B. (1965). *Journal of Urology* **75**, 384.

MacMahon, B. (1960). *Acta Union International Contra Cancer* **16**, 1716.

MacMahon, B. (1962). *Journal of the National Cancer Institute* **28**, 1173.

MacMahon, B. (1966). *Cancer Research* **26**, 1189.

MacMahon, B., Cole, P., Lin, T. M., Lowe, C. R., Mirra, A. P., Ravnihar, B., Salber, E. J., Valaoras, V. G. and Yuasa, S. (1970). *Bulletin of the World Health Organization* **43**, 209.

MacMahon, B., Lin, T. M., Lowe, C. R., Mirra, A. P., Ravnihar, B., Salber, E. J., Trichopoulos, D., Valaoras, V. G. and Yuasa, S. (1970). *Bulletin of the World Health Organization* **42**, 185.

McMichael, A. J. (1978a). *Lancet* **i**, 1244.

McMichael, A. J. (1978b). *Lancet* **ii**, 1099.

McMichael, A. J. (1979). *Nutrition and Cancer* **1**, 82.

McVay, J. R. (1968). *Lancet* **ii**, 1393.

Machle, W. and Gregorius, F. (1948). *Public Health Report* **63**, 1114.

Mancuso, T. F. and El Attar, A. A. (1967). *Journal of Occupational Medicine* **9**, 277.

Mancuso, T. F. and Sterling, T. D. (1974). *Journal of Chronic Diseases* **27**, 459.

Mancuso, T. F., Stewart, A. and Kneale, G. (1977). *Health Physics* **33**, 369.

Maram, E. S., Ludwig, J. and Kurland, L. T. (1979). *American Journal of Epidemiology* **109**, 152.

March, H. C. (1950). *American Journal of the Medical Sciences* **220**, 282.

Martinez, I. (1969). *Cancer* **24**, 777.

Martland, H. S., Conlon, P. and Knef, J. P. (1925). *Journal of the American Medical Association* **85**, 1769.

Maruchi, N., Furihata, R. and Makiuchi, M. (1971). *International Journal of Cancer* **7**, 575.

Matanoski, G. M., Sartwell, P. E. and Elliott, E. A. (1975). *Lancet* **i**, 926.

Matolo, N. M., Klauber, M. R., Forishek, W. M. and Dixon, J. A. (1972). *Cancer* **29**, 733.

Matsunaga, E. (1980). *Journal of the National Cancer Institute* **65**, 47.

Maupas, P., Wener, B., Larouze, B., Millman, I., London, W. T., O'Connell, A. and Blumberg, B. S. (1975). *Lancet* **ii**, 9.

Mettler, F. A., Hemplemann, L. H., Dutton, A. M., Pifer, J. W., Toyooka, E. T. and Ames, W. R. (1969). *Journal of the National Cancer Institute* **43**, 803.

Milham, S. (1971). *American Journal of Epidemiology* **94**, 307.

Mill, J. S. (1859). *On Liberty*. Parker, London.

Miller, A. B. (1977). *Cancer Research* **37**, 2939.

Miller, A. B. (1978). *Cancer Research* **38**, 3985.

Miller, A. B., Kelly, A., Choi, N. W., Matthews, V., Morgan, R. W., Munan, L., Burch, J. D., Feather, J., Howe, G. R. and Jain, M. (1978). *American Journal of Epidemiology* **108**, 499.

Mittra, I. and Hayward, J. L. (1974). *Lancet* **i**, 885.

Modan, B., Barell, V., Lubin, F., Modan, M., Greenberg, R. A. and Graham, S. (1975). *Journal of the National Cancer Institute* **55**, 15.

Modan, B., Ron, E. and Werner, A. (1977). *Radiology* **123**, 741.

Moghissi, K. S., Mack, H. C. and Porzak, J. P. (1968). *American Journal of Obstetrics and Gynecology* **100**, 607.

Mole, R. H. (1974). *British Journal of Cancer* **30**, 199.

Monaghan, J. M. and Sirisena, L. A. W. (1978). *British Medical Journal* **1**, 1588.

Monson, R. R. and Fine, L. J. (1978). *Journal of the National Cancer Institute* **61**, 1047.

Monson, R. R. and Lyon, J. L. (1975). *Cancer* **36**, 1077.

Monson, R. R., Peters, J. M. and Johnson, M. N. (1974). *Lancet* **ii**, 397.

Morgan, C. (1980). *American Journal of Pathology* **98**, 843.

Morgan, R. W. and Jain, M. G. (1974). *Canadian Medical Association Journal* **iii**, 1067.

Mori, W. (1967). *Cancer* **20**, 627.

Morrison, A. S. (1976). *Journal of the National Cancer Institute* **56**, 731.

Morrison, A. S. and Cole, P. (1976). *Urologic Clinics of North America* **3**, 13.

Mosbech, J. and Videbaek, A. (1950). *British Medical Journal* **2**, 390.

Moss, E. and Lee, W. R. (1974). *British Journal of Industrial Medicine* **31**, 224.

Moss, E., Scott, T. S. and Atherley, G. R. C. (1972). *British Journal of Industrial Medicine* **29**, 1.

Movshovitz, M. and Modan, B. (1973). *Journal of the National Cancer Institute* **51**, 777.

Mower, H. F., Ray, R. M., Shoff, R., Stemmerman, G. N., Nomora, A., Glober, G. A., Kamiyama, S., Shimada, A. and Yakakawa, H. (1979). *Cancer Research* **39**, 328.

Mulvihill, J. J. (1975). In *Persons at High Risk of Cancer*, pp. 1–35. Ed. by J. F. Fraumeni. Academic Press, New York.

Mulvihill, J. J., Miller, R. W. and Fraumeni, J. F. (1977). *Genetics in Human Cancer*. Raven Press, New York.

Mustacchi, P. and Millinore, D. (1976). *Journal of the National Cancer Institute* **56**, 717.

Najarian, T. and Colton, T. (1978). *Lancet* **i**, 1018.

Nasca, P. C., Lawrence, C. E., Greenwald, P., Chorost, S., Arbucke, J. T. and Paulson, A. (1980). *Journal of the National Cancer Institute* **64**, 23.

Newell, G. R., Cole, S. R., Miettinen, O. S. and MacMahon, B. (1970). *Journal of the National Cancer Institute* **45**, 311.

Newell, G. R., Rawlings, W., Kinnear, B. K. and Correa, P. (1973). *Journal of the National Cancer Institute* **51**, 1437.

Newhouse, M. L., Pearson, R. M., Fullerton, J. M., Boesen, E. A. M. and Shannon, H. S. (1977). *British Journal of Preventive and Social Medicine* **31**, 148.

Newhouse, M. L. and Thompson, H. (1965). *British Journal of Industrial Medicine* **22**, 261.

Newill, V. A. (1961). *Journal of the National Cancer Institute* **26**, 405.

Nicholls, J. C. (1974). *British Journal of Surgery* **61**, 244.

Nicholls, P., Edwards, G. and Kyle, E. (1974). *Quarterly Journal of Studies of Alcohol* **35**, 841.

Office of Population Censuses and Surveys (1979). *Cancer Statistics: cases of diagnosed cancer registered in England and Wales*. HMSO, London.

Olin, G. R. (1976). *Lancet* **ii**, 916.

Olin, G. R. (1978). *American Industrial Hygiene Journal* **39**, 557.

Olin, G. R. and Ahlbom, A. (1980). *Environmental Research* **22**, 154.

Osborne, R. H. and de George, F. V. (1963). *American Journal of Human Genetics* **15**, 380.

Paddle, G. M. (1980). *Archives of Toxicology Supplement* **3**, 263.

Paffenbarger, R. S., Wing, A. L. and Hyde, R. T. (1977). *Journal of the National Cancer Institute* **58**, 1489.

Paymaster, J. C. and Gangadharan, P. (1967). *Journal of Urology* **97**, 110.

Pearce, M. L. and Dayton, S. (1971). *Lancet* **i**, 464.

Pedersen, E., Hogetveit, A. C. and Andersen, A. (1973). *International Journal of Cancer* **12**, 32.

Peers, F. G. and Linsell, C. A. (1973). *British Journal of Cancer* **27**, 473.

Pell, S. and D'Alonzo, C. A. (1973). *Journal of Occupational Medicine* **15**, 120.

Pernu, J. (1960). *Annales Medicine Internal Fenniae* 49, Suppl. **33**, 1.

Petersen, G. R. and Lee, J. A. H. (1972). *Journal of the National Cancer Institute* **49**, 339.

Petersen, G. R. and Milham, S. (1974). *Journal of the National Cancer Institute* **53**, 957.

Petkovic, S., Tomic, M. and Mutavdzic, M. (1966). *Journal D'Urologie et de Nephrologie* (*Paris*) **72**, 429.

Peto, J., Doll, R., Howard, S. V., Kinlen, L. J. and Lewinsohn, J. C. (1977). *British Journal of Industrial Medicine* **34**, 169.

Peto, R. (1980). *Nature* **284**, 297.

Phillips, R. L. (1975). *Cancer Research* **35**, 3513.

Pincet, J. and Massé, L. (1975). *International Journal of Epidemiology* **4**, 311.

Pinto, S. S., Enterline, P. E., Henderson, V. and Varner, M. O. (1977). *Environmental Health Perspectives* **19**, 127.

Pochin, E. E. (1960). *British Medical Journal* **2**, 1545.

Pochin, E. E. (1967). *Clinical Radiology* **18**, 113.

Polednak, P., Stehney, F. and Rowland, R. E. (1978). *American Journal of Epidemiology* **107**, 179.

Pott, P. (1775). *Chirurgical observations relative to the cataract, the polypuss of the nose, the cancer of the scrotum.* Hawes, Clarke and Collins, London.

Potts, C. L. (1965). *Annals of Occupational Hygiene* **8**, 55.

Pour, P. and Ghadirian, P. (1974). *Cancer* **33**, 1649.

Preston-Martin, S., Paganini-Hill, A., Henderson, B. E., Pike, M. C. and Wood, C. (1980). *Journal of the National Cancer Institute* **65**, 67.

Price, G. H. G. (1962). *Journal of Bone and Joint Surgery* **44B**, 366.

Punnonen, R., Gronroos, M. and Peltonen, R. (1974). *Lancet* **ii**, 949.

Purchase, I. F. H. (1980). *British Journal of Industrial Medicine* **37**, 1.

Rampen, F. H. J. and Mulder, J. H. (1980). *Lancet* **i**, 562.

Ravich, A. and Ravich, R. A. (1951). *New York State Journal of Medicine* **51**, 1519.

Razis, D. V., Diamond, H. D. and Craver, L. F. (1959). *Annals of Internal Medicine* **51**, 933.

Redmond, C. K., Ciocco, A., Lloyd, J. W. and Rush, H. W. (1972). *Journal of Occupational Medicine* **14**, 621.

Registrar General (1971). *Occupational Mortality.* HMSO, London.

Registrar General (1978). *Occupational Mortality.* HMSO, London.

Reid, R., Laverty, C., Coppleson, M., Wiwatwong, I. and Hills, E. (1980). *Obstetrics and Gynecology* **55**, 47.

Reimer, R. R., Clark, W. H., Greene, M. H., Ainsworth, A. M. and Fraumeni, J. F. (1978). *Journal of the American Medical Association* **239**, 744.

Reissland, J. A. (1978). *National Radiological Protection Board Report 79* HMSO, London.

Rimington, J. (1968). *British Medical Journal* **1**, 732.

Rimington, J. (1971). *British Medical Journal* **2**, 373.

Robinette, C. D., Hrubec, Z. and Fraumeni, J. F. (1979). *American Journal of Epidemiology* **109**, 687.

Roe, F. J. C. (1979). *Lancet* **ii**, 744.

Rojel, J. (1953). *Acta Pathologica et Microbiologica Scandinavica* (Suppl. 97) **3**, 82.

Rosdahl, N., Larsen, S. O. and Clemmesen, J. (1974). *British Medical Journal* **2**, 253.

Rose, G., Blackburn, H., Keys, A., Taylor, H. L., Kannel, W. B., Paul, D., Reid, D. D. and Stamler, J. (1974). *Lancet* **i**, 181.

Rose, G. and Shipley, M. J. (1980). *Lancet* **i**, 523.

Ross, R. K., McCurtis, J. W., Henderson, B. E., Menck, H. R., Mack, T. M. and Martin, S. P. (1979). *British Journal of Cancer* **39**, 284.

Rotkin, I. D. (1967). *American Journal of Public Health* **57**, 815.

Rotkin, I. D. (1977). *Cancer Treatment Report* **61**, 173.

Rowland, R. E., Stehney, A. F. and Lucas, J. F. (1978). *Radiation Research* **76**, 368.

Royal College of Physicians (1970). *Air Pollution and Health.* Pitman Medical, London.

Royal College of Physicians (1977). *Smoking or Health.* Pitman Medical, Tunbridge Wells.

Rubin, E. and Lieber, C. S. (1975). *Clinics in Gastroenterology* **4**, 247.

Rubino, G. F., Scansetti, G., Pidlatto, G. and Romano, C. A. (1976). *Journal of Occupational Medicine* **18**, 186.

Rushton, L. R. and Alderson, M. R. (1980). *Carcinogenesis* **1**, 739.

Sadeghi, A. and Behmard, S. (1978). *Cancer* **42**, 353.

Sadoff, L., Winkley, J. and Tyson, S. (1973). *Oncology* **27**, 244.

Sagerman, R. H., Cassady, J. R., Tretter, P. and Ellsworth, R. M. (1969). *American Journal of Roentgenology* **105**, 529.

Sanghvi, L. D., Rao, K. C. M. and Khanolkar, V. R. (1955). *British Medical Journal* **1**, 1111.

Saxen, E. (1961). *Acta Union International Contra Cancer* **17**, 367.

Saxen, E. A., Franssila, K. and Hakama, M. (1969). In *Thyroid Carcinoma*, pp. 98–103. Ed. by C. E. Hedinger. Heinemann, London.

Saxen, E. A. and Saxen, L. O. (1954). *Documenta de Medicina Geographica et Tropica* **6**, 335.

Schimke, R. N. (1976). *Advances in Internal Medicine* **21**, 249.

Schimke, R. N. (1978). *Genetics and Cancer in Man*. Churchill Livingstone, Edinburgh.

Schimpff, S. C., Brager, D. M., Schimpff, C. R., Comstock, G. W. and Wiernick, P. H. (1976). *Annals of Internal Medicine* **84**, 547.

Schmidt, W. and de Lint, J. (1972). *Quarterly Journal of Studies of Alcohol* **33**, 171.

Schneider, R. and Riggs, J. L. (1973). *Journal of the American Veterinary Medical Association* **162**, 217.

Schottenfeld, D. and Berg, J. (1971). *Journal of the National Cancer Institute* **46**, 161.

Schrauzer, G. N. (1976). *Medical Hypotheses* **2**, 39.

Schreek, R. (1944). *Cancer Research* **4**, 433.

Schumann, L. M., Bauer, J., Scarlett, J., McHugh, R., Mandel, J. and Blackard, C. (1977). *Cancer Treatment Reports* **61**, 181.

Schwartz, D., Lellouch, J., Flamant, R. and Denoix, P. F. (1962). *Revue Français* Études Clinique et Biologique **7**, 590.

Searle, C. E. (1978). *British Journal of Cancer* **38**, 192.

Segi, M. and Kurihara, M. (1972). *Cancer mortality for selected sites in 24 countries*, No. 6. Segi Institute of Cancer Epidemiology, Nagoya.

Seidman, H. (1970). *Environmental Research* **3**, 234.

Selikoff, I. J., Churg, J. and Hammond, E. C. (1964). *Journal of the American Medical Association* **188**, 22.

Selikoff, I. J. and Hammond, E. C. (1975). In *Persons at High Risk of Cancer*, pp. 467–83. Ed. by J. F. Fraumeni. Academic Press, New York.

Selikoff, I. J., Hammond, E. C. and Churg, J. (1968). *Journal of the American Medical Association* **204**, 106.

Selikoff, I. J., Seidman, H. and Hammond, E. (1980). *Journal of the National Cancer Institute* **65**, 507.

Shank, R. C. (1977). In *Environmental Toxicology*, pp. 291–318. Ed. by H. F. Kraybill and M. A. Mehlman. Hemisphere, London.

Shennan, D. H. and Bishop, O. S. (1974). *West Indian Medical Journal* **23**, 44.

Shepherd, J. H., Dewhurst, J. and Pryse-Davies, J. (1979). *British Medical Journal* **2**, 246.

Sieber, S. M. and Adamson, R. H. (1976). *Advances in Cancer Research* **22**, 57.

Simon, D., Yen, S. and Cole, P. (1975). *Journal of the National Cancer Institute* **54**, 587.

Sipple, J. H. (1961). *American Journal of Medicine* **31**, 163.

Smith, D. (1976). *Journal of Social and Occupational Medicine* **26**, 92.

Smith, P. G. and Doll, R. (1976). *British Journal of Radiology* **49**, 224.

Smith, P. G., Kinlen, L. J. and Doll, R. (1974). *Lancet* **ii**, 525.

Smith, P. G., Kinlen, L. J., White, G. C., Adelstein, A. M. and Fox, A. J. (1980). *British Journal of Cancer* **41**, 422.

Smith, P. G., Pike, M. C., Kinlen, L. J., Jones, A. and Harris, R. (1977). *Lancet* **ii**, 59.

Sonakul, D., Koompriochana, C., Chinda, K. and Stitnimankarn, T. (1978). *South East Asian Journal of Tropical Medicine and Public Health* **9**, 215.

Spiers, P. S. (1969). *Public Health Reports* **84**, 385.

Stalsberg, H. and Taksdal, S. (1971). *Lancet* **ii**, 1175.

Staszewski, J. (1980). *World Health Statistics Report* **33**, 27.

Stell, P. M. and McGill, T. (1973). *Lancet* **ii**, 416.

Stephenson, J. H. and Grace, W. J. (1954). *Psychosomatic Medicine* **16**, 287.

Stern, E. and Dixon, W. J. (1961). *Cancer* **14**, 153.

Stewart, A., Webb, J., Giles, D. and Hewitt, D. (1956). *Lancet* **ii**, 447.

Stewart, A., Webb, J. and Hewitt, D. (1958). *British Medical Journal* **1**, 1495.

Stewart, H. L., Dunham, L. J., Dorn, H. F., Thomas, L. B., Edgcomb, J. H. and Symeonidis, A. (1966). *Journal of the National Cancer Institute* **37**, 1.

Stocks, P. (1957). *British Empire Cancer Campaign 35 Annual Report*, Suppl. II.

Stocks, P. (1960). *British Journal of Cancer* **14**, 397.

Stocks, P. (1970). *British Journal of Cancer* **24**, 215.

Stott, H., Peto, J., Stephens, R., Fox, W., Sutherland, I., Foster-Carter, A. F., Teare, H. D. and Fenning, J. (1976). *Tubercle* **57**, 1.

Stutman, O. (1976). *Advances in Cancer Research* **22**, 261.

Swerdlow, A. J. (1979). *British Medical Journal* **2**, 1334.

Tabershaw, I. R. (1974). *American Petroleum Institute Project OH-1*, No. 129.

Tabor, E., Gerety, R. J., Vogel, C. L., Bayley, A. C., Anthony, P. P., Chan, C. H. and Barker, L. F. (1977). *Journal of the National Cancer Institute* **58**, 1197.

Teasdale, C., Forbes, J. F. and Baum, M. (1976). *Lancet* i, 360.

Templeton, A. C. (1975). In *Persons at High Risk of Cancer*, pp. 69–83. Ed. by J. F. Fraumeni. Academic Press, New York.

Terris, M. and Oalmann, M. C. (1960). *Journal of the American Medical Association* **174**, 1847.

de Thé, G. (1977). *Lancet* i, 335.

de Thé, G., Geser, A., Day, N. E., Tukei, P. M., Manube, G., Williams, E. H., Beri, D. P., Smith, P. G., Dean, A., Bornkamm, G. W., Feorino, P. and Henle, W. (1978). *Nature* **274**, 756.

Theriault, G. and Goulet, L. (1979). *Journal of Occupational Medicine* **21**, 367.

Thiessen, E. U. (1974). *Cancer* **34**, 1102.

Thomas, T. L., Decoufle, P. and Moure-Evans, R. (1980). *Journal of Occupational Medicine* **22**, 97.

Thorarinsson, A. A. (1979). *Journal of Studies on Alcohol* **40**, 704.

Timonen, T. T. and Ilvonen, M. (1978). *Lancet* i, 350.

Tokuhata, G. K. and Lilienfeld, A. M. (1963). *Journal of the National Cancer Institute* **30**, 289.

Trell, E., Korsgaard, R., Hood, B., Kitzing, P., Nordic, G. and Simonsson, B. G. (1976). *Lancet* ii, 140.

Trichopoulos, D., Tabor, E., Gerety, R. J., Xirouchaxi, E., Sparros, L., Mundz, N. and Linsell, C. A. (1978). *Lancet* ii, 1217.

Tulinius, H. (1977). *Recent Results Cancer Research* **60**, 3.

Turbitt, M. L., Patrick, R. S., Goudie, R. B. and Buchanan, W. M. (1977). *Journal of Clinical Pathology* **30**, 1124.

Tuyns, A. J. and Griciute, L. L. (1980). In *Human Cancer: its characterisation and treatment*, pp. 130–5. Ed. by W. Davis, K. Harrap and G. Stathopoulos. Excerpta Medica, Amsterdam.

Tuyns, A. J., Pequignot, G. and Jensen, O. M. (1977). *Bulletin du Cancer (Paris)* **64**, 45.

Tyroler, H. A., Andjelkovic, D., Harris, R., Lednar, W., McMichael, A. and Symons, M. (1976). *Environmental Health Perspectives* **17**, 13.

Vessey, M. P., Kay, C. R., Baldwin, J. H., Clarke, J. A. and MacLeod, I. B. (1977). *British Medical Journal* **1**, 1064.

Viadana, E., Bross, I. D. and Houten, L. (1976). *Journal of Occupational Medicine* **18**, 787.

Vianna, N. J., Greenwald, P. and Davies, J. N. P. (1971). *Lancet* i, 1209.

Vianna, N. J. and Polan, A. K. (1973). *New England Journal of Medicine* **289**, 499.

Vianna, N. J. and Polan, A. (1979). *Lancet* i, 1394.

Vianna, N. J., Polan, A. K., Keogh, M. D. and Greenwald, P. (1974). *Lancet* ii, 131.

Vogel, C. L., Anthony, P. P., Mody, N. and Barker, L. F. (1970). *Lancet* ii, 621.

Wagner, J. C., Sleggs, C. A. and Marchano, P. (1960). *British Journal of Industrial Medicine* **17**, 260.

Wagoner, J. K., Archer, V. E., Lundin, F. E., Holaday, D. A. and Lloyd, J. W. (1965). *New England Journal of Medicine* **273**, 181.

Wahner, H. W., Cuello, C., Correa, P., Uribe, L. F. and Gaitan, E. (1966). *American Journal of Medicine* **40**, 58.

Wald, N., Idle, M., Boreham, J. and Bailey, A. (1980). *Lancet* ii, 813.

Wallace, D. L., Exton, L. A. and McLeod, S. R. C. (1971). *Cancer* **27**, 1262.

Waller, R. E. (1967). In *The Prevention of Cancer*, pp. 181–6. Ed. by R. W. Raven and F. J. C. Roe. Butterworth, London.

Waterhouse, J. A. H. (1971). *Annals of Occupational Hygiene* **14**, 161.

Wegelin, C. (1928). *The Cancer Review* III, 297.

Weil, C. S., Smythe, H. F. and Nale, T. W. (1952). *Archives of Industrial Hygiene and Occupational Medicine* **5**, 535.

Weiss, N. S. (1978). *Journal of Chronic Diseases* **31**, 705.

Weiss, N. S. and Peterson, A. S. (1978). *American Journal of Epidemiology* **107**, 91.

Weiss, W. and Figueroa, W. G. (1976). *Journal of Occupational Medicine* **18**, 623.

Welton, J. C., Marr, J. S. and Friedman, S. M. (1979). *Lancet* i, 791.

Wennstrom, J., Pierce, E. R. and McCusick, V. A. (1974). *Cancer* **34**, 850.

West, R. O. (1966). *Cancer* **19**, 1001.

Whitaker, C. J., Moss, E., Lee, W. R. and Cunliffe, S. (1979). *British Journal of Industrial Medicine* **36**, 292.

Whorwell, P. J., Foster, K. J., Alderson, M. R. and Wright, R. (1976). *Lancet* ii, 113.

Wicken, A. J. (1966). *Tobacco Research Council Research Paper 9*. London.

Wigle, D. T. (1977a). *American Journal of Epidemiology* **105**, 428.

Wigle, D. T. (1977b). *Archives of Environmental Health* **32**, 185.

Williams, E. H., Day, N. E. and Geser, A. G. (1974). *Lancet* ii, 19.

Williams, E. H., Smith, P. G., Day, N. E., Geser, A., Ellice, J. and Tukei, P. (1978). *British Journal of Cancer* **37**, 109.

Williams, R. R. (1976). *Lancet* i, 996.

Williams, R. R. and Horn, J. W. (1977). *Journal of the National Cancer Institute* **58**, 525.

Woodliff, H. J. and Dougan, L. (1964). *British Medical Journal* **1**, 744.

World Health Organization (1964). *Technical Report Series*, No. 276. World Health Organization, Geneva.

World Health Organization (1978). *Technical Report Series*, No. 619. World Health Organization, Geneva.

Wynder, E. L. and Bross, I. J. (1957). *British Medical Journal* **1**, 1137.

Wynder, E. L., Bross, I. J. and Day, E. (1956). *Cancer* **9**, 86.

Wynder, E. L., Cornfield, J., Schroff, P. D. and Dorarswami, K. R. (1954). *American Journal of Obstetrics and Gynecology* **68**, 1016.

Wynder, E. L., Covey, L. S., Mabuchi, K. and Mushinski, M. (1976). *Cancer* **38**, 1591.

Wynder, E. L. and Gori, B. (1977). *Journal of the National Cancer Institute* **58**, 825.

Wynder, E. L., Hultberg, S., Jacobsson, F. and Bross, I. J. (1957). *Cancer* **10**, 470.

Wynder, E. L., Kajitani, T., Ishikawa, S., Dodd, H. and Takano, A. (1969). *Cancer* **23**, 1210.

Wynder, E. L., Mabuchi, K., Maruchi, N. and Fortner, J. G. (1973). *Journal of the National Cancer Institute* **50**, 645.

Wynder, E. L., Mabuchi, K. and Whitmore, W. F. (1971). *Cancer* **28**, 344.

Wynder, E. L., Onderdonk, J. and Mantel, N. (1963). *Cancer* **16**, 1388.

Wynder, E. L. and Shigematsu, T. (1967). *Cancer* **20**, 1520.

Zack, M. Jr., Heath, W. Jr., Andrews, M., Grivas, A. and Christine, W. (1977). *Journal of the National Cancer Institute* **59**, 1343.

Zeigel, R. F., Arya, S. K., Horoszewicz, J. S. and Carter, W. A. (1977). *Oncology* **34**, 29.

Zur Hausen (1976). *Cancer Research* **36**, 794.

4

Lay and professional beliefs and feelings about cancer

Michael Calnan

The previous chapter focused on an evaluation of the evidence of a relationship between cancer and environmental agents. In this chapter the points of view of the lay person and the medical and paramedical practitioners will be considered. The focus will be on examining the knowledge, definitions and meanings that lay and professional people use in their everyday lives in relation to cancer. Much of the research carried out in this area has focused on examining the point of view of the lay person rather than the professional person, so it is with the lay person that this review will start. Perhaps the reason for this concentration of research on lay rather than professional views is due to an assumption that professionals are more likely to operate with definitions based on scientific knowledge and therefore are operating with the 'correct' definitions so that professionals are less likely to be seen as a research 'problem'.

Lay beliefs and feelings about cancer

Much of the research which has been carried out in this area has focused on public opinion and cancer. These public opinion surveys have been used to provide baseline data for the evaluation of health education campaigns. In addition, information on lay beliefs and feelings about cancer has been derived from studies aimed at trying to understand why people have not complied with health-recommended actions such as taking part in screening programmes or delaying too long before consulting the doctor for a sign or symptom that might be dangerous. The assumption in both these types of studies is that lay knowledge and/or behaviour is in some way idiosyncratic or irrational and needs to be changed. In the case of health education one of the problems is that laymen might hold inappropriate beliefs and these may need to be changed to those beliefs which are officially recommended. In the case of the utilization of services, the problem is that people are not adhering to officially recommended health practices and there is a need to find out why, so these beliefs can eventually be changed. Also, implicit in these approaches is the assumption that teaching individuals health knowledge will lead to the appropriate health-related action. As will be shown later in this section, such an assumption may be misplaced. The other reason for carrying out this type of public opinion survey might be to gain a better understanding of the health needs of the community. The implication of such an approach could be that the health system would be adjusted to meet these needs.

Public opinion and cancer

It is the intention in this section to review the four main public opinion surveys carried out in this country as well as supplementary evidence derived from smaller studies. Similar public opinion studies have been carried out abroad, particularly in the USA and Canada (see Simonds (1970) and Philips and Taylor (1961) for reviews of studies in the USA and Canada respectively). Technical and substantive aspects of each of the studies will be examined which will be followed by a more theoretical criticism with an attempt to formulate an alternative approach.

1953 survey

The first large-scale survey (see Erskine (1966) for review of previous research) of public opinion about cancer in the UK was carried out in the Manchester area (Paterson and Aitken-Swan, 1954). The stated aims were to discover the state of general knowledge about cancer and to throw further light on why women are more reluctant than men to seek advice for symptoms. The study consisted of two samples derived from different sources. The first consisted of 1200 women aged over 21 years, 'systematically' selected from the electoral roll. The second part of the sample came from another study carried out to look specifically at tuberculosis. These people had been randomly selected from households. Four questions were included about cancer in the second study and analysis was carried out only from the answers given by 1203 women who were aged over 21 years. The response rate in the first sample was 99 per cent, but the response rate for the second sample was not reported.

The main findings in the study were as follows.

1. Of five diseases—heart trouble, tuberculosis, asthma, cancer and rheumatism—'over two-thirds of women in the study rated cancer as the most alarming'.

2. A high proportion of women said that cancer was not curable (50 per cent in the cancer survey and a larger proportion in the tuberculosis survey).

3. Nearly three-fifths of the women in the cancer survey said that early treatment increases the chance of cure. The value of early treatment was appreciated by more women in the 'higher than in the lower social classes'.

4. Nearly four-fifths of all the women knew personally someone who had had cancer, but less than a third had heard of anyone who had been cured of it.

A number of questions were asked about the knowledge of symptoms.

5. The women were asked to say which of the following symptoms they would find the most alarming: a constant cough, a lump in the breast which does not hurt, losing weight, seeing a show of blood or discharge ten years or so after the change of life, or frequent pain after eating. Just under two-fifths of the women said that they would find a painless lump in the breast to be most alarming and four-fifths of these women accounted for this because they thought it might be cancer or a growth or a tumour which implied it could be life threatening. A much smaller proportion found that seeing a show of blood or discharge ten years or so after the change of life was the most alarming sign and the majority of these women did not see it as a sign of cancer. This was supported by further evidence that breast lumps are seen by the majority of women (nearly four-fifths) as first signs of cancer, but bleeding or discharge ten years or so after the change of life was only seen by less than a quarter of the women as a sign of cancer. The breast and the womb were given as the most common sites of cancer.

6. Knocks, bumps or falls were given as the main causes of cancer by just over a quarter of the women, but nearly half of the women said they did not know what caused cancer. It is interesting to note that only 2 per cent of women attributed smoking as the main cause of cancer, although this is hardly surprising given the small amount of publicity devoted to this topic by the early 1950s.

7. The women accounted for their worries about cancer as opposed to other diseases mainly in terms of incurability and pain.

To summarize, the vast majority of women found cancer the most alarming disease. Although a majority said that early treatment made a difference, nearly three-quarters had never heard of anyone cured of cancer and a half thought cancer is never cured. Most women said that the most common sites of cancer are the breast and womb and they appear to be more alarmed about signs of breast cancer than about any other symptom. Their knowledge of the symptoms of cancer of the womb was limited. The results also showed that despite cancer of the cervix being more prevalent amongst semi-skilled and unskilled occupational groups, ignorance in these groups was most profound.

The authors concluded:

'The great majority of women realise the possible significance of a painless lump in the breast, but there is no sense of urgency when cancer is so widely believed to be incurable' (Paterson and Aitken-Swan, 1954).

The authors also make a point which is of significance in the assessment of the value of these surveys.

'Certainly the results must be interpreted with caution. Most of the questions in the present survey call for opinion on straightforward matters; direct questions do not reach deeper and more emotional levels of thinking.'

An interviewer, after more in-depth interviewing, identified two important aspects of people's feelings which may have coloured their answers to the direct question. First, when questioned about family incidence the interviewer noticed that respondents felt a certain shame about it and wished to hush it up. The interviewer explains the second aspect which she uncovered (Paterson and Aitken-Swan, 1954):

'Also, several said "No, thank God", not in a relieved way only but as though people with cancer have the plague, which was quite at variance with their assurance in answers to another question that they would willingly visit a friend with cancer.'

This highlights a number of interesting points, not least the nature of the stigma attached to cancer. However, it also shows the limitations of public opinion studies in that they are instruments which serve to support or refute the researchers' constructions of what is meaningful to lay people rather than gaining an understanding of the meaning lay people attach to cancer. In public opinion surveys, it presupposes that researchers' and lay people's definitions are similar.

A follow-up study was carried out by the same authors in 1957 (Paterson and Aitken-Swan, 1958). The aim was to examine any changes in opinion following five years of cancer education, using the previous study as the baseline data. The follow-up study was not carried out on the same population as in the earlier study but on two different populations in two different parts of the region. The educated group consisted of a randomly selected sample of just under 1200 women aged 21 years and over, living in Oldham, Rochdale, Bury and Ashton-under-Lyne. A contrast study was made in a previously defined control area, similar in size and social and industrial structure, centred on Preston, Blackburn and Wigan, in which there was no planned cancer education.

The results from this study were as follows.

1. Cancer was rated the most alarming disease in all the surveys but more so in the control group (1957) than in any of the other groups.

2. In comparison with the 1953 survey, the experimental area shows an increase of 19 per cent in the proportion aware that cancer is sometimes cured against, in the control area, an increase of only half as much (10 per cent). This may be due to health education campaigns which emphasized that cancer is sometimes curable.

3. A painless lump in the breast was regarded as the most alarming symptom by women of all ages, although there was no significant change in the size of the group or the size of the group that was most alarmed by unusual bleeding or discharge.

4. More women in the controls than in the experimental group said that bleeding or discharge was a first symptom or sign of cancer of the womb, and similar findings were found for first signs of a breast lump.

Overall, the results indicated that there had been a change in women's attitudes to cancer. Women in general were more alarmed by it compared with other diseases, although more thought it was curable. This seemed to be the one influence of the health education campaigns as knowledge of symptoms of breast cancer or cancer of the womb had not changed.

1966 study

The second large 'public opinion' study to be carried out in the UK took place on a sample of women aged 21 years and over and living in Lancaster (Briggs and Wakefield, 1967). Like the previous study, a follow-up study was carried out seven years later (Knopf, 1974) which looked at the changes in opinion. Once again the initial study in 1966 was used as the source of the baseline data. In this initial study, 730 women over 21 years were systematically sampled from households on the Lancaster Electoral Register.

The findings were as follows.

1. Almost two-thirds of the women felt that cancer was the disease thought to kill most people. Bronchitis and heart disease each accounted for about a sixth of the responses.

2. Of five diseases—cancer, mental disease, heart disease, bronchitis and TB—cancer was ranked by just over a half of the people as the most alarming and this assessment was being made by all age and social categories.

3. The study showed that cancer was the disease generally thought to be the least curable of the five.

4. Almost nine-tenths of the women felt that early treatment increases the chances of cure, and this was higher than all the other diseases apart from tuberculosis.

5. Women were asked what they thought was the meaning of two symptoms—a lump in the breast and post-menopausal bleeding or discharge. Almost four-fifths of the women gave cancer or a malignancy as an explanation of a lump in

the breast, although only 45 per cent saw post-menopausal bleeding or discharge as a sign or symptom of cancer.

6. Exactly half of the women said that cancer could not be prevented, and about a third said it could. The remainder did not know. The most common preventive measure was to refrain from smoking (14.0 per cent) and then a smear test (8.0 per cent) and check-ups (7.1 per cent). Older women were much less likely to mention smoking than younger ones.

7. Almost a third of the women thought cancer of the womb could be prevented, although only just under a quarter mentioned the smear test as a preventive measure. Only 10.0 per cent of the sample had had a cervical smear test carried out.

8. Thirty per cent of the women said that knocks or falls were the cause of cancer and 18.0 per cent said smoking.

9. Forty-four per cent of women had heard of someone who had been cured of cancer, and 57 per cent said that they had had personal contact with a cancer sufferer. However, only 1 in 8 women had been in contact with a cured case. It appears that contact with a person, whether cured or not, influences beliefs about the curability of cancer. Those who had personal contact with a patient cured from cancer were much more likely to say that cancer was usually curable than those who had no personal contact or had personal contact with cancer sufferers who were not cured.

Briggs and Wakefield (1967) also found some marked variations in opinion by age and social class. Here is a brief summary of the findings.

1. Women from social classes I and II were more likely to say that cancer was curable; that early treatment increases the chance of cure; that cancer is preventable and cancer of the womb is preventable; to know that the smear test is a preventive measure; and to have had personal contact with someone with cancer or to have heard of cancer being cured than women from social classes IV and V. No other social class differences were found.

2. Younger women were more likely to say cancer was curable and cancer was preventable; to mention smoking as a preventive measure and to know that cancer of the womb can be prevented and specifically by a smear test; to have had a smear test; to know that smoking rather than knocks causes cancer and to have heard of someone who has been cured of cancer than older women.

In general, women from social classes I and II appear to be more optimistic about the curability and preventability of cancer than those in other social groups. Younger women, also, were more optimistic and had different ideas about causation than those in older age groups.

Knopf's study (1974) was carried out in Lancaster on different women although, once again, they were samples from the electoral register. This time, however, the age of consent had fallen to 18 years so the sample consisted of women aged over 18 years. In all, 716 households were sampled and 756 women were interviewed (a response rate of 95 per cent). The study was designed to assess changes that have occurred between 1966 and 1973, during which period not only had the educational programme been operating but also there had been increased discussion of cancer in the media.

Knopf's findings showed that the idea that cancer was the main cause of death in the country still persisted as did the view that it was the most alarming. More optimistic views about curability and the value of early treatment were found.

Women in general seem to have a knowledge of the non-malignant nature of breast lumps, although many women had no knowledge at all of the implications of post-menopausal bleeding and discharge. The most significant change occurred about the existence of preventive measures. Forty-six per cent thought that there was something they could do by way of prevention, compared with only 31 per cent in 1966; but there was little change among the over 60s, only a quarter of whom thought prevention possible. More women mentioned smoking as a cause and the cervical smear test as a preventive measure than before. More women also thought cancer of the womb could be prevented than before, the majority of these saying that the smear test could prevent it. Almost a third had had the cervical smear test in 1973 compared with only 10 per cent in 1966. However, age and social class differences still persist in the knowledge, awareness and use of the smear test.

As Knopf points out, there is no way of assessing whether the changes in opinion were due to the educational programme rather than other influences such as the media. The point was also made (Knopf, 1976) that it is difficult to assess whether this increase in information may lead to a change in opinion. She states:

> 'It seems that, if the individual is left to make what he can of the odd facts he picks up from the media, he may well become more pessimistic and doubtful, since he is not also provided with a proper frame of reference within which to interpret his new knowledge, having to rely instead on his pre-existing ideas.'

However, she feels that in the case of cancer the situation is different.

> 'The experience with cancer suggests, however, that when information is deliberately presented as a coherent whole, as in educational programmes, then desirable changes in public opinion may be achieved, albeit very gradually.'

Knopf's optimism about health education programmes may be well founded in terms of changing public opinion, although why the public should be more responsive to messages about cancer is difficult to understand. Also, how this knowledge or opinion is translated into action is altogether a different matter.

1966 study
A parallel study to the one carried out in Lancaster was carried out on Merseyside (Hobbs, 1967). Once again the study was carried out as a baseline for educational work aimed at (i) reducing patient-centred delay occurring either because of a lack of awareness of the significance of symptoms or due to a fear of cancer, and (ii) creating a climate of opinion aimed at enhancing the acceptability of certain preventive health behaviours. The sample consisted of women of 20 years and over and was made up from a series of random samples drawn from the Merseyside area. Of the 836 women sampled, questionnaires were completed by 86.5 per cent. The questionnaire was similar to the one used in the first Lancaster survey. Comparison of these results with those from the study in Lancaster must be made with caution as a small amount of educational work had been carried out in Merseyside before the study was carried out but none had been carried out in Lancaster. The major differences between Merseyside and Lancaster were that although Merseysiders were more likely to impute specific causes of cancer such as knocks or smoking, they tended to be less positive about preventive measures and the value of early detection.

1969 study

The fourth study was carried out in south-east Wales (Williams *et al.*, 1972) in 1969. Random samples of men and women of over 21 years of age were drawn from four separate areas within the region, selected as typifying the main different modes and conditions of life in the part of Wales covered by the education project. A total of 801 women and 203 men were interviewed. Many of the questions were designed to be consistent with those employed in previous similar studies, and particularly those used in surveys in Lancaster and Merseyside in 1966. However, when comparing these studies it must be remembered that they were carried out at different times, that the social class characteristics of the population are different (which might have implications for variation in beliefs), and each area had received its own amount of local public education about cancer. Many of the findings are similar but the most marked differences between the South Wales study and the two others are found in the areas where Knopf (1974), in her follow-up of the Lancaster study, found the most changes. In the south-east Wales study (Williams *et al.*, 1972) more women thought that post-menopausal bleeding was a possible sign of cancer and more women had mentioned the smear test as a preventive measure. More women thought that cancer was preventable and they would take a specific action about it in south-east Wales than in the other studies and more women mentioned smoking as a cause of cancer than in the other studies. Differences were found in beliefs about the curability of the disease between the South Wales study and the others. Women in south-east Wales were slightly more pessimistic about the possibility of cure than the others, which contrasts with Knopf's finding of an increase in optimism.

Other questions were included in the south-east Wales study which were not in the others. For example, women were asked what they would do if they had something wrong with them and they thought it was cancer. Nine out of 10 women said they would go to their own doctor. More women from social classes I and II were more likely to say they would go to their doctor than women from the other social groups.

Of more significance were the marked differences in beliefs according to sex (Williams *et al.*, 1972). It was found that men were more likely than women to:

(i) be aware of the true situation regarding cancer;
(ii) be optimistic about treatment;
(iii) give positive answers rather than 'don't knows'.

Findings about variation in belief according to social class and age were similar to the trends found in previous studies.

This study was followed up by Bluck (1975). The follow-up study was carried out in a comparable area during 1973-74. In all, 357 of the 492 respondents sampled were interviewed. Bluck concludes that the findings from her study substantially confirm those found in the previous south-east Wales study and the studies in Lancaster and Merseyside. However, some differences were found. She states:

'Whilst the Tenovus study results seemed to indicate that among certain groups it was possible to identify a "syndrome of pessimism", there was no evidence in the present study to suggest that respondents were unduly pessimistic about cancer prevention, although a small group could be identified who were pessimistic about prevention.'

Between 1969 and 1973 there was an increase in the use of the cervical smear test and the vast majority of respondents indicated that they were well aware of the dangers of smoking and realized that lung cancer could possibly be prevented by giving up the habit. Once again, marked social class differences were found in knowledge and attitude about cancer prevention, with the least positive attitudes occurring amongst social classes IV and V.

Summary of overall trends in public opinion in the UK

Going back to the study in Manchester in 1953, what have been the most significant changes that have taken place in public opinion between that time and 1973 when Knopf carried out her study? It must be emphasized that these changes refer entirely to changes in women's beliefs. Cancer still rates, for the majority of women, as the most alarming disease, although there has been a change in opinions about the significance of other diseases. There has been a large increase in the number of women who think cancer is curable. The majority of women have always considered a lump in the breast to be an early sign of breast cancer, but more women know about the signs of cervical cancer. More value is placed on early treatment nowadays than in 1954.

Other significant changes have come in the area of prevention and cure. A much larger proportion of women say cancer can be prevented, and more know that cervical cancer can be prevented by a smear test. More women are having smear tests, as might be expected; however, over half of the women still had not had one carried out by 1973. There were also changes in the explanations of the causes of cancer. In 1953, smoking was cited by only 2 per cent as being a cause of cancer, but this figure had increased to nearly 33 per cent in 1973. However, still just over a quarter of women when asked what causes cancer give a spontaneous answer of knocks, blows or falls.

Social class and age differences in health belief about cancer still persist and the older women and the working-class women are less likely to hold beliefs that are congruent with those held by official health authorities. One study found marked differences in beliefs between males and females.

Trends in public opinions towards cancer in other countries

How do these trends compare with those in other countries? A vast amount of research on this subject has been carried out in the USA and it is the intention to concentrate here on those American studies. On the whole, compared with the UK studies, the studies in the USA have tended to be more broadly based in terms of sampling and in terms of questions asked. According to Simonds (1970) seven major national surveys about cancer were carried out in the United States between 1948 and 1970. All of these studies, apart from one, were sponsored by or carried out by the American Cancer Society.

Simonds (1970) shows that, as in the UK, in the period 1939–66 cancer was still believed to be the most serious disease an individual could contract. Simonds also found that between 1948 and 1966 there seemed to be a decrease in the population who thought that examinations would detect presymptomatic conditions and there was little change in public opinion about the curability of cancer since 1939. These findings appear to differ markedly from the results from the UK studies, although there was greater optimism about the curability of some forms of cancer in the US.

Simonds concludes (1970) that:

> 'There is less squeamishness about cancer, as evidenced by the greater per cent who indicate that they would be willing to work next to someone who has cancer. There are fewer misconceptions about cancer, as shown by the smaller per cent who believe that one person can catch cancer from another.'

However, despite the improvement in beliefs and attitudes, the public still does not do enough to protect itself against cancer.

A further series of opinion studies was carried out in the US during the 1970s. Some studies have concentrated on specific forms of cancer such as attitudes to breast cancer (American Cancer Society, 1974) and others have covered the whole area of cancer (Holleb, 1978; James and Lieberman, 1979). It is the most recent study (James and Lieberman, 1979) that will be described here. This study, sponsored by the American Cancer Society, was an update of their previous study carried out in 1966. It was a national study, carried out in 1978 and based on a sample of 1553 men and women aged 18 years of age and above.

The results showed that the proportion of people going regularly for physical examinations increased from 26 per cent in 1966 to 36 per cent in 1978. Respondents were asked about their images of check-ups and the person who regularly goes for them. On the whole, there was a positive image of check-ups and people saw them as worthwhile, necessary, thorough and effective, although many people feel that medical check-ups are expensive. Not surprisingly, those who regularly go for check-ups saw those who go for check-ups as intelligent, responsible and well organized by comparison with non-goers, who saw those who go for check-ups as worriers, scared and hypochondriacal.

The study also showed that the public feel a great deal of fear and anxiety about cancer and they are pessimistic, at least compared with medical knowledge, about its curability. The American public knew, on average, 4.6 of 7 cancer warning signs and this figure was similar to that found in 1966.

A number of questions were asked about the use of early detection tests. The proportion of women who had the Pap test (cervical cancer) increased from 64 per cent in 1966 to 86 per cent in 1978. In 1978, 67 per cent of women reported performing breast self-examination in the past year, although only 27 per cent did it once a month on average. In 1978, 71 per cent of the sample reported having had a digital rectal examination and 34 per cent reported having it done regularly. Four per cent reported as having a proctoscopic examination and 14 per cent said that they had had one at some time.

Finally, cigarettes top the list of nineteen possible causes of cancers in the minds of both smokers and non-smokers in the American population. Although smokers more than non-smokers said they had more likelihood of getting lung cancer, about 71 per cent believe that, if lung cancer is detected early, there is a good chance that it can be cured.

In summary, this most recent study carried out in the US suggests that whilst there has been an increase in people's knowledge about cancer and an apparent increase in the use of early detection tests, cancer still provokes considerable fear and anxiety.

Young people's beliefs and feelings about cancer

Following the recent trend of health education focusing on the young rather than the adult, a number of studies have been carried out examining school children's beliefs and feelings about cancer. Perhaps the most comprehensive study was carried out by Charlton (1977) on pupils and teachers in comprehensive schools in Manchester. The aims of the research were to educate young people correctly about cancer:

'with no overtones of emotion and mystery so that these negative attitudes to cancer will not be perpetuated and these pupils, when they are older, will seek medical help quickly if necessary ...'

The research was set up:

'first to find out what ideas the pupils already had about cancer, where these ideas had come from and if these young people wanted to know more about cancer ...'

The first part of the project was a fact-finding survey. Using the results of this as a baseline, teaching materials were designed and, in the third and final stage, lessons were evaluated in schools. In all, 3537 pupils and 191 teachers took part in the first stage of the survey. It is the pupils' answers that will be examined in this section. Like the adults in the previous opinion studies, the pupils were asked, of road accidents, cancer, heart disease, bronchitis and TB, what kills the most people in this country. Nearly 3 out of every 5 pupils said that road accidents kill the most people and just over 1 in 4 said cancer. Only just under a third said cancer was usually or sometimes curable. Nine out of 10 pupils mentioned smoking as a cause of cancer and 1 in 10 mentioned knocks/falls. Three out of every 5 pupils had heard of a medical test to find cancer early.

As a result of a health education exercise, there was a substantial increase in the percentage of pupils who thought cancer was curable and there was also an increase in the percentage of those who thought that cancer was more curable if treated early.

The evidence from this study suggests that school children are less likely to say that cancer is the disease that kills most people than adults, although they are less likely to think cancer is curable than adults. Whilst young people are more likely to pinpoint smoking as a cause of cancer than adults, some still hold the belief that knocks or falls are causes of cancer.

Methodological problems in 'public opinion' studies

Other studies in this country have concentrated on one particular cancer site and looked at why some people use the screening and treatment services more than others. More recently, many of these studies have attempted to examine beliefs and behaviour in a more systematic and detailed manner and these studies will be used to illustrate the argument that a different perspective should be adopted.

However, before this is discussed some further 'technical' points need to be made about these 'public opinion' studies. The ideal method of discovering changes in opinion is to follow a series of national cohorts over time. As has already been mentioned, the samples in the studies carried out in the UK up until now have not always been equivalent and thus changes in opinion may be due to changes in the composition of the sample and not to real changes in opinion. The second point refers to the type of questions asked and how question formation makes an important difference in the nature of the data. This point is ably made by Simonds (1970) commenting on the American opinion studies, but this also applies to the British studies. He gives an example from a survey carried out in the US in 1963. Results showed that:

> 'Respondents answered in the affirmative that tests or check-ups would show that a person had cancer before he noticed something was wrong, and responded in the negative to a similar question when it was applied to them personally.'

These opinion poll surveys may produce unreliable information because instead of producing actual beliefs they elicit 'normative' or 'ought' statements, particularly when there has been some educational exercise carried out previously.

The fixed response questionnaire approach, which was a common tool in these studies, gives respondents little opportunity to express their definitions, which may be different to those expressed in the questionnaire. Thus the questionnaire may reflect only the researchers' judgements about what concepts are significant in this area (see Harrison and West, 1976).

Marsh (1979) has a more fundamental set of criticisms of 'public opinion' studies in general. She argues that the notion of public opinion is essentially individualistic. The respondents are not allowed in the interview situation to discuss the issue with others as the interview concentrates on the individual. This individual approach may be completely different to the way the respondent makes decisions in everyday life, as the precursors of action or behaviour may be an 'opinion' developed through social interaction. The second point Marsh refers to is that public opinion studies assume everybody has an opinion about everything. Thus it is assumed that everybody knows and has an opinion about cancer. Marsh further argues that, in these studies, opinions all seem to be fixed and latent. A refined survey instrument will identify the true underlying feelings and beliefs.

It is evident, as Marsh points out, that this is a 'perversion' of the way people think about topics and the way people change their views. She states, in her concluding remark about the value of public opinion studies, that whilst there are some topics about which people are willing to express clear opinions, too frequently questions tend to create rather than reflect public opinion. Marsh suggests that this process of creating what everybody thinks may exert a strong conformist influence on what the public actually do think.

Public opinion about cancer and the use of services

A more fundamental criticism of this type of study is that it is predominantly atheoretical. A variety of questions, predominantly testing people's medical knowledge about cancer, is asked and analysed in relation to a number of sociodemographic factors. What is lacking is some underlying model or framework which explains the nature or the hypothesized nature of the relationship between the variables. The assumption which appears to be inherent in these 'public opinion' approaches is that correct knowledge leads to correct health behaviour. Wakefield (1976), in describing the functions of health education, clearly illustrates this by defining the aims of public education as follows:

'To inform and educate about treatable forms of cancer and to reassure people that treatment is to their advantage.'

In addition, public education should also seek:

'To persuade people, particularly those at special risk, to undertake preventive action, to accept tests so that cancer can be detected at an earlier stage, or to seek appropriate medical advice quickly when recognizable signs of ill health occur.'

Thus, Wakefield sees knowledge as the key to people adopting appropriate forms of health and illness behaviour. However, more recent studies which have concentrated on examining specific factors related to preventive and illness behaviour have suggested that 'correct' health knowledge is not enough. For example, in a study of what makes women seek advice for breast conditions, Eardley (1974) found that the majority of women consult someone else before they see a doctor and might be influenced by that advice. Similarly, in a breast screening study, Hobbs *et al.* (1978) showed that response to a letter of invitation to attend for mammographic examination was influenced by the opinion of others. This evidence suggests that decisions to take part in screening or to consult a doctor are not just a reflection of individual attitudes or knowledge but are also social in nature and involve consultation with lay others.

Breast cancer has received a large amount of attention from researchers in recent years and some of this research illustrates a shift in the approach to understanding illness and health behaviour. Many more factors, both psychological and social, have been considered and examples from some of these studies may illustrate the complex nature of laymen's health beliefs and feelings. Some studies have concentrated on explaining why women delay in consulting with a doctor when they have breast conditions (Greer, 1974; Margarey and Todd, 1976). Whilst these studies concentrated on women with breast conditions, they do illustrate beliefs and feelings about cancer. Explanations of delay have varied. Some have emphasized that these women are more likely to be threatened by a cancer diagnosis or the loss of a breast. The anxiety or distress generated by these fears tends to cause delay, although the threat may, according to some authors, lead to denial. Other explanations emphasize the lack of awareness of the implications of a breast condition. So, these studies suggest that the negative image of cancer and its consequences may influence delay in consultation amongst some women. However, the relationship between knowledge of cancer, the threat of cancer and adoption of officially recommended health actions is not as simple. Some studies have shown that those who believed that their symptoms might be cancer were just as likely to delay as those who did not suspect this (Aitken-Swan and Paterson, 1959).

Other studies have concentrated on explaining the uptake of early detection programmes for breast cancer. These studies, too, illustrate women's prevailing beliefs and feelings about breast cancer. For example, women who participate in screening programmes are more likely than non-participators to see the disease as being serious, more likely to feel susceptible to it, less likely to have been highly anxious about it, although they were more likely to have a good knowledge of the disease and its risk factors (Van Den Heuval, 1978). Van Den Heuval (1978) also showed that other factors apart from health beliefs and feelings about cancer were influential on participation, such as social class, education and age.

Studies of factors associated with the practice of breast self-examination also illustrate women's prevailing beliefs and feelings about breast cancer. For example, one study (Manfredi et al., 1977) showed that women's belief in the efficacy of early detection of the disease to reduce the danger from the disease was found to be the strongest correlate of the ability to perform breast self-examination. Haran et al (1979) found that awareness of breast self-examination (BSE) was found to be related to use of other preventive health measures, such as the use of chest x-rays or cervical smears. They also found that those who practise breast self-examination are more likely to view breast cancer as the most worrying illness to which women are prone. On the other hand, awareness of breast self-examination appears to bring with it a greater optimism about care. Perhaps of more interest are the findings of Stillman (1977), who found 97 per cent of 122 women scored high in perceived beliefs of breast self-examination in reducing the threat of breast cancer, and 87 per cent scored high in perceived susceptibility to breast cancer. Forty per cent practised BSE monthly, but over 20 per cent of the sample had high beliefs and were non-practisers. Stillman states that it cannot be concluded that beliefs cause behaviour, but that other factors such as embarrassment or religious upbringing influence health beliefs and practices.

The point of discussing these studies, although many of them could be defined as being in the secondary prevention area, is to show not only how women feel about breast cancer but also to show that obtaining information about lay health knowledge concerning cancer is not sufficient to explain health beliefs or health behaviour. The stated objectives of many of the 'public' opinion studies were to increase knowledge so as to influence health and illness behaviour. From this evidence it is suggested that knowledge is one component of health beliefs. Health beliefs alone are not necessarily strong predictors of behaviour.

Theoretical approaches to health behaviour

More coherent models of health behaviour have been developed (see Becker et al., 1977) but have yet to be empirically tested. Becker's model attempts to predict compliance with official health-recommended actions such as screening, immunizations, diet, exercise, personal and work habits as well as entering or continuing a treatment programme. So it covers not only the take up of health services but also compliance with actions recommended in health education campaigns about health behaviour. The model consists of a number of factors which comprise the concept 'readiness to undertake recommended compliance behaviour' and these include motivation, value of illness threat reduction, and probability that complaint behaviour will reduce the threat. In addition, a number of modifying and enabling factors are suggested which might influence action; these are demographic, structural, attitudes, interaction and enabling. A number of studies have used parts of the model and have concentrated on utilization or illness behaviour.

No study has tested the whole model or examined its relationship to primary prevention such as dieting or exercise or giving up smoking.

More recently, modifications have been suggested for this model so as to incorporate a more collective and less individualistic approach to compliance with health-recommended actions. Becker (1979) has suggested that patients' 'locus of control' may be a further important factor in predicting health behaviour. He suggests that the more the patient feels powerless to control his or her life or the more fatalistic the person is, the less likely he or she is to comply. In addition, social support, whether through the family or other lay network, has been identified as a factor in influencing the maintenance of health behaviour. Antonovsky and Anson (1976) suggest that the health belief model approach with its emphasis on rational action based on weighing up the costs and benefits will only appeal to the needs of the rational-goal-directed woman. He argues that three other types of women exist: the conformist woman, the complacent–stoic woman and the ambivalent–anxious woman. Each is an ideal type constructed by Antonovsky and Anson (1976) from their data and is a sociological type formulated in terms of women's orientation to health behaviour. Each type of health orientation is associated with various patterns of preventive health behaviour.

More fundamental criticisms have been made which apply to all of the studies received so far, from the simple 'public opinion' approach to the 'health belief models' and the more recent attempts to develop collective approaches. These criticisms have been aimed primarily at studies of illness behaviour and the use of health services for illnesses rather than at health and health behaviour.

Dingwall (1976) suggests that the major weaknesses in the previous approaches to illness behaviour are that they are 'scientistic' and 'absolutist'. Dingwall argues that it is assumed that natural scientific phenomena are the same as social phenomena and thus these studies have depended on the methodological procedures of the natural sciences. For Dingwall, such an approach is mistaken, and whereas natural phenomena merely behave, human beings act and they have intentional action and a meaningful language system. Dingwall emphasizes the need for sociological work to examine individual action and the meaning of that action and not to assume that actors are empty organisms responding passively either to their 'predispositions' or to the wider social system. Thus, whilst it may be useful to relate social class or family size to utilization or compliance, the important question to ask is why such a relationship is found. Some authors have tried to explain the 'why' question in terms of psychological dispositions such as vulnerability or a propensity to use the health services or in terms of social forces or cues. In each of these cases the implicit assumption is that individuals' action occurs as a response to stimuli emanating from internal or external forces. There is no room for a theory which emphasizes the critical and active powers of individuals.

Dingwall also states that this dependence on natural scientific methods in social enquiry also reflects a specific orientation towards knowledge. This approach claims that its theories and explanations and bodies of knowledge have a unique access to truth. This is an absolutist version of knowledge in contrast to a pluralist approach in which all accounts of the world are of equal status. Therefore, medical theories and lay theories are, from a sociological point of view, of equal interest and status.

Dingwall suggests that previous studies of illness behaviour, through their reliance on natural scientific methods, have failed to develop a truly sociological theory of illness. They have concentrated on behaviour without attempting to understand the meaning of that behaviour and thus have failed to develop a sociological theory of action. Implicit in this dependence is an acceptance of an absolutist version of knowledge and this acceptance has meant that many of these studies have based their assumptions about lay and patient behaviour on a version of the social world which has been derived from official medical knowledge. These studies have treated this definition itself as unproblematic. Thus lay theories of illness are treated as idiosyncratic or reflect some pathological irrationality. Lay theories are treated as in some way inferior to biological medical explanations.

Dingwall's criticisms of the studies of illness behaviour also apply to those which have concentrated on health and health behaviour. For example, those looking at opinions on cancer have taken it for granted that the way in which lay people think, talk and act about cancer is very similar to the way in which official medical practitioners think about cancer or think that lay people should think about it. No research has attempted to examine lay beliefs about cancer and the way cancer is interpreted in terms of lay knowledge, which may be vastly different to medical knowledge.

In the field of illness behaviour the emphasis has shifted away from focusing on the social problems of patient delay or under- or over-utilization, towards exam-ination of illness and how it is interpreted by lay people. As a result, help-seeking behaviour is seen as one of many possible and legitimate responses to the proble-matic experience of illness. Similarly, such a change in approach could take place in the field of health and health behaviour. Instead of concentrating on why people do not comply with officially recommended health practices, the concept of health should be considered to be problematic and a topic for study. Thus, research might concentrate on what health means to lay people within different social contexts and might see preventive practices or health behaviour as one possible response to lay evaluation.

Such an ethnographic approach, which is commonly employed in anthropol-ogical work, has yet to be systematically applied in the field of health and illness. However, its importance as a research tool to complement the more traditional approaches is beginning to be recognized. For example, Cohen (1979) identifies the value of this approach in 'hypothesis' generation and for discovering new relationships.

Professional beliefs and feelings about cancer

The beliefs and feelings of those in the medical and paramedical professions about cancer have recently become the focus of attention for two reasons which are interrelated. First, there is the suggestion that these groups may fulfil an important educative function for their patients and the negative images of cancer held by the general public may merely reflect the negative images of professionals (Hen-derson et al., 1958). Second, it has been suggested that non-compliance with health-recommended practices is due in part to the nature of the communication between doctor and patient. Patients dissatisfied with the amount and nature of the information given in their encounters with doctors are defaulting from doctors' instructions (Korsch et al., 1968). So it is claimed that not only do medical and paramedical professionals fail to communicate to the patient information that the patient requires, but also that they are communicating the 'wrong' image of cancer. Evidence to support the latter proposition is difficult to find. However, in matters of health, medical personnel (whether it be doctors, nurses or others) play as significant a part as any, at both the informal and formal level, in providing knowledge and advice. While for some people the doctor is the first person to whom they turn as a source of expertise or knowledge about health, for others the nurse, who is the neighbour or friend, may be the person who is turned to. So it is the potential influence of the medical and paramedical professionals which is the basic reason for the attention given to their beliefs and feelings. Once again the theory seems to be that given the 'right' information, the 'right' message should come across to the patient.

The numbers of studies of professional or paramedical beliefs and feelings about cancer are much less numerous than those carried out on public opinion. Perhaps, the three important 'professionals' in the cancer area are doctors, nurses and teachers.

Doctors' beliefs about cancer

Some studies of doctors have been specifically concerned with examining doctors' beliefs and feelings about cancer (see Easson, 1974) and others have looked at encounters between doctors and patients in cancer wards. Both types of study can be used to elicit information about the way doctors feel about cancer and cancer patients. The most recent study of general practitioners' beliefs and procedures with regard to cancer and its prevention was carried out by Bluck (1975) in south-east Wales. She outlines her reasons for focusing GPs (see also Wakefield, 1972).

'It seemed important that the medical profession, or its representatives, should be the object of study as well as the public because members of the profession play an important role as initiators and legitimators of appropriate behaviour in the face of health or illness.'

She continues:

'Thus it seems obvious that doctors have an important part to play in encouraging the public to take preventive action, and indeed to regard preventive action as appropriate. The general practitioner, as the member of the medical profession most people see most often, could play a leading role in providing this encouragement.'

Bluck (1975) sampled 153 general practitioners in three different areas in south-east Wales and, in all, 127 responded to the postal questionnaire. The questionnaires were orientated to preventive practices in general but a large part focused on cancer. A large majority of doctors said they advised their patients about smoking, but about a half carried out cervical smears in their surgery and discussed breast self-examination with patients. Whilst the vast majority of the general practitioners had 'No Smoking' signs in their surgeries, only about a third carried cancer education leaflets.

The general practitioners were asked what could prevent lung cancer and cervical cancer. Most doctors were optimistic about prevention of lung cancer, although not so optimistic about cervical cancer. The smoking habit was most frequently referred to as a way of preventing lung cancer. Other measures commonly referred to were control of air pollution, regular chest x-ray and improved industrial health measures. With cervical cancer, the most common preventive measures mentioned were cervical smears, the importance of early detection of symptoms, and the examination of women at risk.

The majority of the general practitioners were positive about the importance of preventive medicine in their work and about health education, particularly in relation to prevention of lung cancer.

General practitioners were also asked how they would react to a healthy person asking for a general examination. In response to this question, a large number of general practitioners indicated that they assume that a person requesting a general examination 'for his or her satisfaction' has a further reason—a real reason for making this request. This implies a type of psychoanalytic approach when the patient's request is seen to be irrational or idiosyncratic and the real motives are hidden. Thus, these patients are evaluated on the grounds of temperament or character before examination takes place. This suggests that the practice of preventive medicine is still seen by some general practitioners to be outside of what they see as their appropriate work roles.

With regard to the general 'attitude' of general practitioners towards cancer, Bluck (1975) states:

'There is no evidence however to suggest that the doctors who deliberately avoid discussing cancer for such reasons constitute more than a small minority of the respondents. But there is evidence to suggest that many general practitioners are reluctant to discuss topics or actions relevant to cancer.'

She found that small groups of doctors displayed a 'pessimistic' attitude to cancer, but then qualified it by stating:

'However, although it is possible to delimit small groups of doctors, at least in the city and valley areas, who appeared pessimistic about cancer prevention, and were reluctant to discuss preventive measures, the evidence to suggest that these doctors had a particularly pessimistic attitude to cancer is insubstantial.'

The importance of the attitudes and beliefs of general practitioners cannot be overemphasized, particularly in relation to preventive medicine. Hospital doctors, in their formal capacity, are in a different position; they are normally faced with people with a problem of some sort, and their role would be concerned with helping people to cope with cancer rather than with prevention. So the images put over by hospital doctors may influence the way their patients cope with cancer.

Studies directly focusing on hospital doctors' beliefs about cancer are rare. Some evidence can be derived from studies which have focused on other aspects of hospital life. McIntosh (1977) carried out a predominantly observational study of a cancer ward in a Scottish hospital. He concentrated on how the medical staff communicated information to the patients about their medical conditions.

McIntosh found that the doctors followed the routine policy of only telling patients who want to know the diagnosis of their condition. McIntosh (1977) suggests that while doctors believed most patients did not want to know they also believed some could and should be told. He states:

'The problem was they had no way of ascertaining with any certainty whether patients genuinely wanted to know or how they would respond to disclosure. In response to these uncertainties they adopted the only safe course of action open to them; they avoided disclosure to all patients.'

One of the reasons why this routine policy of 'not telling' is adopted could be that the doctor shares with the patient the negative image of cancer and any disclosure of information that might imply cancer is seen by the doctors as 'bad news'. Other reasons such as concern about upsetting the patient, concern about unpleasant interaction or concern about the loss of professional credibility due to the failure to cure the disease may be of equal importance.

Nurses' beliefs about cancer

Several studies of nurses' beliefs and attitudes to cancer have been carried out in the UK. Davison (1965), in a study of public health nurses' opinions on the treatment and curability of cancer, found that 20 per cent of the sample maintained that hospital treatment was not worthwhile. This 'pessimism' was compounded by the fact that nurses underestimated the survival rates of lung, mouth, cervical and breast cancer. Knopf-Elkind (1979), in a more detailed study of nurses' knowledge and views about cancer, found that there was an association between nurses' training and experience and their attitudes towards cancer. She states:

'In general, then, the greater the nurses' training and experience the more likely one will be to make a balanced assessment of cancer.'

This finding points to the importance of personal experience of cancer on beliefs and attitudes about cancer. These findings support those from the public opinion studies (Briggs and Wakefield, 1967) that personal experience leads to more optimistic beliefs about curability of cancer.

Teachers' beliefs about cancer

The least researched of these professional groups in relation to beliefs and feelings about cancer are teachers. Charlton (1977) has recently carried out a study on a sample of 191 teachers. Almost half of the teachers said that cancer was the most alarming disease, although 9 out of 10 said it was usually or sometimes curable; almost the whole sample said that early detection increases the chance of a cure. Smoking was given most frequently as the cause of cancer, followed by chemicals. It appears that teachers, as a group, are well informed about cancer and appear to have a more optimistic approach to cancer than other professional groups.

Summary

The research on the health beliefs and cancer in the medical and paramedical professions has been minimal and there is a need for much more, particularly focusing on how these groups influence the way the layman views cancer. Certainly, it is difficult to make any general statements from the evidence presented here. The evidence does suggest that some doctors hold negative beliefs about cancer and its treatment, although the vast majority are in favour, at least in theory, of utilizing methods for cancer prevention. The relative importance of nurses compared with doctors in influencing patients' images of cancer is also difficult to judge. While the nurses' role in communication of diagnosis and prognosis may be minimal (McIntosh, 1977), the relationship between their beliefs and feelings about cancer and the effectiveness of their caring practices may be important.

Conclusion

A series of studies on public opinion and cancer has been carried out in this country since the Second World War. Such studies have been generally motivated by the belief that lay opinion can be altered to meet the requirements of official medical opinion, which will create the 'right' environment for the public to adopt the 'appropriate' health practices. The studies have been regional as opposed to national, and have been funded by various local authorities and voluntary bodies. The studies have suggested that with regard to knowledge about cancer, most people still find it the most alarming of the diseases, although beliefs about curability and the value of early detection and prevention have become more positive. The public's explanations of the causes of cancer have changed from identifying knocks or falls as the primary cause to identifying the primary cause as smoking.

Apart from the technical and methodological weaknesses in these studies previously outlined, there have been considerable gaps in the substantive material collected. These studies have almost entirely focused on female beliefs about cancer. In addition, the studies have been fragmented and atheoretical in nature and have been dominated by official assumptions about what lay people believe and should believe and how they should behave. What is needed is a detailed examination of the way lay people think, feel and interpret cancer within their own cultural and social setting. These studies should involve both qualitative and quantitative methodology with as much emphasis given to in-depth, small-sample studies as to the large-scale survey approach. In addition, the relationship between knowledge and behaviour should be seen as a problematic one and as much emphasis should be given to the examination of social influences on behaviour as to psychologistic or individual motives.

Some studies have examined professional beliefs and feelings about cancer. Further research is needed to examine this area in a more detailed and comprehensive fashion; the relationship between professional beliefs and professional practices should be examined. In addition, the assumption that professionals have a significant influence on the lay public's image of cancer has to be empirically examined.

It was also evident from the studies, which examined both lay and professional beliefs and feelings about cancer, that one of the justifications for carrying out these studies was that both groups were believed to be unduly pessimistic about cancer. It was felt that this pessimism was due to both these groups, lay and professional, having incomplete or inaccurate knowledge about the chances of cancer being successfully prevented, treated or cured. There are a number of problems attached to the assumption that the more an individual's knowledge of cancer is congruent with medical 'facts' then the more likely it is that the individual will be optimistic about cancer. In none of these studies were the respondents asked if they were optimistic or pessimistic about cancer and thus there was no way of identifying whether the definitions of pessimism of lay or professional people were similar to official definitions. In addition, it is necessary to ask why a percentage increase in survical rates should have an influence on feelings about cancer. Finally, the optimism–pessimism conceptual framework may be not the only way of explaining feelings about cancer. Within their own framework of perception of risks and vulnerability, individuals' feelings about cancer may be realistic.

References

Aitken-Swan, J. and Paterson, R. (1959). *British Medical Journal* **1**, 708.

American Cancer Society (1974). In *Public Education about Cancer*, pp. 68–73. Union Internationale Contre le Cancer, TRS, Geneva.

Antonovsky, A. and Anson, O. (1976). In *Cancer: The Behavioural Dimensions*, pp. 35–44. Ed. by J. W. Cullen, B. H. Fox and R. W. Isson. Raven Press, New York.

Becker, M. H. (1979). In *New Directions in Patient Compliance*, pp. 1–32. Ed. by S. J. Cohen. Lexington Books, New York.

Becker, M. H., Haefner, D. P., Kasl, S. V., Kirscht, J. P., Maiman, L. A. and Ronnstock, I. M. (1977) *Medical Care* **5** (Suppl.), 27.

Bluck, M. E. (1975). *Public and Professional Opinion on Preventive Medicine*. Tenovus Cancer Information Centre, Cardiff.

Briggs, J. E. and Wakefield, J. (1967). *Public opinion on cancer, a survey of knowledge and attitudes among women in Lancaster*. Department of Social Research, Christie Hospital and Holt Radium Institute, Manchester.

Charlton, A. (1977). *Research Report—Teaching Children about Cancer*. Manchester Regional Committee for Cancer Education.

Cohen, S. J. (1979). In *New Directions in Patient Compliance*, pp. 153–64. Ed. by S. J. Cohen. Lexington Books, New York.

Davison, R. L. (1965). *British Journal of Preventive and Social Medicine* **19**, 24.

Dingwall, R. (1976). *Aspects of Illness*. Martin Robertson, London.

Eardley, A. (1974). *International Journal of Health Education* **17**, 256.

Easson, E. C. (1974). The role of the doctor in public education. Union Internationale Contre le Cancer, *Technical Report Series* **10**, 14.

Erskine, H. G. (1966). *Public Opinion Quarterly* **30**(2), 308.

Greer, S. (1974). *Proceedings of the Royal Society of Medicine* **67**, 470.

Haran, D., Hobbs, P. and Pendleton, L. L. (1979). Research in Psychology and Medicine, Vol. II. *Social Aspects, Attitudes, Communication, Care and Training*, pp. 101–9. Ed. by D. J. Osborne, M. M. Grumebery and J. R. Eiser. Academic Press, London.

Harrison, R. M. and West, P. (1976). In *Public Images of Epilepsy* (unpublished paper). Presented to BSA Annual Medical Sociology Conference, York.

Henderson, J. G., Wiltkower, E. D. and Longheed, M. N. (1958). *Journal of Psychosomatic Research* **3**, 27.

Hobbs, P. (1967). *Public opinion on cancer—a survey of knowledge and attitudes among women on Merseyside*. Merseyside Cancer Education Committee, Liverpool.

Hobbs, P., Eardley, A. and Wakefield, J. (1978). In *Public Education about Cancer*, pp. 75–80. Ed. by J. Wakefield. Union Internationale Contre le Cancer, TRS, Geneva.

Holleb, A. I. (1978). In *Public Education about Cancer*, pp. 53–5. Ed. by J. Wakefield. Union Internationale Contre le Cancer, TRS, Geneva.

James, W. G. and Lieberman, S. (1979). In *Public Education about Cancer*, pp. 66–79. Ed. by P. Hobbs. Union Internationale Contre le Cancer, TRS, Geneva.

Knopf, A. (1974). *Changes in opinion after 7 years of public education in Lancaster*. Manchester Regional Committee on Cancer.

Knopf, A. (1976). *Social Science and Medicine* **10**, 191.

Knopf-Elkind, A. (1979). *Nurses' knowledge and views about cancer*. Department of Social

Research, Christie Hospital and Holt Radium Institute, University Hospital of South Manchester.

Korsch, B. M., Gozzi, E. K. and Francis, V. (1968). *Pediatrics* **42**, 855.

McIntosh, J. (1977). *Communication and Awareness in a Cancer Ward*, pp. 58–80. Croom Helm, London.

Manfredi, C., Warnecke, R. B., Graham, S. and Rosenthal, S. (1977). *Social Science and Medicine* **11**, 433.

Margarey, C. J. and Todd, P. B. (1976). *Australian and New Zealand Journal of Surgery* **46**, 391.

Marsh, C. (1979). In *Demystifying Social Statistics*, pp. 268–88. Ed. by J. Irvine, I. Miles and J. Evans. Pluto Press, London.

Paterson, R. and Aitken-Swan, J. (1954). *Lancet* **ii**, 857.

Paterson, R. and Aitken-Swan, J. (1958). *Lancet* **ii**, 791.

Philips, A. J. and Taylor, R. M. (1961). *Canadian Medical Association Journal* **84**, 142.

Simonds, S. K. (1970). *Health Education Monograph* **30**, 3.

Stillman, M. (1977). *Nursing Research* **26**(2), 121.

Van Den Heuval, W. J. A. (1978). In *Public Education about Cancer*, pp. 18–25. Union Internationale Contre le Cancer, TRS, p. 31. Geneva.

Wakefield, J. (Ed.) (1972). In *Seek Wisely to Prevent*, pp. 68–107. HMSO, London.

Wakefield, J. (Ed.) (1976). In *Public Education about Cancer*, pp. 71–93. Union Internationale Contre le Cancer, Geneva.

Williams, E. M., Cruickshank, A. and Walker, W. (1972). *Public opinion on cancer in South East Wales*. Tenovus Cancer Information Centre, Cardiff.

5

A review of government policies aimed at primary prevention

Michael Calnan

Introduction

In this chapter, government policies aimed at controlling the various agents which were identified in Chapter 3 as potential carcinogens will be described and evaluated. The following agents will be considered: tobacco, alcohol, food and medicines and drugs. Environmental and genetic agents are not considered in this review. Each agent will be considered separately as each has more unique than common features in relation to their implications for prevention. Although this review will focus on policies which have been proposed and used in the United Kingdom, some comparison will be made between these policies and those developed in other countries. The intention is to draw out the specific qualities of the UK economic, political and cultural setting which inhibit or enhance the success of cancer prevention policies, rather than to carry out an extensive internationally based analysis of prevention policies. The basic approach in this review involves an examination of both the policies for cancer control that have been adopted by the UK government and those alternative policies that have been developed through experiment and field trial and which may have been used in other countries. From this it may be possible to see what the UK government has done and is doing about cancer control and what it could be doing. However, it is important not to divorce government policy from its social, economic and historical circumstances, so the analysis will include an attempt to explain why governments have adopted certain policies where others have used alternatives or done nothing at all. The latter approach will throw some light on the practical possibilities of certain prevention policies being adopted as well as the degree of social and economic change which is necessary before a government can pursue specific policies.

Cancer prevention: whose responsibility?

Western capitalist countries place great emphasis on individual rights and freedom. Men and women should think and act as they wish to and their behaviour should only be restricted when it infringes other's freedom and rights. The role of the State or central government is to protect individual freedom and rights and to protect the safety and well-being of the individual. The inclination is to minimize State involvement.

On the other hand, in socialist countries the emphasis is placed on the collective well-being of the country's population. The role of the State is seen as the major instrument through which the population's well-being can be enhanced. Thus, emphasis is placed on the maximum amount of State involvement.

The United Kingdom, although predominantly a capitalist country, has seen direct government involvement particularly in health and social services. The development of the welfare state after the Second World War can be seen as an attempt to counteract the diswelfares created by the capitalist system. However, these welfare and public health measures did not arrive without a battle over the right of the State to intervene in individual affairs.

These different positions on the relationship between the individual and the State are ideological. However, when it comes to developing policies for prevention which incorporate one or other of these ideological principles, then difficulties arise. For instance, in recent years there has been considerable debate and controversy over proposals to make it an offence not to wear a seat belt in the front seat of a car. The discussion is concerned, at least partially, with whether the State has the right to intervene in areas which should be a matter of personal choice. Similarly, in the case of smoking, discussion has occurred over the right of the State to try to regulate individual smoking behaviour and the activities of the tobacco industry, which once again should be a matter of personal choice. The approach to prevention which is favoured by exponents of this position is education. Individuals should be given the relevant information about health risk and should be free to make their own decision about the costs and benefits of their actions. They should be allowed to choose according to what is important to them. Concerns about health, pleasure, inconvenience, life and death, are all matters which should fall within the individual's range of responsibility. The State provides the information through education.

The problem with this approach is that it is based on the assumption that an individual's beliefs and actions are entirely free of external influences or forces. Thus individuals are in control of their own health. However, such an approach is rather naïve and simplistic. First, some agencies in a society have a vested interest in patterns of behaviour which might lead to injury or ill health. So methods are used to persuade the individual to continue to act in this particular way. As will be seen in the section on smoking, the advertising campaigns sponsored by the tobacco industry counteract the health education campaigns which emphasize the dangers of smoking. In fact, the former advertising campaigns have much greater financial support than health education campaigns and on the whole are more sophisticated. They do not just concentrate on giving out information on which the individual can base a judgement, but emphasize images to which the individual may be unconsciously attracted. Thus, health education is not given in a vacuum but has to compete, at present unequally, with other forms of communication strategies. Therefore, the individual may not be totally in control of the decisions that he makes in terms of matters of health. Second, there is considerable evidence of an association between socio-economic circumstances and incidence and prevalence of ill-health (Brenner, 1972; Draper *et al.*, 1977; McKeown, 1979). This clearly suggests that socio-economic forces play a significant part in the causation of various illnesses. Thus an individual's control over his own health is significantly influenced by his social and economic circumstances. In addition, the lack of available economic and social resources may severely limit people's accessibility to services, accessibility to information and also limit the ability to which people can adopt their preferred pattern of behaviour. Also, variation in lifestyles according to socio-economic group and other socio-demographic characteristics means that for some groups, health risks receive a low priority compared with other aspects of life which might contain greater risk but less compensatory pleasure. Thus, individuals will vary in the way they make decisions about health risks because of the variation in experience due to socio-economic circumstances. The policy implications of this, given the concern with individual freedom, is that the State should step in to ensure that individual rights and freedom are protected from the excesses of the economic and social system. Thus, either the government can educate the population into understanding that social and economic forces might be responsible for some of their ill-health and they should pressure for changes, or the government can intervene directly through the regulation or eradication of these social and economic forces that are at the root of an individual's problems. The latter could be conceived as a type of public health approach which, as shall be seen, has not been adopted very frequently by British governments.

This brief discussion is not meant to be exhaustive but to highlight some of the difficulties involved in basing policies entirely on the principle of maintaining individual freedom by minimizing State involvement. In addition, a further problem arises with the point about the legitimacy of personal freedom when no harm comes to others. The problem here is how 'harm to others' is defined. Certainly, individual decisions to smoke and risk life may not directly harm others. However, it has been argued that smokers use a percentage of scarce health care resources which could be used in other non-preventable areas of medicine (Lancet Editorial, 1980). Thus, according to this argument, the general public or the potential patient is being influenced by the individual's decision to risk life. Accepting the principle that the individual's right to freedom is of overriding importance (many people would not accept this), it is evident from this discussion that the State has an important part to play in regulating the distortions in individual freedom generated by a capitalist economy. Certainly, without such an approach the notion of individual freedom is meaningless.

Tobacco and the United Kingdom

How many smokers?

The statistics presented here show the trends in smoking amongst the population in the UK from the end of the Second World War up to the present time. The sources of national statistics are mainly the Tobacco Research Council (Todd, 1975; Lee, 1976)—now the Tobacco Advisory Council—and since 1972 through the General Household Survey (GHS) (OPCS, 1978); and also from 1971 the health departments have commissioned *ad hoc* surveys by National Opinion Polls. Figure 5.1 shows that since the war there has been a different pattern of change in the prevalence of smoking for males and females. For males over 16 years the figures show an overall decline in the proportion of manufactured cigarette smokers from 62 per cent in 1950 to 47 per cent in 1975. The latest GHS figures (OPCS, 1979) show that by 1978 45 per cent of the male population were cigarette smokers. During this period the most marked decline occurred in the second half

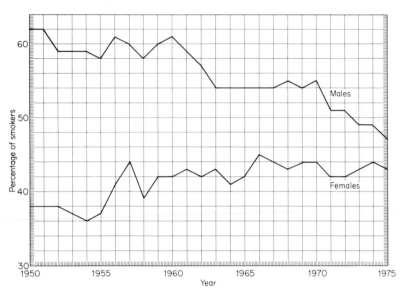

Fig. 5.1 Percentage of males and females aged 16 years and over who smoked manufactured cigarettes in the UK, 1950–75. (Source: Tobacco Research Council, see Lee, 1976.)

of the twenty-five years. In contrast, for females over 16 years of age the proportion of cigarette smokers rose steadily since the war, reaching 44 per cent in 1957. For a time since then there has been little variation, although GHS (OPCS, 1979) figures show there was a decline between 1972 and 1978 from 41 per cent to 37 per cent.

There have also been marked changes in the prevalence of smoking between the different social classes (see Figs. 5.2 and 5.3). At the end of the Second World War and up to the end of the 1950s there was no marked social class difference in cigarette smoking, but today there is a steep social class gradient. In 1978 (OPCS, 1979) figures showed that 25 per cent of professional males smoked, compared with 60 per cent of males in unskilled manual occupations. Twenty-three per cent of professional females smoked, compared with 41 per cent of females in unskilled manual occupations.

There has also been a decline in the prevalence of smoking amongst most socio-economic groups over recent years, although the most marked decline occurred amongst professional groups (OPCS, 1979); even amongst unskilled females, a group which showed a marked increase during the post-war period, there appears to be a levelling off in the prevalence of smoking. The groups with the lowest prevalence of smoking are found amongst professional people, particularly amongst doctors although hospital nurses are similar to the general populations of working age in their proportions of smokers (DHSS, 1976).

More recent figures (OPCS, 1979) show that between 1972 and 1978 the proportion of smokers fell among all age groups, although the extent of the fall and the peak period of its occurrence vary for different age groups. However, a more marked and consistent decline took place among men aged between 16 and 24 years.

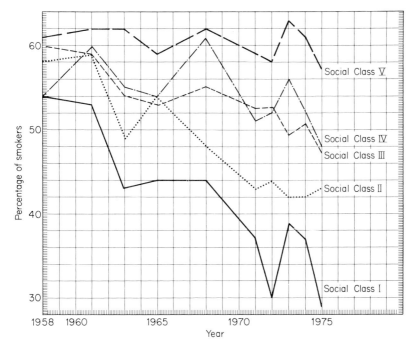

Fig. 5.2 Percentage of males aged 16 years and over smoking manufactured cigarettes in the UK, by social class, 1958–75. (Source: Tobacco Research Council, see Lee, 1976.)

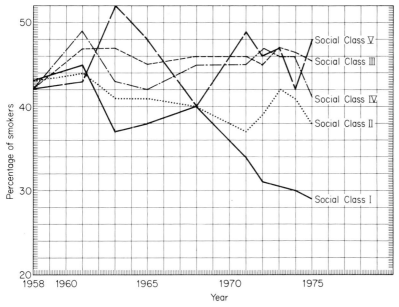

Fig. 5.3 Percentage of females aged 16 years and over smoking manufactured cigarettes in the UK, by social class, 1958–75. (Source: Tobacco Research Council, see Lee, 1976.)

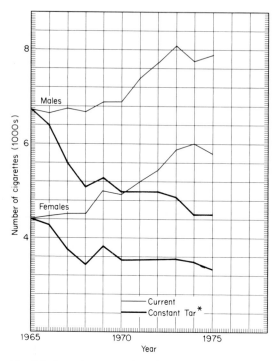

Fig. 5.4 Annual consumption of current and constant tar cigarettes, for males and females aged over 16 years in the UK, 1965–75. (Source: Tobacco Research Council, see Lee, 1976.) * Constant tar cigarettes represent the number of cigarettes which would have been smoked per adult if, during the years after 1965, they had drawn the same total weight of particulate matter (i.e. tar) into their mouths, but had been smoking cigarettes which were the same as the average cigarettes smoked in 1965. It is calculated by multiplying actual cigarette consumption by index of standard tar.

Since the war, the type of cigarettes smoked has changed. There has been a swing towards filter-tipped cigarettes. For instance, in 1968 70.7 per cent of manufactured cigarettes smoked were filter-tipped and five years later, by 1973, this percentage had increased to 83.0 per cent (Todd, 1975). There has also been a change in the prevalence of different types of 'minor' tobacco goods that are smoked. Cigars have become more popular and pipe smoking less popular, although the sales of all these minor products seem to have remained stable (Todd, 1975; Lee, 1976). The tar/nicotine content of cigarettes has been reduced over the last forty years. In 1935 the standard tar content was 32.8 mg per cigarette and the nicotine content was 3.0 mg per cigarette. By 1973 the tar content was 18.7 mg per cigarette, a drop of 57 per cent, and the nicotine content was 1.4 mg, a drop of 47 per cent (Todd, 1975). Figure 5.4 shows that, in spite of the growth in consumption of cigarettes amongst men and particularly amongst women, the quantities smoked per adult male and female in terms of constant tar cigarettes were considerably less in 1973 than they were in 1965. The male figure declined by 33 per cent between 1965 and 1973 and the female figure by 18 per cent (Todd, 1975). Since the publication of the tar/nicotine government league tables in 1973, there has also been a switch from high- to low-tar cigarettes. In 1977, 12 per cent of manufactured cigarettes sold were low tar. The sales of high-tar cigarettes and middle-to-high tar cigarettes fell from 18 per cent in 1972 to 9 per cent in 1977. Middle tar still accounted for the highest percentage, 70 per cent in 1977, although this was down on the 77 per cent in 1972. Low-to-middle tar cigarettes in 1977 accounted for 9 per cent of sales of manufactured cigarettes compared with 5 per cent in 1972 (Central Statistical Office, 1979).

The fall in prevalence between 1972 and 1978 appears to be mainly due to a consistent decrease throughout the period in the very similar proportions of both sexes who were 'light' smokers (fewer than twenty cigarettes a day). Between 1972 and 1978 the proportion of male heavy smokers increased and then declined to the original level of 1972, but the proportion of female heavy smokers seems to be still increasing although the 1978 figures show a slight decline (OPCS, 1979). This increase in the number of heavy smokers, at least pre-1977 (see Fig. 5.5), is

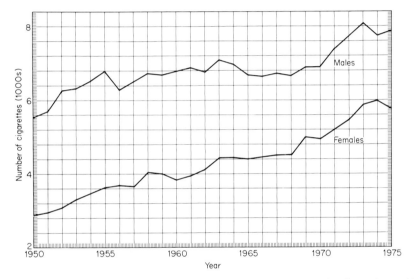

Fig. 5.5 Annual consumption of manufactured cigarettes per smoker for males and females aged over 16 years in the UK, 1950–75. (Source: Tobacco Research Council, see Lee, 1976.)

supported by other evidence (Capell, 1978). Capell showed that between 1972 and 1976 the number of smokers smoking over thirty per day increased by approximately half a million. Ball (HMSO, 1979a) in his minority report to the Hunter Committee on tobacco constituents and additives, suggests that more attention should be paid to this apparent rising consumption.

Ball argues that given the fall in the prevalence of smokers since 1978, if the majority of the smokers who gave up were light smokers, then one would expect an increased average consumption. He suggests that this could account partially for the rise in average consumption of women but was not correct for men. He suggests that the rise in average consumption for men is an underestimate as, prior to quitting, the average consumption of ex-smokers during the period 1968 to 1975 was 22.1 cigarettes per day, whereas the average consumption for all male smokers during that period was 20.8 cigarettes per day. Thus, according to Ball, this suggests that the heavier smokers may have been giving up and the present rise in consumption is more marked than it appears.

Such an increase in consumption may not be as worrying as Ball makes out. It may be due to a switch from high- to low-tar cigarettes and smokers may be consuming more low-tar cigarettes to maintain the level of nicotine absorption that they are used to (Russell, 1976). Alternatively, this increase in consumption of cigarettes may not reflect a similar increase in tobacco consumption and may only reflect a change in the nature of the cigarette smoked. The total weight of tobacco sold in the form of cigarettes fell during the 1960s and, apart from increases in 1972 and 1973, fell again in 1975 (HMSO, 1977b). Now, this might merely reflect the fall in the prevalence of smokers but it could also mean that less or the same amount of tobacco is being smoked even though cigarette consumption per smoker has risen. As has already been shown, there has been a marked swing towards filter-tipped cigarettes.

Given that less than half the population of both males and females in the United Kingdom are smokers, then it could be argued that since the war and particularly in recent years the United Kingdom has moved from a smoking society to a non-smoking one. This change in smoking behaviour suggests an overall change in public opinion, although it may only reflect a change by some particular groups. What is the evidence to suggest that public opinion as a whole has shifted towards non-smoking as a value in itself? Evidence to show whether or not the non-smoking population has become more concerned about smoking and its influence on their lives is difficult to find. However, amongst smokers, 3 out of every 4 wish to have or have tried to stop smoking (Royal College of Physicians, 1977) and for Russell (1971) this is one indicator of a significant change in the social climate against smoking.

In summary, the trends in tobacco use since the war appear to have been dominated by the fall in the prevalence of smoking amongst men and the increase in smoking amongst women. The latter trend can be accounted for in terms of the continuing changes in the status and image of women in Western society. Further evidence which supports the theory that smoking habits cannot be divorced from their cultural setting are the increasing social class differences in the prevalence of smoking. Some occupational differences in the prevalence of smoking have been presented and further information is needed on smoking habits of groups according to ethnicity and by economic activity. It may be that those who are not economically active through unemployment or social isolation, brought about by economic inactivity, may play a part in determining levels of cigarette consumption.

Two other points of importance are first, that if public health measures are to be effective, there is a need to understand how cigarette consumption behaves at a general level. It is necessary to know whether by controlling consumption of cigarettes the incidence of all levels of consumption of cigarettes is influenced or whether only 'light' smoking is changed. If the latter pattern is the more accurate, then this not only has considerable implications for explanations of smoking behaviour but also for public health control policies. The second point is a methodological one and refers to the problems and biases associated with statistics on smoking. Both the Tobacco Research Council and the General Household Survey, quite understandably, use self-definitions of smoking (see OPCS (1972) for comparison of 'definitions'). For example, the Tobacco Research Council (Lee, 1976) used the following definitions.

Smokers 'are current smokers of manufactured cigarettes, hand-rolled cigarettes or pipe, by self-definition, or of cigars (at least one cigar of any size a week) or any combination of these'.

Ex-smokers 'are people who are not "smokers" but who claim to have smoked in the past at least a cigarette a day, or a pipe a day, or a cigar a week, for as long as a year'.

Non-smokers 'are people who have never smoked cigarettes, pipes or cigars at this rate'.

The problem with using self-definitions is one of the under-reporting of smoking habits. The problem is stated clearly in a report by OPCS (1978) on the General Household Survey. In analysing changes in smoking habits over time, they have assumed that response bias, such as under-reporting, remains constant but, as they point out, there is an area of considerable uncertainty.

'Given the apparent shift in public attitudes to smoking in recent years, the possibility that response bias may have changed cannot be ruled out; there is, however, no means of assessing this.'

Difficulties of under-reporting may also arise when smoking is discussed in the context of diseases popularly believed to be related to smoking and where respondents might feel that some 'moral' evaluation of their behaviour is taking place (OPCS, 1972).

The economic and political importance of tobacco to the UK

To explain the presence or the lack of government policy towards the prevention of cigarette consumption in terms of solely health concerns would be an inadequate representation of the way public policy is generated. There are a variety of theories available which attempt to explain the process of policy making and development (for example, see Friedman, 1975). However, what is evident in all these theories is that a variety of groups representing different interests will influence the form or substance of the policy itself. Tobacco is no exception and to explain governmental policy or the lack of it adequately it is necessary to examine the interests that are represented in the continuation or the cessation of cigarette consumption.

In terms of its economic value, tobacco varies in its significance from country to country. In the United States, for instance, where tobacco is grown, manufactured and consumed domestically and exported, a number of different groups have vested interests in the persistence of its use, particularly for cigarette consumption. Thus the consumption of tobacco contributes to the income of tobacco growers and tobacco manufacturers as well as providing a source of revenue through taxation for the government. Also tobacco exports contribute substantially to the US balance of payments with other countries.

As Friedman points out (1975):

'Together, these four factors form an impressive economic rationale for governmental inaction. A structure of economic incentives has developed that benefits both the tobacco industry and the government and any decline in the consumption of cigarettes would produce negative consequences for governments as well as for industry.'

In Britain, according to Friedman (1975), in spite of the presence of three large cigarette manufacturing companies, the economic and political importance of tobacco is based primarily on cigarette taxation. Tobacco is imported, which in itself is a drain on the balance of payments, and the only other interests, apart from the manufacturing industries and the government, in the maintenance of cigarette consumption are the retailers and distributors of tobacco.

Government revenue from tobacco comes from two sources, the largest source being the tax on the retail price of cigarettes and the other source being import duty on tobacco. It has been estimated that tax revenues make up over 80 per cent of the retail price of cigarettes in Britain in contrast to federal, state and local taxes in the United States which made up about 47 per cent in 1973 (Friedman, 1975).

UK government policy and the control of smoking

In the light of this background information, government policy will be outlined. As will be shown, governmental policy can take many forms, ranging from active intervention through legislation to passive support of the *status quo*. Obviously, such political stances are influenced by ideological assumptions about the responsibility of the State not only in matters of health but also in broader areas of economic and social policy. It must also be remembered that the lack of an explicit policy or an apparent non-policy position is as much a statement of the interests of the government as is the presence of a positive policy. Finally, government strategies aimed at influencing smoking must not be seen in isolation but must be examined in the context of their policies in other areas of preventive medicine.

The last decade has shown a marked development in the Government's interest in preventive medicine as a whole and smoking in particular. Before that time, policy as regards the prevention of smoking was fragmented and incoherent. The Government had taken two initiatives. First, in 1933 the sale of cigarettes to persons aged under 16 years was prohibited. Second, in 1965 all cigarette advertising on Independent Television was banned and this ban was extended to commercial radio in 1973. Apart from byelaws of the Transport Act giving agencies such as British Rail the right to prohibit smoking in some parts of its trains, and the powers conferred on the Government through the 1965 Food and Drugs Act, 1970 Food Hygiene (General) Regulations, which requires that people employed in the direct handling of foods should not smoke, these are the only legislative measures that the Government has passed up to this present time.

In spite of the scarcity of direct intervention through legislation, the Government has on some occasions attempted but failed to introduce legislation, although in the main it has concentrated its efforts through more indirect measures such as through support for programmes of persuasion of the population of smokers, through propaganda in the mass media, or through voluntary agreements with industry.

The bulk of government activity occurred during the 1970s and consisted of a series of voluntary agreements between industry and government (see TACADE/ASH 1977, for full details). These voluntary agreements have involved the tobacco industry agreeing to publish a government health warning on cigarette packs and advertisements. The warning states 'Government Health Department's warning: cigarette smoking can seriously damage your health'. The tar/nicotine content of brands of cigarettes was also published and levels of tar content are now published on cigarette packs and advertisements. The content of advertisements was not to be attractive to the young and in the late 1970s advertising of high-tar cigarettes was to be phased out. During the 1970s, these voluntary agreements between government and industry contained increasingly tougher controls, at least on paper. The effectiveness of the controls was difficult to estimate and there were claims that their impact was being minimized. The Government also allocated resources to various health education agencies to carry out campaigns aimed at informing the public of the dangers of smoking. The Government, coupled with these other measures, began to pursue a policy which attempted to develop a safer cigarette. In 1973 the new Independent Scientific Committee on Smoking and Health was set up to advise on scientific matters concerned with smoking and health (HMSO, 1979a). Its first priority was to produce guidelines for, and to adjudicate the testing of, tobacco substitutes and additive materials. In 1978 a new 'high tar tax' was introduced in the Budget which involved the levy of a supplementary duty on cigarettes with a tar yield of 20 mg or more. Finally, the Government, in the form of the Minister of Sport, forged another voluntary agreement with industry which contained controls on advertising at sporting events.

A new voluntary agreement between the Government and the tobacco industry was recently negotiated (1980) and the agreement is to last for eighteen months, when the intention is to discuss the possibilities of a legal ban on advertising.

In summary, over the last ten years there has been an increase in government activity in the area of smoking control. Proposals have been made, by individuals or government departments, to introduce legislation in some form but none of these proposals reached the statute books. However, the stance of the Government has predominantly been one of attempting to persuade both the population of smokers and the tobacco industry to control their activities with regard to smoking on a voluntary basis. Progress has been made towards the creation of a safer cigarette. The predominant policy approach has been one which has emphasized the need to prevent people from taking up smoking and to persuade smokers to give up or switch to a safer cigarette. The effectiveness of these policies will be discussed later, but it is of value to examine the Government's overall strategy for prevention and health and examine the priority given to smoking control.

It was not until the second half of the 1970s that the Government attempted to produce a specific policy for prevention. In 1976, a consultative document was published by the Department of Health and it was entitled 'Prevention and Health: everybody's business' (DHSS, 1976). In this document this statement is made about smoking:

'No one can seriously doubt any longer that the habit of cigarette smoking has been directly responsible for an enormous amount of preventable disease and untimely death in this country.'

In the discussion that follows in the document there is a suggestion that health education which has given publicity to the hazards of cigarette smoking and the other attempts which have been made to assist smokers to stop may not be enough and they state:

'We must therefore consider the adoption of other lines of attack if we are serious about preventing smoking-related disease.'

They conclude with the suggestions that government intervention through the Medicines Act of 1968 may be the best policy. They argue that this would enable the control over the:

'yield of tar and other noxious substances, health warnings on advertisements and packets, restriction of promotion of sales, and the use of substitutes and additives, to be based on advice from an expert and independent advisory committee after consultation with interests likely to be substantially affected'.

The perception of the role of government legislation which is advocated by the document is difficult to elucidate from this statement as it is uncertain as to the degree to which the Government would use the Act to control advertising etc. in the face of opposition from the 'interests likely to be substantially affected'. The ambiguity of this statement about legislation or active government intervention is understandable in the light of the consultative document's general approach to government intervention.

For example it states:

'There is much potential for prevention in health education aimed at altering people's attitudes towards such things as tobacco, alcohol and exercise—persuading them in effect to invest in their own health.'

The document further states how the Government could influence people's attitudes:

'by altering the structure of incentives facing people, by reducing the cost of, for example, investing in physical recreation or by acquiring information about the dangers of cigarette smoking through health education, but the onus of making decisions in order to safeguard health must necessarily rest on the individual'.

This statement clearly suggests that the responsibility for health lies predominantly with the individual and not the Government, which implies that direct government intervention should be minimal. For example, Macfarlane *et al.* (1978) state:

'The authors of "Prevention and Health: Everybody's Business" have tried to show that prevention is technically possible and there is a need for it, but that it is the responsibility not of the state but of the individual.'

Macfarlane *et al.* (1978) offer an explanation for this approach. They state:

'Preventive medicine and health education are particularly important when resources are tightly limited as they can often lead to savings in resources in other areas.'

Similarly, Davis (1979) describes this approach as an attempt to control the rising tide of demand for medical care by shifting the responsibility for illness on to the individual.

These authors argue that too much emphasis is placed on the individual habit of smoking and not enough attempt is made to identify or control the forces or pressures which are created and reinforced by the social and economic environment (McKinlay, 1974). This approach has been referred to as victim blaming, where the individual is blamed for behaviour which is outside his control (Crawford, 1977).

Given the consultative document's approach towards government intervention in the control of smoking, it was surprising to see the recommendations of the House of Commons' Expenditure Committee which reported in March 1977 (HMSO, 1977a) that:

> '(i) legislation should be introduced to *ban* the advertising of tobacco and tobacco products, except at the point of sale;
>
> (ii) as an interim measure, there should be stricter control of advertising through sponsorship, such as is at present being discussed between government and the industry;
>
> (iii) an increase in duty to achieve a price increase sufficient to reduce cigarette consumption should be imposed annually;
>
> (iv) cigarette coupons should be abolished;
>
> (v) cigarette machines should be available only on premises to which children do not have ready access;
>
> (vi) there should be a much stronger health warning on packets and tins stating that smoking, especially cigarette smoking, is a major factor in the causation of lung cancer, bronchitis and heart disease;
>
> (vii) that the present trend to provide non-smoking areas in public places be encouraged to continue;
>
> (viii) anti-smoking education should be directed to specific target groups;
>
> (ix) more attention should be given to the problems of people who fear they will put on weight if they stop smoking;
>
> (x) that more research should be done into the causes of and solutions to the problem of physiological addiction (to smoking).'

The Government's response to the Committee's recommendations (HMSO, 1977b) came in December 1977, in the form of a White Paper. Only two of the recommendations (nos. ii and vii) were accepted without reservations. The recommendation to ban cigarette advertising was not accepted on the grounds that there was insufficient evidence of its effects on consumption. The Government also suggested that, given the lack of evidence, it would be an unnecessary restriction on individual freedom. The White Paper stated further:

> 'Moreover, a ban would detract from that part of the government's strategy which encouraged smokers, who cannot or will not give up smoking, to smoke cigarettes in the relatively less harmful lower-tar groups; and it would remove an important vehicle for the health warning.'

It is also noticeable that the Government considered but did not accept the annual use of taxation to influence changes in the consumption of cigarettes. The Government recommend, with its EEC partners' agreement, that a supplementary tax should be imposed on brands with high levels of noxious yields which 'would provide an additional financial incentive for persistent smokers to transfer to lower-tar yield cigarettes'.

Also, the document outlines the Government's plans for placing the control of tobacco substitutes and additives under the 1968 Act and in the 1977 voluntary agreement with industry these powers would be used only if the need arose.

One again the policy of the Government was one of emphasizing:

'that present trends towards a non-smoking society can be sustained and reinforced by a consistent strategy of education and persuasion of the individual and co-operation with the tobacco industry' (HMSO, 1977b).

Finally, the Royal Commission on the NHS reported in 1979 (HMSO, 1979c). Once again emphasis was placed in the report on prevention although, as Draper points out, the same philosophy as before was proposed (Draper *et al.*, 1979). He argues that, although some of the adverse influences on health are clearly described:

'there is no doubt that T.V. and radio, certainly in their commercial forms, do a great deal of harm by promoting excessive consumption of alcohol, tobacco and sweets for example'.

He suggests that the Commission's recommendations do not challenge strong influences on health and therefore they advocate more TV time for health education.

In summary, although government policy towards smoking control has become more substantive in the last few years, direct intervention through public health measures has not been advocated. Emphasis has been placed on preventing or reducing the smoking habit through co-operation with the tobacco industries and on health education.

Have these policies been operating effectively?

This section will consider if and how the policies, which were described in the latter part of the previous section, have been implemented by the Government. First, the various ways that the Government has gone about attempting to influence the general public will be considered. It must be remembered that these proposals placed emphasis on preventing young people taking up smoking and persuading smokers either to stop or switch to a brand with a lower tar/nicotine content. Second, an examination of how far the voluntary agreement between the Government and the tobacco industry is operating effectively will be given.

With regard to the first point, the agencies through which the Government has attempted to implement its policy are the Health Education Council and its equivalent in Scotland. Both are government-supported agencies with quasi-independent status to which the Government has given extra financial support for various education campaigns in smoking control. In addition, the Department of Health gives a grant which provides partial support to an independent body 'Action on Smoking and Health' (ASH) which fulfils the general function of keeping the debate about smoking and health in the public eye.

Beginning in the late 1960s and carrying on throughout the 1970s, the health education agencies have launched a series of national campaigns through the mass media—i.e. newspapers, posters, and television and radio. An identifiable shift in emphasis in these campaigns has taken place during the period, with the earlier campaigns emphasizing the relationship between lung cancer and smoking and the later campaigns attempting to change the social climate about smoking with their emphasis on the social undesirability of being a smoker, particularly aimed at the young or highlighting the rights of non-smokers. These campaigns were supported directly by the Government.

The second point refers to how the agreement between government and the tobacco industry was operating. Before this is discussed, it is necessary to look at how the present-day legislation is functioning. Perhaps the weakest part of the legislation falls in the area of prohibiting the sale of cigarettes to those under 16 years old. In 1975 a survey conducted for ASH by the Opinion Research Centre showed that 80 per cent of tobacconists surveyed were selling cigarettes to under-age children. ASH pressed for firmer enforcement of the 1933 Children and Young Persons Act. This Act did not cover Ulster and in 1977 the Government decided to introduce legislation to prohibit the sale of cigarettes to children under 16 in Northern Ireland. The legislation concerning the advertising of cigarettes on television and radio is obviously more clear-cut although, as shall be seen, there has been an over-proportionate investment in advertising for other tobacco products on television (see TACADE/ASH, 1977).

A lack of available information is one of the many difficulties involved in assessing whether the voluntary agreements between the Government and industry have worked or are operating effectively. It was argued that the industry breached the agreements of 1977, or the spirit of the agreement, on a number of counts. For example, it was argued that the government health warning was designed in such a way as to minimize its impact. It was also claimed that a disproportionate amount of advertising on television of cigars relative to sales had occurred.

Why did the Government adopt these policies?

In this section, two interrelated questions will be examined. First, why did the Government show an interest in policies for smoking control at this particular time? Second, why were these policies as opposed to the alternatives adopted by the Government?

With regard to the first question, it is evident that the Government's involvement with the issue of smoking and health came before it had developed an overall policy for prevention and health and before involvement in other specific areas of preventive medicine. Apart from the availability of epidemiological evidence which, compared with other environmental agents, was relatively strong, two specific influences have been identified (Friedman, 1975). One of these influences has been hinted at previously—i.e. the publication of the series of three reports on Smoking and Health by the Royal College of Physicians (1962, 1971, 1977). The impact of these reports is difficult to assess, although it is noticeable that some action directly followed the publication of the first two. In both cases it involved industry anticipating government action and thus adopting self-regulatory procedures voluntarily. However, it was only after the second report that the Government became involved with industry on a voluntary basis. Each of the three reports received wide publicity throughout the media and in each of the three the Government was exhorted to take stronger and more direct action. Their recommendations included urging the Government to prohibit cigarette advertising and gift-coupon schemes, and impose differential tax on tobacco products that are more harmful and enforce restrictions on smoking in public transportation.

The second strong pressure against cigarette smoking which may have acted upon the British Government, according to Friedman, came in the form of an individual—the then Chief Medical Officer of Health, George Godber. Friedman (1975) described the verbal war of Sir George Godber in this way:

> 'He acted on this issue as the moral conscience of the nation and publicised the dangers of cigarette smoking and continued to pressure for government action. In his yearly messages on the state of the public health in Britain, he progressively increased his criticisms of cigarette smoking.'

Throughout the 1960s Sir George Godber continually came out with statements about the dangers of smoking—and the need to change Britain into a non-smoking society. However, in 1970 Sir George Godber acknowledged that the reasons why British society and its government are unwilling to control smoking (Friedman, 1975):

> 'With so much involved in commerce and agriculture, and so much government income from taxation, it isn't surprising that the voice of reason is indeed a still small voice in a bubble of advertising and social behaviour, all encouraging the use of the cigarette.'

Friedman has identified these two pressures (the reports of the Royal College of Physicians and the verbal war of Sir George Godber) as playing a significant part in producing government action in smoking control. However, these proposals are purely speculative and what is needed is a detailed study of how and why policies are formulated and more specifically who played a part in influencing the formulation of government policy towards smoking control. Of particular interest is finding out the part public opinion played in the development of policy. How far did smokers support the idea of smoking control?

The second question to be examined is why did the Government adopt the policies that it did? Why did it go for a voluntary agreement with industry which involved some curbs on cigarette promotion in combination with investing funds in propaganda aimed at persuading people to give up smoking or not to start?

One possible explanation for the voluntary agreement between industry and the Government is the political strength of the tobacco industry and other vested interests. How strong is the tobacco industry and the other vested interests which make up the pro-tobacco lobby? With regard to the economic strength of the tobacco industry *vis-à-vis* its contribution to the British economy, its contribution to employment on a national scale is small. As Friedman (1975) points out, there is no reason why these employees could not be absorbed into the other industrial interests of the tobacco companies. However, an economic contribution does not necessarily dictate a group's political strength. Certainly, the small number of large companies in the tobacco industry in this country makes it easier to have a united front. However, this has not always been the case and there was considerable intra-industry conflict and competition in the second half of the 1960s over the proposal to drop coupon schemes. The political strength of the tobacco industry is also enhanced by its links with other countries through overlapping ownerships or output control of one company by another. Thus, companies can pressure governments from other countries to influence British government policy.

It could also be argued that the tobacco industry's co-operation with the Government could be interpreted as an action which reflects its vulnerable position *vis-à-vis* the threat of government intervention. Thus the tobacco industry's acceptance of self-regulation is not only an attempt to retain its authority and therefore pursue its goal to maintain and increase profits but also reflects its acceptance that it is in no position to fight with the Government over this issue. Compared with the US, the tobacco industry's response has appeared to be much more muted.

Friedman has accounted for this 'muted response' in a number of ways. He argues that the tobacco industry seeks, 'almost above all else, a stable predictable business environment as does the tobacco industry in the US and Canada'. He argues that in Britain, (i) the Government's tradition of negotiation and co-operation with industry as opposed to direct intervention through nationalization, and (ii) the centralization of British Government decision making, have created a less confused and less threatening business environment than in the United States or Canada.

The tobacco industry has accepted self-regulation because it staves off direct government intervention and does not directly threaten a stable business environment. In addition, it assumes that government intervention will not go any further and thus conflict with the Government has been muted. Further evidence of co-operation by the tobacco industry can be found in their support for research, particularly in the area of developing a safer cigarette. Friedman (1975) makes the important point that support by the tobacco industry in the US for this kind of research has never occurred, mainly because of their fears of alienating the tobacco growers.

The tobacco industry has reacted in other ways to the 'inevitability' of increasing government control of cigarette sales and promotion. There is evidence of diversification by tobacco companies into other areas of industry. This diversification has been shown to have been occurring in Britain, the United States and Canada (Friedman, 1975). However, it is difficult to know whether the amount of diversification has increased in recent years as the cigarette market appears to have become more uncertain. As Friedman has pointed out, there is no available evidence to examine whether there is a disproportionate amount of diversification in the tobacco industry compared with any other industry. The other way the tobacco industry is dealing with the restrictions in potential domestic markets is by increasing the proportion of cigarettes manufactured for export. This has happened in the United States in particular. These markets are usually those in the Third World where governments have imposed no restrictions on the type of cigarette sold and how it is promoted (Muller, 1978).

Perhaps the most surprising feature of the picture in the United Kingdom is the lack of government involvement or intervention over smoking control. Compared with Canada and the US, where the tobacco lobby appears to be much stronger, government involvement in this country has been limited. As Friedman (1975) points out:

'British governmental involvement in the present smoking–health controversy can best be understood by keeping in mind the underlying desire of the government for industry self-regulation and discipline. Nevertheless, the reality of reluctance to regulate is in sharp contrast to the almost unlimited ability of the British government to act.'

He goes on to suggest that potentially Britain had more opportunity than the US Government. But he states:

'There is a sharp contrast between the ability to act and the actual action that may be due in part to an accepted tradition that mitigates the use of government power. If there were no strong economic or political interests affected, this tradition might have found an exception.'

Is Friedman correct in thinking that the passive government stance is due to a combination of traditional British governmental practice of negotiation and co-operation and the influence of strong economic and political interests? Have we underestimated the strength of the tobacco lobby or is it a matter of confusion of interests in the Government itself?

Certainly, with regard to the strength of the tobacco lobby, a number of other bodies apart from the tobacco companies have been cited as being involved. For example, a recent article in the *Guardian* (Dean, 1980) states:

'Much of the popular press refused to criticise the industry, not least because of the £30 million which this industry spends on advertising each year.'

Thus, it is claimed the media has an interest in the maintenance of cigarette advertising. However, its dependence on such revenue may have been exaggerated. According to a recent article (Ferguson, 1976) throughout the mass media, in newspapers both daily and Sunday, monthly magazines and posters, there is evidence of an increasing decline in he proportion of advertising revenue gained from tobacco advertising. Only in areas such as cinema advertising is there a significant dependence. Whilst this evidence does not suggest that the media does not still support cigarette advertising it does suggest that it is trying to ease itself out of a position of dependency and thus reduce its strength as a vested interest. As Ferguson concludes (1976):

'So although nobody in the media welcomes the idea of a ban, it will clearly be less felt today, across the board, than it would have been five to six years ago. The preparations have been made.'

The strength of the pro-smoking lobby is also enhanced by the representation of its interest in Parliament and in Government. For example, according to information presented in an article by Turner (1980), in the present Parliament, apart from the sixty MPs who have a constituency interest in tobacco, another thirty-two have links with advertising and public relations companies which may have, or wish to obtain, tobacco accounts.

The constituency interests in tobacco of a number of MPs reflect the importance of the opinion of the voting public on the activities of politicians and the Government itself. Not only must the MPs take into account the employment interests of their constituents, but to propose a general policy of smoking control the Government may need to take into account the climate of opinion amongst the public as a whole and in particular amongst smokers. If smokers are in the majority and a large majority of them does not wish to stop smoking, then the Government may

not wish to risk alienating a large proportion of the voting population by introducing regulatory policies. On the other hand, if the smokers are in a minority
and of these a large group say they would like to give up smoking or are against
cigarette promotion, and the non-smoking population begin to take an interest in
smoking control, then the climate may be right for introducing legislation or more
interventionist policies. However, the influence that public opinion has on the
formation of government policy (Manis, 1976) is difficult to assess, as is the relative
importance of public opinion in the debate over smoking control compared with
other issues involving other aspects of government policy. There is also the more
fundamental question of whether politicians' concept of public opinion is based in
empirical reality. There is no evidence to say whether politicians' beliefs about
the state of 'public opinion' actually reflect what the electorate really feels.

This confusion of interests does not only exist in Parliament amongst MPs but
within the Government itself. It appears that the Government has no overall
policy for smoking control and each government department pursues its own
objectives in the light of its own policy interests. This, as shall be seen, leads to a
conflict of interests—i.e. one department pursuing a policy enhancing smoking
control and the other inhibiting it. In the United States, according to Friedman
(1975), this fragmented approach has enhanced the smoking control programme
because agencies working independently of other government agencies have
managed to grasp the issue as a whole and pursued regulatory policies without
being deterred by the interests of other agencies. In the UK, no department or
agency is independent enough to pursue such an aggressive policy and, even
though government departments do have their own interests and objectives, the
centralization of policy making makes for a greater amount of control.

Friedman (1975) argues that one of the most significant explanations of the
lack of a positive government policy towards smoking control is the Government's
dependency on the revenue derived from tobacco. As Turner (1980) estimated, in
1980 the Treasury received approximately £3000 million from VAT and duty on
tobacco. Whilst the interests of the Treasury are probably the most important
influence on government policy, there are other government departments with
interests in the reservation of the tobacco industry. This quote from Turner (1980)
clearly illustrates the point:

> 'The Department of Employment has a strong interest in keeping the 36 000
> people employed in tobacco manufacture in work. To support that, the De-
> partment of Industry has given £30 million grants for re-equipment and
> regional development since 1972.'

Turner gives further details of the Department of Industry's support for the
tobacco industry. She states:

> 'In the last year the department has given regional grants totalling £217 000 to
> Imperial Tobacco for factories in Newcastle, Liverpool and Glasgow; £61 000
> to British American Tobacco for a factory in Liverpool; and £1 107 000 to
> Carreras/Rothman for a factory in Darlington.'

Turner then goes on to discuss the interests of the Department of Trade. She
states:

> 'The Trade Secretary is aware that tobacco (expected to value £4300 million

this year) is important to 350 000 retail outlets in this country and that last year we exported cigarettes to over 150 countries, for £464 million.'

She describes the Overseas Development Administration's activity thus:

'The Overseas Development Administration and the Commonwealth Development Corporation have paid three countries (Zambia, Malawi and Belize) £3½ million since 1974 to develop their tobacco-growing industry. The EEC subsidises tobacco farming in France and Italy by £100 million a year.'

Turner then discusses the position of the Sports and Arts Ministries. First, she discusses sport:

'Both Benson and Hedges and John Player have dreamed up links with cricket, Marlboro' with motor-racing, State Express 555 with darts, and Embassy with snooker. Labour's Sports Minister, who has interests in sponsorship companies, showed little interest in closing the loopholes in the government's agreement governing sponsorship.'

She goes on to the Arts Minister:

'Action by his counterpart at the Arts Ministry suggests otherwise. The 14 strong "committee of honour" set up last week to double the £4–£5 million currently provided by business sponsors, includes both the external affairs executive and the former head of public affairs of Imperial Tobacco.'

In summary, from the evidence presented we can speculate on some of the more significant influences which have caused the British Government to be so inactive in smoking control compared with other countries. Certainly, the strength of the tobacco lobby and the divided interests within the Government have supported such a 'non-policy' position. Perhaps, too, the general public's lack of interest due to the lack of publicity given to the issues may not have helped towards government action. Without a clear framework for understanding government policy making, we can go no further in attempting to explain why the Government had adopted such a stance. It must also be emphasized that governments may vary in their approach to the importance of legislation according to their convictions about the responsibility of the State. Countries where the predominant government ideology is the preservation of individual freedom in combination with a free enterprise economy expect the minimum of State involvement in the social and economic life of society. On the other hand, in countries where the economy and political and social institutions are controlled by the State, the possibilities of State intervention are much greater. However, the commitment to a smoking-control policy (whether it be through legislative action or self-regulation) will depend in any country, irrespective of policitical persuasion, on the priority given to the public health over competing economic and political needs. One would assume that in countries where the government puts great emphasis on collective needs rather than individual needs, the public health would be given a high priority. However, even in these countries economic interests may dominate health needs. In the UK, with its mixture of a free economy and state intervention, one would expect that a Labour government would be more likely to lean towards direct government intervention rather than the Conservative party. Despite Friedman's statement (1975) that the tradition of British Government is one of co-operation with industry and other groups, it is evident that attempts to nation-alize industry are more likely to come under a Labour government than a Conservative government. In the area of smoking control, it is difficult to know whether the gradual movement towards government intervention or the increas-ing activity of the Government is due to an increase in public interest about the 'problem' of smoking, or reflects the political persuasions of government in power over the last ten years. Certainly, there is no evidence to suggest that the involve-ment of the Government in concerted action about smoking control has occurred either under a Labour or Conservative government. It may be that individuals, particularly health ministers, determine the degree to which their department becomes involved in action. Although, as was shown under the last Labour government, attempts to push for legislation such as the inclusion of tobacco under the Medicines Act may not always be successful.

How effective are government policies?

In this section, the policies proposed by the Government in Great Britain will be evaluated using the evidence available. In addition, evidence of the efficacy of the proposed policy will be discussed using evidence obtained from implementation in other countries and from experiment and field trial. Thus, the questions to be asked in this section are:

(i) how effective have the Government's policies for smoking control been?

(ii) how effective have these policies been in other countries and what is the evidence for their value from research studies?

(iii) what alternative policies are available to the Government?

Education and smoking control in the mass media

One policy proposed and implemented by the Government, mainly through financial support given by the Department of Health to the Health Education Council, was the introduction of a number of campaigns in the mass media directed at the general public. The nature of these campaigns changed and so did their objectives. The earlier campaign attempted simply to make the general public aware of the dangers of smoking. Lately, the campaigns have shifted towards attempting to change the social climate of opinion about smoking by emphasizing the anti-social nature of smoking behaviour. The target group also shifted from the general public as a whole, through to the smoking population and then on to those not smoking and, finally, education was aimed at the young. This change reflected a recognition that knowledge alone would not dissuade people from smoking and that smoking was attached to certain attractive images in society. These images, the sources of which which are difficult to identify, are particularly attractive to the young and the idea of the campaigns was to try to change the images attached to smoking from attractive to being unattractive. Russell (1971) supports this shift and states:

'Repeated associations of smoking with maturity, success, toughness, attrac-tiveness and sophistication, etc., appeals to both conscious and unconscious needs. A recent survey has shown that schoolboys are indeed partly motivated to smoke by the image of toughness, sexiness and precocity that smoking provides.'

The success of such a change will be discussed below, but it must also be remembered that the size of the financial support given to these campaigns is minuscule compared with the money spent by the tobacco industry on promotion. For example, the tobacco industry spends £80 million a year on promotion, which the Government counters with £1 million on anti-smoking campaigns.

To assess the effectiveness of a campaign involves the evaluation of a population before and after a campaign in the light of the aims and objectives of the campaigns. Perhaps the most ideal technique of evaluation is the employment of the classical experimental method. This involves a before-and-after study of a cohort of the population comparing it with a control sample without any intervention. Thus it would be possible to compare any change which may have been produced by the campaign with any change which occurred 'naturally'. In this instance, both the characteristics of population in the group exposed to education and the control group should be comparable and so should exposure to the influences which may produce change over the period of evaluation.

It is only recently that these health education campaigns, particularly the ones aimed at a mass audience, have attempted to employ the minimum requirements for evaluation. Certainly, in large mass campaigns it is particularly difficult to employ a vigorous methodology in that there may be a wide variety of potentially influential factors. However, in 1972 the British Health Education Council launched an anti-smoking campaign on national TV. The aims of the campaign were fourfold.

(i) To publicize the introduction of health warnings on cigarette packets.

(ii) To stimulate a belief that smoking is undesirable.

(iii) To encourage smokers to give up smoking.

(iv) To discourage non-smokers from starting to smoke.

Populations were interviewed pre-campaign and immediately post-campaign with a follow-up after seven weeks. The results showed (Research Bureau Ltd, 1972):

(i) 87 per cent at all stages were aware of the existence of the packet warning;

(ii) recall of part of the actual statement was by 65–74 per cent in each campaign;

(iii) about 60 per cent were aware of TV adverts;

(iv) no change was reported in smoking behaviour;

(v) there was no significant change in attitudes to smoking in the national campaigns;

(vi) after seven weeks, non-smokers tended towards greater disapproval, while smokers became more favourable.

There seems to be an increase in awareness of the propaganda but no change occurred in attitudes to smoking or smoking behaviour. It is also interesting to note that after the campaign smokers were more favourable to smoking. Other HEC campaigns were also evaluated. An evaluation of anti-smoking adverts in cinemas in 1972 showed no change in attitudes to smoking, although there was a slight increase in awareness of cancer risk but not of bronchitis or heart disease risk (Research Services Ltd, 1972).

More optimistic results were found from an evaluation of an HEC Adolescent Anti-smoking campaign through advertising in 1976. Whilst neither smoking habits nor attitudes to smoking changed, specific *attitudes* to *smokers* changed—i.e. 'I do not like boys/girls who smoke'. Agreement increased from 36 per cent to 51 per cent; strong agreement from 17 per cent to 33 per cent (Research Surveys of GB Ltd, 1976).

Results from a short-burst anti-smoking campaign on TV (Research Surveys of GB Ltd, 1977) showed that, in the experimental areas, those who saw smoking as an anti-social habit increased by 17 per cent to 39 per cent compared with 12 per cent to 15 per cent in the control areas. Those who said they might give up smoking increased from 26 per cent to 37 per cent.

The HEC also carried out campaigns in 1974, 1975 and 1976 to test the efficacy of information about the tar and nicotine content of manufactured cigarettes. The results showed that smokers' knowledge increased and was more realistic but behaviour was little affected except in relation to the selection of cigarettes *for their tar yield* (Research Surveys of GB Ltd, 1974, 1975, 1976).

In summary, the campaigns so far show at the most a change in knowledge and a small change in attitudes about smokers but little evidence of change in behaviour, although some people select cigarette brands according to their tar yield.

The evidence suggests that these campaigns have had little effect on smoking behaviour. What does the other evidence show about the effectiveness of mass communication campaigns for smoking control?

One study by Warner (1977) analysed the cigarette consumption in he USA over time to determine the effect of anti-smoking campaigns carried out since 1964. It suggested that the following activities caused drops in consumption.

(i) Health scares in the 1950s reduced smoking by about 3 per cent in 1953 and by 8 per cent in 1954.

(ii) The Surgeon-General's report in 1964 reduced smoking by 5 per cent.

(iii) Anti-smoking adverts from 1968 to 1970 reduced consumption by about 8 per cent.

(iv) Predicted consumption for 1975 was approximately 22 per cent above the reported actual consumption.

These findings suggest that anti-smoking propaganda may have long-term effects.

A number of other studies have attempted to evaluate TV's influence on smoking. Three different studies have been carried out, each with a different set of aims. First, Eiser *et al.* (1978a) carried out an evaluation of two TV programmes which aimed to emphasize the health hazards of smoking. Evidence shows no difference in increase in awareness of health hazards in viewers as compared with non-viewers, and the same was true for the intention to give up smoking. However, a majority of smokers already considered smoking harmful. Therefore, a purely educational programme attempting to drive home this message is bound to be ineffective.

A second study, also by Eiser *et al.* (1978b), evaluated two TV programmes designed to help those who wish to give up smoking. Results showed that immediate and long-term effects were insignificant, although there was a 'slight but not significant' tendency to be successful at giving up between viewers and non-viewers.

The final study, by Vuylsteek *et al.* (1977), involved an evaluation of a Belgian TV programme which screened a single anti-smoking version.

Results show that of 186 who stopped smoking during the period, 23 per cent had done it on family advice, 20 per cent because of illness, 18 per cent due to the TV programme and 13 per cent on medical advice.

In summary, the effectiveness of mass communication campaigns on TV or other medium seems limited, especially in the short term. (Long-term effects of propaganda are yet to be examined.) The value of mass media campaigns in general in health education has been summed up by Gatherer *et al.* (1979):

'Increase in knowledge appears in most campaigns to be a short-term result.'

Only small changes in attitudes were found, although some studies show a shift in direction opposite to the one hoped for. However, Gatherer *et al.* (1979) state:

'Where behaviour is a single action, mass media campaigns appear to be most effective—e.g. in producing clinic attendance or use of the telephone. With general change in behaviour patterns, the outcome is much less dramatic.'

Overall, Gatherer *et al.* (1979) found that individual instruction is the best form of education, followed by groups; with impersonal, generalized instruction the least effective. Whilst it might be possible for the Government to invest in measures to increase the availability of individual instruction, any effort at a national level is limited to mass media campaigns through education which appear to be ineffective in changing behaviour.

The apparent failure of these mass media campaigns could be put down to the lack of a large investment by the Government. However, given a larger investment, would the outcome be more effective and what can be expected from mass media communication? Certainly, there seems to be a commonsense assumption that the mass media has considerable persuasive and influential powers and this is apparently supported by the considerable amount of money that goes into commercial advertising. In a review of the evidence, McCron and Budd (1979) argue that the mass media has a limited influence. They suggest that as early as 1960 researchers had accepted:

'that if the mass media have any influence on their own it tends to be in the direction of reinforcing existing beliefs and opinions, rather than in changing or converting them. Only where opinions on an issue are not yet formed or crystallised are the mass media likely to play a more directly influential role.'

McCron and Budd (1979) make a similar point with regard to commercial advertising. They state:

'It can be said fairly safely that little commercial advertising has as a primary objective the conversion of behaviour, or the production of qualitatively different forms of behaviour. In fact, most advertising is geared to mobilising and channelling existing predispositions playing on various social and individual needs and wants.'

McCron and Budd (1979) suggest an alternative framework of explanation of the influence of the mass media to the 'direct effects' model. They argue for a shift in perspective which sees the audience as active and critical rather than as a passive receptor of mass communication techniques. They attempt to move away from the individually orientated explanations of previous theories towards a perspective which sees:

'the media influence process as part of our general cultural environment, and we would argue that the impact as instruments of health education can only fully be grasped from such a perspective' (McCron and Budd, 1979).

They identify three mechanisms or modes of influence:

(i) the presentation of images and models of approximate or desirable behaviour;

(ii) the promotion of the climate of opinion;

(iii) the shaping of the debate or agenda about health.

Whilst it is not the intention to go into any greater depth about approaches to mass communication research, it is evident that the failure of much of the health education anti-smoking campaigns which have utilized mass media campaigns may be due in part to their high expectations about the persuasive power of the media. It may also be due to a lack of understanding of the communication process itself and its effects.

Before other health education approaches are discussed later in this chapter, a number of points about the ethical and political nature of health education need to be emphasized (see p. 102). First, much of health education, irrespective of topic and method, has been individually orientated. As has been shown with government policy towards prevention, the emphasis has been placed on attempting to modify individual attitudes and behaviour in relation to health. The assumption is that individuals are responsible for their health and so they should be responsible for changing their life style. However, as has been shown with tobacco, there is a variety of vested interests which support the maintenance and persistence of cigarette smoking and some of them actively promote the habit. So health education, according to some writers (see Cust, 1979), should refocus attention on the political and economic forces involved in the production of ill-health (Draper et al., 1980). Thus, health education

'might also be concerned with helping people to understand the details of the relationship between smoking and vested interests and this with making more likely collective action to reduce the pressure to smoke' (Tuckett, 1979; see also Brown and Margo, 1978).

The second point refers to the desirability of getting people to give up smoking. The value of 'good health' defined in conventional health education terms might be of limited significance in a number of social contexts and cigarette or alcohol consumption is based on rational rather than idiosyncratic premises. Tuckett (1979), in this example, emphasizes the influence of material circumstances on behaviour and comments on the relationship of social class differences and smoking:

'Whether this is due to a failure to appreciate the risk of cigarette smoking or a generally low level of morale and self-esteem among people forced to undertake and adjust to dangerous, dirty and repetitive jobs, with restricted life chances, is unknown.'

This leads on to the argument that individuals should be left to choose their own priorities for health. In this context, the aim of health education is to inform the individual of how to maintain health if he opts for that choice. The problem with this argument is that it might underestimate the social and economic forces that act on an individual's freedom and the choices available to him, so that health education may be only attempting to counteract the anti-health influence produced by political and economic forces.

The importance of this discussion is that it is necessary not to lose sight of what health education is attempting to do and why it is attempting to do it, and that there are political and ethical assumptions which are implicit in each of the policy positions.

Government restrictions on cigarette promotion

In the previous section we looked at governmental attempts to counteract the apparent effects of cigarette promotion. In this section we will look at more direct measures of government control through the use of legislation banning cigarette advertising. In the UK, as has been shown, some controls on advertising have been agreed on a voluntary basis between the Government and the tobacco industry which are in the hands of the Advertising Authority.

Before we discuss the impact of government controls on cigarette promotion, we need to clarify what is meant by cigarette promotion. It can be defined as any form of sales promotion which encourages smoking. In Great Britain the techniques used include direct advertising through mass media, posters, cinemas, gift coupon schemes, special offers of discounted cigarettes, incentives to retailers, television advertising of 'same name' cigars and pipe tobacco, sponsorship of sport and the arts, and a host of minor promotional activities. In addition, there are the public relations activities of the tobacco industry which are a less direct but important form of sales promotion.

As might be expected, there has been considerable dispute about the effects of cigarette promotion between the tobacco industry and those in the anti-smoking lobby. Gray (1977) clearly illustrates these conflicting propositions. First, he outlines the arguments about the effects of promotion put forward by the anti-smoking lobby. He suggests that promotion acts to redistribute the existing market; secondly, the tobacco industry recruits smokers through the portrayal of attractive images in advertising; thirdly, cigarette promotion can be seen as a public relations activity and a means for maintaining support; fourthly, Gray argues that cigarette promotion

> 'undermines government or school-based educational activities and establishes in the minds of the young people the view that tobacco smoking is an acceptable habit, espite the fact that health warnings are widely applied to it' (Gray, 1977).

On the other hand, Gray (1977) outlines the arguments of the pro-smoking lobby in support of the maintenance of cigarette promotion. First, there are the arguments that advertising is only directed towards smokers and is aimed at increasing the brand's share of the market (see Kirkwood, 1980). Second, there are the arguments that cigarette advertising enables promotion of health messages such as health warnings on packets and helps to promote low-tar cigarettes. Third, there are the arguments that refer to general principles which suggest that the anti-smoking lobby is a kind of anti-advertising lobby which sees cigarette advertising as being the first of many targets. Fourth, an advertising ban might damage the interests of the media. Fifth, an advertising ban would not be effective and it would be difficult to apply to imported publications. Finally, some cigarette manufacturers argue that cigarettes are not proven hazards.

Whilst a large number of these arguments have been contested by Gray (1977), some of these arguments have been supported by the UK Government in its most recent White Paper on prevention (HMSO, 1977b), justifying their decision not to ban cigarette advertising. One of the arguments emphasized the importance of cigarette advertising in not only advertising the government health warning but also advertising low-tar cigarettes. Obviously, as Gray stated, health education could perform this function but there are a number of assumptions which have recently been questioned. Firstly, that a switch to low-tar/nicotine cigarettes necessarily reduces the risk of ill-health. (More will be said about that when the low-tar nicotine programme is discussed.) Secondly, implicit in this position is the assumption that dependence is predominantly a physiological or pharmacological phenomenon. It has been suggested that dependence consists of a number of other dimensions, which are equally crucial, one of which is a social dimension. Cigarette advertising may reinforce this social element and its elimination may help reduce dependence.

In the light of this discussion, what available evidence is there which has shown whether legislation to ban cigarette advertising is effective or not? Afghanistan, Singapore, Italy, Norway, Finland, Hungary, Czechoslovakia, USSR, Iceland, Saudi Arabia and Turkey have introduced advertising bans. Cigarette advertising in Poland and Rumania has never been allowed. In Italy an advertising ban was introduced in 1962 in order to protect the State tobacco monopoly against aggressive American and other foreign companies. This apart, advertising bans have normally been imposed to protect the public health. Three Scandinavian countries—Norway, Finland and Sweden—have introduced comprehensive tobacco acts entailing a strategy focusing not only on one aspect of the problem such as cigarette advertising but also—as in Finland—on taxation and the allocation of 0.5 per cent of revenue frm tobacco duty to anti-smoking campaigns and research (see Elo (1979) for a detailed description). In 1978, legislation enabling control over promotion was introduced in Eire. Legislation in France prohibits advertising and publicity on TV and radio and certain other media, and smoking is prohibited in public places.

To date, only two studies have evaluated the ban on cigarette advertising. Hamilton (1972) compared figures from 11 countries, 8 of which had some sort of ban plus adverse publicity about smoking. Results showed advertising bans have no effect, although adverse publicity does. He argues that the more effective smoking control policy would be to increase investments in anti-smoking messages rather than banning advertising. More recently, Bjartveit (1977) analysed smoking habits during the first year after implementation of the Norwegian Tobacco Act, 1975. The Passing of this Act included:
  (i) a total ban on all advertising of tobacco products;
  (ii) legislation to label all packets with symbol and text pointing out damages;
  (iii) prohibition of sale or handover to persons under the age of 16 years.

The results showed that in Norway the adult per capita consumption fell by 2.7 per cent in 1975/76. This change was most marked among males, with a drop from 52 per cent to 48 per cent of smokers within a period of six months. No change in per capita consumption was found for women. In Oslo, there was a fall in smoking amongst men from 60 per cent to 45 per cent and daily consumption fell from 16.7 units to 14.4 units. The drop was most marked amongst the female population who were aged 15 to 21 years. These results suggest that the Act is having an impact even at this early stage.

This evidence appears to support a relationship between cigarette advertising and the demand for cigarettes. Other evidence from research carried out in the

United Kingdom has confirmed this relationship (McGuiness and Cowling, 1975). McGuiness and Cowling found advertising has had a statistically significant effect on the expansion of sales. They state that in the period before the Royal College of Physicians' report:

'A 10% increase in advertising is estimated to have caused sales to expand by 0.14% within the period of adjustment to the desired level of sales ...'

They state further:

'The ability of advertising to influence decisions not only in the current period but also in future periods causes the ten per cent increase in advertising to lead to an eventual 2.8% increase in sales ... this magnitude probably reflects the role that advertising plays in attracting potential customers into the market.'

They also suggest that health publicity in the form of a Royal College of Physicians' Report may have had an effect countering advertising. They state:

'In the period following the report, a 10% increase in advertising is estimated to have raised sales by about 0.1% in the period.'

In summary, whilst it is too early to assess the impact on the cigarette consumption and the numbers of smokers, of limitations that have been placed on the form of advertising of cigarettes through the voluntary agreement, available evidence suggests that government control of cigarette advertising in other countries, in combination with other control measures, has had the effect of reducing the demand for cigarettes. However, if this is due to a ban on advertising or mainly due to the impact of the other measures is unclear. Whether a ban on cigarette advertising which is voluntarily agreed between government and the tobacco industry would have the same impact is difficult to assess from the available evidence. The difficulty in interpreting these data and those from the Norwegian study is that it is impossible to isolate the effects of advertising from the effects of health publicity. Certainly, in Norway it must be remembered that the advertising ban is coupled with an education campaign, and how far the reduction in smoking is due to one or the other is difficult to know. It has been argued that advertising responds to, rather than generates, consumer spending (Schmalensee, 1972).

The Government health warning

In the United Kingdom, since 1972, all cigarette packs and advertisements have to carry a government health warning. This idea was also based on a voluntary agreement between the Government and the tobacco industry.

How far this warning has been effective is difficult to estimate, given the wide range of health education techniques used during this period. Certainly, there is some evidence which suggests that people are aware of the message (see Gatherer et al., 1979), but the implications of this for changes in attitudes and behaviour are not known. The Third Report of the Royal College of Physicians (1977) implies that it has been ineffective:

'Although Government spokesmen claimed that the warning was effective, 82 per cent of smokers stated in a public opinion survey that it had had no effect on their smoking.'

Gray (1977) speculates on the value of the warning. He identifies four different advantages:

(i) it opens doors to other actions by the Government;

(ii) it opens doors of schools to health education;

(iii) it politically commits the Government to the official view that smoking is dangerous;

(iv) the absence of the warning may be regarded by children and the public as reflecting the absence of an opinion by the Government which is detrimental to an anti-smoking programme.

He does identify one minor disadvantage, which is that the warning on the packet may sometimes provide an insurance policy for the tobacco industry against court action for compensation.

The safer cigarette

In this section, a consideration of different types of measures to the ones described previously is presented. In contrast to the attempts to control the usage of the harmful products through the use of anti-smoking propaganda or control of smoking propaganda, this is a public health measure which attempts to make the product less harmful through the control of its constituents.

Now, in this country this policy has been developed in a number of different forms. First, as has already been mentioned, the Government in 1972 published its low-tar/nicotine tables which have been modified on a number of occasions since then. These tables have been publicized by the Health Education Council. The objective of the campaign was to show that smokers of high-tar cigarettes have higher death rates than those who smoke low-tar cigarettes. This would make the general public aware of the relative harm of the cigarettes that they are smoking and encourage them to switch to a less harmful brand. In support of this policy, the advertising of high-tar brands was to be phased out immediately and middle-to-high brands were to be phased out by 1978. Advertising was to be concentrated on low-tar brands. Cigarette packets and advertisements would carry a description of the tar groups to which the advertised brand belongs.

There is some doubt as to whether this policy of concentrating advertising on the low-tar groups has been adhered to by the tobacco industry. However, results from an evaluative study of the Health Education Council advertising campaigns (1974, 1975 and 1976) showed that by the third campaign there was an increase in the proportion of smokers who mentioned tar yield as a factor in choosing between brands. Further data showed that between 1973 and 1976 the size of the low-tar market increased from 0.5 per cent to 7.2 per cent. Since that time the statistics have been compounded by the introduction by the Government, in September 1978, of a supplementary tax on all cigarettes with tar yields of 20 mg units or more. By November 1978, the proportion of the cigarette market occupied by such cigarettes had fallen to 3 per cent from 15 per cent (Lancet, 1979), while during the preceding year there had been no material change in the tar yield structure of the market. So there is some evidence to suggest that there has been a shift towards low tar amongst smokers, although more detailed statistics need to be made available. Certainly, there has been a drop in the average tar yield. Between 1965 and 1973 tar yields fell from 31.4 mg/cigarette to 18.7 mg/cigarette. Since 1973 the rate of fall has dropped (HMSO, 1979a). However, a number of doubts have been expressed about the value of this policy.

First, it is argued that the relative shift towards low-tar cigarettes has not been significant and the trend to lower tar and nicotine yields seems to have flattened off. Further evidence to support this is the failure of so many low-tar brands to sell when put on the market in 1973. The reason for this apparent barrier at an average nicotine yield towards 1.0 mg units or more suggests that smokers go no lower because to do so deprives them of satisfaction. The argument runs like this (Russell, 1976):

> 'Tar and nicotine yields of cigarettes available in Britain today correlate 0.93, and further reduction of tar intake is limited by the reluctance of smokers to tolerate similar reductions in nicotine.'

Russell (1974) argues that the crucial factor in understanding cigarette smoking is dependence on nicotine. He states:

> '... after initiation to smoking has been mediated by various psychosocial motives, the pharmacological effects of nicotine take over as prime reinforcers of such strength and universal appeal that eventual dependence is almost inevitable.'

Russell (1974) suggests that the idea that adult smokers persist in smoking because of the need to maintain the right image is misleading. They continue to smoke because they are dependent.

It is argued that even when smokers switch to low-tar/nicotine cigarettes, they smoke more cigarettes or inhale more deeply which means that they take in more tar and carbon monoxide (CO) per unit of nicotine (Russell et al., 1980).

Whilst Russell feels that a movement towards a safer cigarette is a more realistic goal than anti-smoking propaganda because of this dependence aspect, he suggests that the safest cigarette would have a high (relative) nicotine yield so smokers puff and smoke less but with low-tar and a low CO yield. He has shown (Russell, 1976) that it is possible within the present tar/nicotine tables to change to a brand which lowers the smoker's tar intake but maintains the nicotine level. He suggests that whilst such a cigarette (ideally) does not exist, it is certainly not beyond the technical skills of the tobacco industry. He argued (Russell, 1976):

> 'This motivation (tobacco industry's) might be provided if the Government, in their six-monthly tar and nicotine tables, would focus attention not so much on the tar yield (which is the current practice) but on the nicotine yield and the ratio of tar to nicotine.'

This, according to Russell, would enable smokers to find a brand that meets their nicotine needs but also has the least amount of tar.

Secondly, the arguments about lowering tar yields exclude the possibility that there are other constituents which could be harmful. Whether nicotine is harmless is uncertain, but the other main component of tobacco smoke apart from tar and nicotine is carbon monoxide (CO) which is probably an important factor in the cause of cardiovascular disease, including coronary heart disease, as well as influencing child development when women smoke during pregnancy. Whilst CO levels in cigarettes have been reduced, as have tar and nicotine levels, by the introduction of ventilated filters, it is still advocated that CO be added to the league tables. A study (Russell, Wilson et al., 1973) comparing the effect on tobacco consumption of changing to high- and low-nicotine cigarettes found that as nicotine levels went up or down CO levels fell. This was due to low-nicotine cigarettes having low CO yields and, when smoking high-nicotine cigarettes, was attributable to reduced consumption.

Three other disadvantages of the policy of switching to low-tar cigarettes have been identified by Gray (1977). He proposes the following three arguments.

1. The suggestion that low-tar cigarettes are 'safer' has frequently been developed in the media into a suggestion that they are 'safe' when they are not.

2. The launching of some low-tar cigarettes has been the excuse for a substantial amount of promotional activity in both America and Britain.

3. The implication that 'safer' cigarettes are available may well reassure long-term smokers who might otherwise be persuaded to give up smoking completely.

Now, even within these limitations, it is argued that the safer cigarette approach is more realistic than the anti-smoking approach, given the assumption that smoking can involve dependence. These advocates might say that their approach was justified given the lack of success of anti-smoking propaganda. The Government has also been involved in other activities which involve the tightening up on controls to limit the constituents in cigarettes. In this country, the marketing of tobacco substitutes and additives is carried out subject to the controls required by the Secretary of State on the advice of the Independent Scientific Committee on Smoking and Health (the Hunter Committee). All advertisements for tobacco substitutes and brands containing substitutes must specify the proportion of substitute material in the brands (normally 75 per cent tobacco) and all advertisements for part-substitutes are subject to the same controls as ordinary cigarette advertisements. Marketing of the part-substitute brands is subject to long-term human health studies under the guidance of the Hunter Committee. Subsequently, the White Paper on Prevention and Health discussed the recommendation to put the powers to control tobacco substitutes and additives under the 1968 Act, in the same way that controls are exercised over medicinal products under the Medicines Act. In the voluntary agreement the Government said that these powers would be used only if the need arose.

Two tobacco substitutes, NSM14 and Cytrel 361, were given a conditional go-ahead by the committee, but since that time the hoped for long-term epidemiological study monitoring the impact of their introduction was not possible due to a fall in sales to under 2 per cent of the market share (HMSO, 1979a).

The second report of the Hunter Committee (HMSO, 1979a) discussed the developments and possibility of creating a 'lower-risk' cigarette, although perhaps of more significance was the minority report which suggested that the committee's recommendation lacked urgency. This minority report suggested that there was already sufficient evidence to justify recommending maximum limits for tar and carbon monoxide (see also Jarvis and Russell, 1980). Dr Ball (the author of the minority report) also suggests that in recommendations for the development of a safer cigarette it is important that consumption is reduced as well as toxicity:

'If the average tar and carbon monoxide levels are reduced in the next 5 years by, say, 30% and the consumption rises by 30%, the health of persisting smokers is unlikely to improve. Increases of this order have been recorded in recent years.'

Fiscal policy

Gray (1977) has suggested that a government can attempt to control tobacco consumption through fiscal policy by adopting three potential legislative targets.

1. An overall progressive increase in taxation with the clear health-related objective of reducing consumption.

2. A differential system of taxation which favours cigarettes which are low in tar, nicotine and carbon monoxide.

3. The inclusion in the tax structure of a levy to finance a smoking education programme.

The first two have been tried. It is too early to know whether the differential system of taxation which was introduced in 1978 has led to a shift in demand from high- to low-tar cigarettes. However, the tobacco companies, in anticipation of this occurring immediately, reduced 4.5 mg of tar/cigarette in about twenty brands (HMSO, 1979a).

Some studies have been carried out to examine the relationship between cigarette price and consumption in the UK, although none has concentrated specifically on government-inspired price changes that were motivated for reasons of health. Of three studies which examined this relationship between price and consumption of cigarettes, two found a positive relationship (Russell, 1973; Peto, 1974) and the other found a negative relationship (Atkinson and Skegg, 1974). Russell compared annual changes in consumption and price between 1946 and 1971. He found that 22 of 25 consumption changes coincided with price changes of opposite direction. In contrast, Atkinson and Skegg (1974) examined the nature of the relationship between 1951 and 1970; allowing for both the Royal College of Physicians' report in 1962 and the ban on cigarette advertising in 1965, they found that changes in price had an insignificant effect on the consumption of cigarettes. According to their results, the most significant influence was income, with publicity being more important than price. Peto (1974) re-analysed Atkinson and Skegg's data and came up with some different results. He found that male cigarette consumption between 1951 and 1970 showed a marked response to price changes. He suggested that the evidence of the response of consumption to income changes was mainly attributable to the large increases in consumption and income in 1960, without which the estimated effect is minimal. According to Peto's evidence, the publicity generated by the RCP's report of 1962 led to a significant fall of about 5 per cent in consumption but the TV advertising ban had a smaller and insignificant effect.

Whilst the balance of evidence seems to support the existence of an inverse relationship between consumption and price, the degree of change both in the short and longer terms caused by different increases in the price of cigarettes is difficult to predict and so is the impact of price changes on 'heavy' and 'light' consumers of cigarettes.

It appears that the influence of price rises is to generate an initial fall in demand which then slowly increases to the original level. It is evident, therefore, that consistent annual increases in the prices of cigarettes through taxation may produce consistent decline in consumption. The problem is estimating how large these price increases should be. Peto (1976) argues that, based on the assumption that a 10 per cent increase in real price reduces consumption by 5 per cent, the outcome of increasing the real price of cigarettes by 10 per cent per year for ten years, then maintaining it at that level, would be a reduction in at least 12 000 premature deaths a year among persons aged under 65 years, coupled with a substantial increase in revenue. The price elasticity of demand for tobacco, however, might be smaller than 0.5 and, as Atkinson and Townsend (1977) point out, this would need large increases in price. They state that when the price elasticity of cigarettes is 0.5:

> 'A 56% increase would be needed to effect a 20% reduction. Very large increases in price would probably have proportionately greater effect than the relatively small changes observed in the past, but in general it seems that increased taxation can only form part of a strategy to reduce consumption.'

Their package aimed at producing a 40 per cent decrease in consumption involves a 56 per cent price rise which leads to a 20 per cent fall in consumption, restrictions on cigarette promotion which leads to a 10 per cent fall in consumption, and a further 10 per cent fall in consumption which is due to investment of £10 million on health education. The 'costs' of reduction in consumption of tobacco specifically caused by large increases in price are, first, that tobacco is one product which contributes to the Retail Price Index (RPI), and to increase the price of tobacco would be inflationary and would be acting against latterday government economic policy. National Consumer Council (1979) statistics show that in 1978 both the price and tax on cigarettes were lower than in the years 1968 to 1972, 1974 and 1975, and since 1968 the retail index for tobacco rose by 162 per cent and the general price index by 220 per cent. So it appears that even with successive increases in taxation on cigarettes, the real price of cigarettes has fallen on frequent occasions during the period 1968–78 and the tobacco component of the RPI has increased at a slower rate than general prices.

Secondly, another argument against large increases in prices of cigarettes is that such a policy is socially regressive in that poorer groups would be hit harder by price increases. This is further compounded by the marked social class differences in the prevalence of smoking at the present time. The dependent nature of cigarette smoking, be it pharmacological, psychological or cultural, might mean that smokers might give up other goods to continue smoking at the same level.

The final 'cost' of price rises in cigarettes is in the loss of government revenue obtained by the taxation of cigarettes. However, as Peto (1976) and Atkinson and Townsend (1977) show, the low price responsiveness of the demand for cigarettes means that large increases in price produce a gain rather than a loss in revenue.

Atkinson and Townsend (1977) also identify another 'cost' to the Government of a significant decrease in smoking. They estimate that savings to the Government in terms of costs of hospital in-patient stay, general practitioner consultations, sickness benefits and widows' benefits of a 40 per cent in cigarette smoking are greater than the costs incurred in increases in expenditure on retirement pensions and health education.

Smoking in public places

One other measure which the Government might introduce to control smoking is to restrict smoking in public places. The British Government has put pressure on hospital and health authorities to control smoking on health premises as well as on British Rail and London Transport to increase the provision for non-smokers. They had had some success in relation to the latter in that in 1977 British Rail had 50 per cent of its carriages given over to non-smoking on Inter-city and 60 per cent of carriages on most surburban lines. London Transport have 75 per cent of its carriages as non-smokers.

Apart from the irritation, discomfort and distress caused by smokers, there is evidence to show that passive smoking can be a small but real health risk (Russell, Cole and Brown, 1973).

MH
Summary

The Government in the UK has played a very limited role in smoking control compared with other governments in the Western world. Even compared with the USA and Canada, where vested interests in tobacco are stronger, the United Kingdom's Government is out of step (Friedman, 1975). European countries such as Finland, Norway and Sweden have developed a comprehensive anti-smoking package incorporating a combination of legal and educational measures. In the UK, legislation has been almost confined to the elimination of cigarette advertising in the broadcast media. Some funds have sponsored health education campaigns and research into the smoking–health linkage. Much emphasis has been placed on voluntary agreements with the tobacco industry, particularly in relation to restrictions on advertising.

The measures that the Government in the UK has instigated since 1975 are a negotiated voluntary agreement with the tobacco industry which involved agreement to reduce and eventually stop the advertising of high-tar cigarettes and a voluntary agreement between government and the tobacco industry over advertising at sports meetings. In addition, a supplementary tax has been brought into operation which discriminates against high-tar cigarettes.

Apart from the lack of clear evidence on the value of a number of legislative policies (which is not usually the criterion for not bringing in legislation), it appears that the reasons why the Government in the UK has pursued such a non-intervention policy lie with the interests vested in tobacco. Not only is there doubt about whether the Government has the political strength to intervene even if it wanted to, but there is also doubt about whether it would be in its own interests to intervene.

There has been a drop in the number of smokers, although this has mainly occurred amongst males and amongst the middle classes. However, there is some doubt as to whether consumption per head of smoker is dropping. Whether any of the government strategies were instrumental in this decrease in smoking is difficult to tell. Certainly, the mass health education campaigns seem to have done no more than change people's knowledge. However, this may be all that would be expected, given the nature of the campaign, and all that is necessary in that it creates the right social environment for the acceptance of other control measures. There has been a switch to low-tar brands, although whether this is due to the introduction of the supplementary tax, the publication of tar/nicotine tables or the switch in promotion towards low-tar brands is not clear. The idea of a safer cigarette seems to be one policy that the Government has endorsed, particularly for smokers who are dependent. However, as has been shown, there are problems involved in the policy of endorsing a safer cigarette, for example the lack of information about carbon monoxide levels given to consumers. It is also doubtful whether there would be any value in providing the consumer with further information—that is, information on carbon monoxide levels—upon which the smoker has to make a judgement about which is the safer cigarette. At the moment the smoker has to check the tar:nicotine ratio and this would be further complicated by details of the carbon monoxide levels. Further research evidence could give the Government the ability to control the range of cigarettes available to the consumer.

The evidence on the impact of advertising is conflicting. Certainly, in Norway the ban on advertising in combination with other measures has led, at least initially, to a drop in smoking. It appears that no government smoking control measure alone can significantly influence smoking behaviour and what is required is a comprehensive strategy of smoking control aimed at different levels. This control strategy should be viewed as a long-term policy aimed at controlling the incidence of new cases of smokers. The short-term concerns should also include how to develop a safer cigarette for the dependent smoker.

Fiscal policies can also be effective in controlling consumption but, as has been noted, this tends to penalize the disadvantaged.

In conclusion, it appears that the Government's future long-term smoking control policies should be aimed at the development of a package of measures which include: intensive health education to the young; controls on cigarette promotion; controls on cigarette smoking in public places in combination with large increases in the tax on cigarettes. In addition, the Government could radically reorganize its economic policy so as to minimize the social and economic consequences of the phasing out of tobacco manufacture and distribution in this country completely.

Alcohol and cancer: policies for prevention

In this section, past, current and future policies aimed at the prevention of ill-health from the use of alcohol will be examined. It must be emphasized that the focus will be on those government policies aimed at controlling excessive alcohol use so as to influence physical health rather than those aimed at controlling the social and psychological effects of alcohol such as drunkenness and driving, drunkenness and public and domestic violence and the impact of the state of alcoholism on the individuals' lives and the lives of their families. To make such a distinction is in some ways artificial, particularly when the aim is to control excessive drinking whatever effect of drinking is the specific target of the policy. Even policies aimed at controlling drinking in specific situations, such as the legal control of drink when driving, may have spin-off effects on excessive drinking by reducing the range of circumstances in which drinking is legitimate. So the policies considered here will be those aimed at controlling excessive alcohol use with a specific focus on implications for physical ill-health. Certainly, cancer has been one of the least mentioned of the harmful effects of alcohol and thus has not had a priority in policies for control (see Royal College of Psychiatrists, 1979).

How many drinkers?

There are a number of different sources of data which are used to assess overall consumption. They can be broadly divided into two different groups. Those data derived from survey data and those from sales and production figures for alcohol. Both approaches have weaknesses, as will be shown.

Some studies of alcohol consumption have used the sales of alcohol as their measure. Lint and Schmidt (1968) reported a study on consumption derived from sales in localities in Ontario. Forms have to be completed on purchasing alcohol in that Province, and such data were used for one month (repeated a year later) to identify the consumptions of wines and spirits; the purchase slips included the individual's address and only those addresses within a defined locality were accepted; the names were then aligned to identify repeat purchases by the same individual within one month. For a smaller locality, comparable data were available for beer consumption. One of the problems about such data is that purchase is obviously not synonymous with consumption; however, the majority of individuals who were 'high purchasers' in the month obtained their alcohol from multiple purchases throughout the month—which did not suggest they were so doing in order to have a particular party, but that the drink was being bought for their own use. Obviously this is a real weakness of such data, and without the use of special enquiry to determine this factor does leave a question mark against the material.

Single and Giesbrecht (1979) commented on two aspects of sales data. They point out that it is necessary to convert the type of beverage to alcohol and that if the type of drink sold changes over time, the conversion factor requires amendment. They point out that in Ontario there had been a shift to the sale of weaker table wines and a change from 16 per cent to 12 per cent conversion was required for wine sales. They point out that without this correction there was an overestimation of total alcohol consumption by about 2 per cent. The other problem involves the home production of beverage; they estimate from sales of raw materials and equipment that wine and wine brandy production at home might lead to an overall underestimation of consumption by about 67 per cent (in Ontario there were no hard data on other forms of unrecorded production, though they were not thought to be appreciable compared with wine and wine brandy).

Sales and production figures are also used as measures of national alcohol consumption, particularly for international comparisons in the form of per capita consumption of pure alcohol per person aged 15 years and over. However, this measure is subject to a number of similar weaknesses. For example, Davies (1979) states:

'This measure, therefore, tells us nothing about illicitly produced alcohol, legal sales that are not recorded (such as cider in France), licit home production, alcohol purchased and brought into a country through duty free customs allowances, or the quantities held in stock by wholesale and retail merchants or state alcohol monopolies.'

Davies (1979) suggests, therefore, that figures for per capita consumption based on production and sales figures should be treated with caution, particularly in that they may suffer from under-reporting.

By European standards, the per capita consumption of pure alcohol in the UK is low. For example, in 1976 the per capita consumption of pure alcohol in litres per person aged 15 years and over was 9.1. In France, the equivalent figure in the same year was 22.3, in Italy 17.2, in West Germany 16.7, in Belgium 12.8, in Denmark 11.6, Netherlands 10.9 and Ireland 9.1 (Davies, 1979). So, no other EEC country has a lower per capita consumption than in the UK. However, when the rate of change in per capita consumption is considered, a different picture emerges. For example, in 1950 the per capita consumption of pure alcohol in litres per person aged 15 years and over was 4.9. By 1970 it had risen to 7.0 and by 1976 it had risen to 9.1. The overall percentage change in per capita consumption between 1950 and 1976 was 86 per cent, and between 1970 and 1976 it was 30 per cent. As Davies reports (1979), this makes the UK the fourth highest amongst EEC countries for percentage increase in per capita consumption of pure alcohol for the period 1970–76. Some European countries have actually witnessed a fall in per capita consumption. For example, in France between 1950 and 1976 the overall percentage change in per capita consumption of pure alcohol was a fall of 6 per cent. In Italy, between 1970 and 1976, per capita consumption fell by 8 per cent.

Norway and Sweden are the European countries with the lowest per capita consumption of pure alcohol. As will be seen, these countries appear to have more restrictive alcohol control policies than others in Europe. In 1976, the per capita consumption of pure alcohol in litres per person aged 15 years and over was 5.7 in Norway and 7.3 in Sweden. However, both these countries had witnessed an increase in per capita consumption, although in Norway the increase was more marked (Davies, 1979).

Figure 5.6 shows trends in alcohol consumption in the UK by beverage type for the period 1927–79. These data show that whilst beer still remains the preferred type of beverage there have been more marked increases in the consumption of spirits and wine compared with beer. This change has been particularly significant over the last twenty-five years. Thus, in terms of the distribution of alcohol consumed in the UK, wine and spirits account for a higher percentage in 1976 than they did in 1950 and the percentage of pure alcohol consumed in beer has fallen (Davies, 1979). In 1950, of pure alcohol consumed in the UK, 12.8 per cent was in the form of spirits. By 1976 this figure increased to 23.0 per cent. In 1950 the percentage of pure alcohol consumed in the UK in the form of wine was 3.2 per cent and by 1976 it was 10.8 per cent. Consequently, whilst 83.9 per cent of the pure alcohol consumed in the UK in 1950 was in the form of beer, by 1976 this figure had been reduced to 66.1 per cent. In summary, whilst overall consumption of alcohol has increased in the UK, the greatest increases have been in wine and spirit consumption. As a result of this, nowadays wine and spirits account for a larger proportion of the overall consumption of pure alcohol in the UK. A similar trend to the one described in the above, where the traditional beverage remains the preferred type although there has been a more marked increase in consumption in alternative beverages, has occurred in other countries (Bruun et al., 1975). For example, in France, although wine remains the preferred beverage, there has been an upsurge in the consumption of beer. In Poland, where spirits remain the preferred beverage, there has been an upsurge in wine consumption (Davies, 1979).

Consumption data related to frequency of alcohol use are difficult to find. Some survey data are available, although here too there are problems. Pernanen (1974) shows that only a half of total alcohol sales are accounted for in data collected through surveys. Under-reporting may occur due to problems of recall or social and moral pressures on the respondent which may lead to deliberate understatement (OPCS, 1978). Another reason may be the incomplete coverage of surveys in that non-respondents may be more likely to be heavy drinkers (OPCS, 1978)

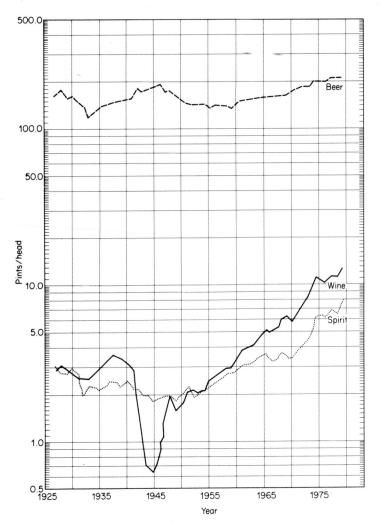

Fig. 5.6 Beer, wine and spirit consumption per head of population in the UK, 1927–79. (Source: Brewers' Society, 1980.)

and thus be more difficult to contact as they more often live in institutions such as doss-houses (Plant, 1979).

The overall validity of some surveys has been assessed by comparing the national consumption of alcoholic beverages with that which would be indicated from small-sample surveys—these in general indicate that the sample survey may underestimate the total consumption by 50 per cent. The estimates for this underestimation vary; the important point to consider is whether this is a biased underestimate of those at the high end of the intake or is consistent under-reporting at all levels of consumption.

Plant and Pirie (1979) reported surveys on alcohol consumption in four Scottish towns. The variation will be discussed in a later subsection, but there was internal inconsistency between the percentage of drinkers, the percentage of heavy drinkers, and the mean intake for all individuals in the locality. Also, their results were contrasted with those obtained in an earlier Scottish study (Dight, 1976). There was quite marked variation in the results obtained in these two different Scottish studies; unfortunately, the organizations carrying out the study, the wording of the questionnaires, and the general frameworks of the enquiries were rather different—and it is impossible to tell to what degree this method difference in the surveys had generated the difference in results. It is, however, indicative of the kind of problem that occurs between two surveys.

Orrego et al. (1979) assessed the reliability of information on alcohol consumption through interviews with patients attending a liver clinic. Over a six-month period, thirty-seven patients had their urinary alcohol measured daily, and each week the patients were questioned, amongst other things, about their alcohol consumption in the past week. The patients convincingly denied alcohol intake on 52 per cent of occasions when they were questioned, when their urine contained alcohol. A quarter of these subjects denied drinking on every occasion. Those who admitted drinking intermittently had urinary alcohol values about double those who denied it (1001 mg per litre in comparison with 538 mg per litre). Orrego and his co-workers point out that the 'deniers' appeared to consume less alcohol than those who admitted their drinking but that caution is obviously required in assessing the interview data.

The other form of data which are collected through surveys is purchase data. For example, in the Family Expenditure Survey in the UK, detailed information is collected from households on the total and specific expenditure over a period of a week. This survey also suffers from the weakness of not sampling from the whole population. Also, there is a question mark against the accuracy of the respondents' answers about the other members' of the families expenditure on alcohol.

Data collected in the General Household Survey (OPCS, 1978) are analysed in terms of a classification which incorporates both quantity and frequency of drinking. The scale was divided up into occasional, infrequent light, frequent light, moderate and heavy. Their results showed that the drinking patterns for males and females were completely different. Men were more likely to be heavy (25 per cent) or moderate drinkers (15 per cent) than women (2 per cent) and women (25 per cent) were more likely than men (9 per cent) to be occasional drinkers. This pattern was maintained through all age groups. For both sexes, the older the person the less heavy the drinking pattern. These differences in drinking habits according to sex are supported by studies in Scotland (Dight, 1976) and in South London (Robinson, 1976).

The GHS data (see OPCS, 1978) also show socio-economic group differences in patterns of drinking. Each socio-economic group was standardized for age to allow for variations in age distribution within groups. Even after this standardization, about 33 per cent of men in manual socio-economic groups were shown to be heavy drinkers compared with less than 15 per cent in non-manual occupations and less than 10 per cent in professional groups. There was little difference between manual and non-manual groups in the proportion of abstainers among men, but the highest proportion of abstainers was in the unskilled group.

More women heavy drinkers were found in the manual as opposed to the non-manual group, although frequent light drinkers were higher among women in non-manual groups than amongst manual groups. Women in the unskilled manual group were twice as likely as women in non-manual groups to be abstainers.

These data suggest significant variations in drinking patterns according to age, sex and socio-economic group. The GHS data (OPCS, 1978) also pointed to marked regional variations in male heavy drinking. There was a general steady gradient from south to north, although Scotland was not as high as the northern counties of England.

The studies provide important cross-sectional data on drinking habits but they need to be complemented by longitudinal data or follow-up studies on changes in drinking habits. This is of particular importance in the light of the consumption data presented earlier which have shown an increase in overall consumption and differential increases in consumption according to beverage type in the UK over the last thirty years. Questions such as: has the increase in consumption occurred throughout the population? or is it confined to specific groups? need to be answered.

Bruun *et al.* (1975), in a discussion of hazardous consumption levels, argue that consumption is 'heavy' or excessive when it has the effect of significantly reducing life expectancy. They conclude that:

'The lowest level of chronic alcohol consumption which constitutes a significant hazard to longevity has yet to be determined. It is almost certainly substantially less than a daily equivalent of 120 g and quite possibly below 60 g' (120 g is equivalent to 15 centilitres).

The South London Survey (Robinson, 1976) showed 61 per cent of drinkers consume between 1 and 10 centilitres per week, 16 per cent of drinkers consume between 10 and 20 centilitres per week and 23 per cent of drinkers consume in excess of 20 centilitres per week. In Scotland (Dight, 1976), 56 per cent of drinkers consume between 1 and 11.25 centilitres per week, 18 per cent of drinkers consume between 12 and 22.50 centilitres per week and 26 per cent of drinkers consume in excess of 22.50 centilitres per week.

The GHS classification (OPCS, 1978) defined heavy drinking as when seven or more units (equivalent to 9 g of absolute alcohol) were drunk at *least* on one or two occasions per week. According to their definition, 25 per cent of males aged over 16 years were heavy drinkers and 2 per cent of females aged over 16 years (13 per cent in all).

Davies made his estimations from the data collected in the Scottish survey, which shows that nearly all the 26 per cent who consume more than 22.50 centilitres per week are males. Also Davies states:

'It may be estimated that 7% of Scottish regular drinkers consume a mean number of 12.87 centilitres of pure alcohol daily, a level that is within the range considered to be "heavy", "excessive" or injurious to health and/or longevity!'

The percentage of persons in the UK consuming more than 15 centilitres of pure alcohol per day is 2.13 (Davies, 1979) which means that out of fifteen European countries the UK ranks tenth highest.

Davies also presents estimates of the number of persons who are alcoholics (variably defined) or who have alcohol-related problems in the United Kingdom and selected countries of Europe. Using three different sources, each with their own different definitions, he shows that in a report of the Royal College of Psychiatrists (1979) 300 000, or 7.1 per 1000 population, in the UK were persons with drinking problems sufficient to warrant the label of 'alcoholism'. The DHSS (1976) estimated that 500 000, or 11.9 per 1000, people in the UK were 'persons with a serious drinking problem'. OPCS (1977) estimated 740 000, or 17.6 per 1000 population, in the UK were 'alcoholics, based on GP consultations'. Even though there is this wide variation in estimates of alcoholism in the UK, as Davies points out, all of these estimates for the UK are lower than those available in other European countries.

The role of the government in alcohol control policies

The efficacy of government control policies

Before various control policies are considered, it is necessary to examine the theoretical evidence upon which various governmental policies could be based. The important question is whether governmental policy should focus on controlling the level of consumption of alcohol in society, whether it should focus on changing societal values about alcohol or whether it should allocate its resources to the treatment and rehabilitation of heavy drinkers. The first two are genuine prevention policies and the last is a form of secondary prevention in that it may reduce ill-health through treatment.

Now, each of these approaches is based on a different theory about the causes of heavy drinking. The argument that policies should focus on the heavy drinkers alone is based on the assumption that heavy drinkers are a group apart from normal drinkers and the two are not related in any way. The argument is that alcohol is not the cause of alcoholism in that alcoholics have an intrinsic pathological disorder of which heavy drinking is only a symptom (Schmidt, 1977). Thus a public health approach aimed at controlling overall consumption would be irrelevant as alcoholics are not social drinkers. On p. 218 the various theories of the causation of drinking problems will be discussed and it will be shown that although biological or psychological attributes may play a part in the process of becoming an alcoholic, they cannot be divorced from the environmental or social context in which drinking occurs. Certainly, from a practical point of view the most realistic approach is to focus on social and environmental influences in prevention policy rather than psychological attributes.

The two other approaches to alcohol control are based on theories of drinking behaviour which are more sociological in nature. The approach which places an emphasis on the need to change the social values or norms in relation to drinking has been termed the integration theory of drinking. This approach suggests that the reason for drinking problems in many cultures is due to the negative and mystical value put on the use of alcohol. Alcohol use is divorced from normal everyday life practices and thus becomes seen as an unhealthy practice. According to this approach, there is a need through education and legislation to integrate drinking practices into people's everyday lives and thus 'normalize' drinking. The policies suggested are, amongst others, the lowering of the legal drinking age, relaxing of the licensing laws on availability of alcohol by increasing hours of drinking time, and educating young people in the use of alcohol in their everyday lives such as at mealtimes etc.

Further examples of the types of policy are illustrated by Wilkinson (1970). He suggests a five-point programme for alcohol control:

(i) a low level of emotionalism about drinking and a lack of ambivalence;

(ii) a clear distinction between drinking *per se* and drunkenness;

(iii) drinking in situations of restraint;

(iv) drinking on occasions when drinking itself, being only one of several integrated activities, does not become an overwhelming focus of the group's attention;

(v) drinking with food.

Wilkinson (1970) outlines more specific proposals for the attainment of the above goals. These proposals include reduction of the legal age for the purchase and consumption of alcohol, education promoting moderate drinking patterns, commercial advertising to emphasize moderate and safe drinking, a differential taxation system discriminating against strongly alcoholic products, and the integration of the family into taverns.

The evidence to support such an approach is derived from cross-cultural studies which have attempted to show that in countries where drinking is integrated into everyday life, such as at mealtimes, the rates of alcohol problems are low.

However, judging from the evidence presented by Davies (1979) on rates of heavy drinking and rates of death from cirrhosis of the liver in sixteen European countries, this integration approach does not seem to be supported. In the countries where drink appears to be integrated with everyday life, such as in France, Italy and Spain (see Davies, 1979), compared with other European countries where there are stronger controls on the availability of alcohol, the rates of heavy daily alcohol consumption and the rates of death from cirrhosis of the liver are relatively high. For example (Davies, 1979), in 1970, 9.05 per cent of the population in France consumed more than 15 centilitres of pure alcohol per day; 7.39 per cent of the population in Italy consumed more than 15 centilitres of pure alcohol per day, whereas in the UK and Sweden the percentage figures were 2.13 per cent and 1.99 per cent respectively. The rate of deaths per 100 000 population from cirrhosis of the liver in 1974 in France and Italy was 32.8 and 31.9, respectively, whereas in the UK and Sweden it was 3.8 and 7.4, respectively.

Schmidt (1977) suggests that in countries such as France and Italy the reasons for this high consumption and associated problems are due to the fact that alcohol use, far from being restricted to mealtimes, is an integral part of other activities, such as work and recreation. However, what is not evident is whether these countries witness the degree of drunkenness and associated problems which is found in countries with more stringent licensing laws.

This highlights another important question. What type of drinking practices lead to heavy drinking with its associated problems? As has been shown, the so-called 'integrative' drinking practices of the Italians who regularly drink with their meals do not necessarily lead to a low prevalence of drinking problems. Conversely, the Irish have been characterized as having a utilitarian attitude towards drink because of their use of liquor to alleviate physical and emotional discomfort (Lint and Schmidt, 1971). Given the theory that drinking practices with a non-integration approach to drink are much more likely to be related to high prevalence of heavy drinking, one would expect the Irish attitude of seeking intoxication would be associated with a high prevalence of heavy users. In fact, the evidence is to the contrary (Lint and Schmidt, 1971). This evidence suggests that drinking practices are important predictors of the prevalence of heavy use when they influence the range of opportunities in which drinking is legitimized. Evidence of frequent intoxication does not necessarily imply excessive use.

In support of this integration theory, Clayson (1977), in examining the role of licensing, suggests that one of the more valid comparisons is between England, Wales and Scotland. He argues that these countries have many common features in terms of influence on alcohol consumption, such as taxation on alcoholic drink, advertising and marketing strategies and common language, tradition and customs. He argues that the major difference between the two countries is in the licensing laws (pre-1976 Act in Scotland).

Clayson (1977) suggests that, according to the argument that greater availability leads to increased consumption and therefore more drinking problems, one would expect a much higher level of alcohol consumption and associated problems in England and Wales than in Scotland. He shows, however, that the average weekly consumption of alcohol in Scotland is the same as in England and Wales, and Scotland has a higher rate of alcoholism and a higher rate of deaths from cirrhosis. Scottish people drink less at home than those in England and Wales and thus, Clayson (1977) argues, the evidence suggests that it is the licensing laws which place drinkers in Scotland under social pressure and thus generate the associated problems.

The final approach suggests, in contrast to the integration theory described in the above, that the level of consumption of alcohol in a society is directly associated with the prevalence of heavy drinking. The implications of such an approach are that central government can influence heavy drinking by attempting to control overall consumption of alcohol. It is this approach that recently has received increasing support (Bruun et al., 1975; Schmidt, 1977; Robinson, 1977).

The basis of the argument is derived from the work of Ledermann (1956), a French mathematician, on the distribution of alcohol consumption. The technical question with which Ledermann was concerned was the nature of the relationship between the mean alcohol consumption of a population and the proportion of the population consuming an excessive amount.

Using data from populations with different mean consumptions, Ledermann (1956) found that the distributions of drinkers, according to consumption, in the various populations were similar. The distributions were highly skewed, with the majority of the population being moderate drinkers and a small proportion being heavy drinkers. The implications of Ledermann's findings were that it might be possible to estimate the proportion of individuals in a population who had an alcohol intake of a certain level from the overall consumption of alcohol in the population. The distribution of alcohol consumption in any population followed the lognormal distribution described previously. The mean and the variance are the two parameters which describe this distribution. As Duffy (1977a) points out, as two parameters need to be determined and only one empirical quantity is available which is total alcohol consumption, then further information is needed about the distribution. Duffy (1977a) states how Ledermann tries to overcome this problem. He states that:

'Very few individuals will drink more than an extremely large daily quantity of alcohol, and substituting the values one per cent and one litre for "very few" and "extremely large" a second relation is obtained, thus identifying the parameters uniquely.'

Bruun *et al.* (1975) have adopted an amended version of Ledermann's approach. They have argued that not only do empirical data indicate that the distribution of consumption is similar in all populations, but that the dispersion parameter does not change significantly when total consumption changes (Chilvers, 1980). Thus, the prevalence of heavy drinkers can be estimated from mean per capita consumption in a population.

The theory of drinking behaviour which explains the phenomenon is essentially sociological in nature. The emphasis is on the social nature of drinking and the influence of other people on the individual's pattern of drinking. Thus, an increase in one person's consumption may lead to increases in friends' and acquaintances' consumption, primarily because these people are essentially social drinkers and an increase in one person's consumption increases the opportunities to drink. Thus the consumer who drinks much more than his friends will be given further opportunities to increase his drinking and thus will become a heavy drinker. Schmidt (1977) puts it more clearly:

> 'An increase in the consumption of "normal" drinkers may induce changes in the drinking habits of near-heavy drinkers which may in turn lead to an increase in the prevalence of heavy users.'

Schmidt (1977) makes the point that this theory, whilst explaining the snowballing effects of drinking behaviour, does not explain either why individuals start to drink more or why populations in general increase their consumptions. Schmidt explains the adoption of new drinking habits in terms of expansion of drinking habits which in turn are fostered by increasing geographical mobility, media presentation of alternative drinking habits, and new habits generated by the industry to sell their products. According to Schmidt (1977), drinking becomes routinized in the population's everyday lives. This is what the integration theorists would expect as it would lead to healthy drinking. According to Ledermann's theory (1956), such a process has the opposite effect.

In recent years there has been growing controversy over the value of the Ledermann theory. Ledermann's theory has its supporters and a number of empirical studies have presented evidence which, according to the authors, confirms the value of such an approach (Lint and Schmidt, 1971). For example, Lint and Schmidt state:

> 'Whatever arbitrary definition of alcoholism is employed, the distribution of individuals according to consumption quantities illustrates clearly that the prevalence of alcoholism is invariably determined by the overall level of consumption in the population.'

Their contention is supported by the presentation of the distribution of the consumption of alcohol in Ontario in 1968 which showed the distribution to be lognormal and to fit the Ledermann theory (Popham *et al.*, 1975). This study has itself come under criticism (Duffy, 1977a) but, before these are examined, other criticisms of the Ledermann theory will be outlined. The whole question of the Ledermann approach has been discussed at a meeting in London in 1977 (Alcohol Education Centre, see Davies, 1977).

The importance of this model is that it is not only descriptive but might be used as a predictive tool (Miller and Agnew, 1974).

Miller and Agnew (1974) divide their criticims of Ledermann's model into those that apply to it as a descriptive tool and those that apply to it as a predictive tool.

The deficiencies of the model as a descriptive tool, according to these authors, are as follows.

1. Problems of application due to:

(i) the unreliability of alcohol consumption statistics;

(ii) the unreliability of estimates of drinking populations;

Heterogeneous populations are not applicable for the Ledermann theory as they will include different drinking habits. Groups with different drinking habits are different populations.

2. The data base:

(i) small and non-representative populations used for empirical studies;

(ii) no empirical support for assumption on the upper limit of alcohol consumption.

3. Empirical validation:

(i) studies carried out suggest the distribution of alcohol consumption is log-normal, but no statistical tests have been carried out to compare the expected results with the actual results.

4. The model and its relationship to alcoholism:

(i) the substitution of 'alcoholics' for heavy drinkers is not empirically or theoretically substantiated.

5. The model and beverage difference:

(i) There is no empirical evidence to test Ledermann's assumption that all alcoholic beverages are equally implicated in 'alcoholism' or that beverage differences do not affect consumption.

Miller and Agnew's (1974) assessment of Ledermann's model as a predictive tool, in terms of its value for predicting a change in the proportion of heavy drinking after a change in the mean consumption within a country, is as follows.

1. Longitudinal rather than cross-sectional data should be used to test the Ledermann model.

2. There is a question about which of the variables, prevalence of heavy drinkers or mean consumption of alcohol, is the cause and which is the effect. This factor may be important.

3. It may not be possible to predict drinking behaviour with accuracy at the extremes of the range. Also the heavy drinking group may consist of two populations: (i) social drinkers, and (ii) alcoholics. Small differences could be masked in the overall sample.

4. There is uncertainty about the effects of changes in mean consumption and they may have different effects across the whole range of consumption.

5. There is no clear explanation of how the lognormal distribution is generated.

In conclusion, Miller and Agnew (1974), whilst accepting that there is some evidence to suggest that alcohol consumption may be lognormally distributed, state that there is little evidence that consumption is Ledermann distributed. They suggest there are major problems in applying it to real populations and at the predictive level there is considerable doubt about its power, particularly as there is little evidence on within-population changes. Miller and Agnew (1974) therefore suggest the Ledermann theory should be used with extreme caution.

Duffy (1977a) in an analysis of the Ledermann approach, suggests that the major error in the model is a statistical one. He suggests that Ledermann made the mistake of assuming that an attribute must follow a simple mathematical distribution in a population. Duffy suggests that Ledermann's assumption that the lognormal distribution of alcohol consumption can be found in all homogeneous populations at all times with such goodness of fit that predictions may be made about size of the population at the extreme range is misguided. With the population sizes that Ledermann used coupled with the poorness of fit of the mathematical distribution to the tails of the distributions (a common occurrence in this work), Duffy (1977a) is not surprised that Ledermann's data did not support his theory.

In addition, Duffy (1977a) examines data used by Lint and Schmidt (1975) which the latter authors use as evidence to confirm the value of Ledermann's model. Duffy (1977a) shows that the distribution of alcohol purchases found by Lint and Schmidt did not match the distribution obtained from application of the Ledermann model.

Duffy (1977a) in his conclusions is stronger than previous critics. He suggests that the answers Ledermann's methods provide about excessive drinking are wrong. More important, he suggests that if Ledermann's methods and his distributional assumption are discarded, the value of using total consumption figures in the study of alcoholism is brought into question. Duffy (1977a) goes on:

> 'In particular, the idea that alcohol control policies aimed at reducing total consumption in a population will undoubtedly produce a reduction in the prevalence of excessive drinking is seen to be incorrect.'

Finally, two other points identified by Miller and Agnew (1974) about the implications of the Ledermann model need to be presented. First, the authors suggest, although implicit in the Ledermann model is that heavy consumers and alcoholics differ only in the degree of drinking, it does not mean to say that alcoholics cannot be distinguished from heavy consumers using other criteria. Secondly, if Ledermann's theory holds, this doesn't necessarily imply that for preventive measures to be effective all consumers must be affected. It may be possible to redistribute use of alcohol amongst consumers. Unfortunately, Miller and Agnew do not offer a means for doing so.

Chilvers (1980) also questions the statistical logic of the amendments to Ledermann's approach made by Bruun et al. She argues that dissimilar distributions can have equal means and dispersions. Chilvers also suggests that even in populations with relatively small differences in per capita consumption, dispersions may be dissimilar. Duffy (1977b) has shown that quite large differences in the estimated proportion of 'excessive' drinkers may arise from small differences in dispersions. Previous supporters of the Ledermann approach also increasingly began to express caution about the validity of the approach. Lint (1977), in a clear and cautiously worded discussion of this topic, emphasized that alcohol consumption was only likely to approximate to a lognormal distribution and that there were major difficulties in the validity of data to test the model. He stressed that the use of the curve to estimate the prevalence of excessive use was a different matter which would require a precise mathematical description well beyond the general characteristics of the approach. Ledermann himself had used the word 'provisoirement' and some other curve may be more appropriate. He also suggested that the evidence to date did indicate that an increase or decrease in average consumption would imply an increase or a decrease in excessive consumption. Skog (1977) also emphasized the speculative nature of the fixed upper limit as selected by Ledermann; he also indicated that social interaction is an important factor in determining the drinking behaviour, and could have introduced heterogeneity which created problems with the application of the model. A lognormal model was essentially the result of a number of multiplicative factors together influencing the result; he suggested that the fit was by no means ideal to population consumption and that a gamma- or chi-square curve might provide a better fit. As with Lint, he emphasized that the change in consumption would tend to be associated with a change in the proportion of individuals consuming excess alcohol. However, he emphasized that it was quite wrong—neither scientific nor appropriate—to suggest that the only way to control excess consumption was by altering the average population consumption. Lint (1978) replied to these criticisms, ending with an opinion that is very similar to that already quoted from his earlier (1977) paper. Skog (1980) also responded to an article by Duffy and Cohen (1978); he raised a whole series of specific criticisms of some of the points in their earlier paper, presented some data that had been published by others and commented upon by Duffy, and indicated that an appropriate degree of fit occurs with the lognormal curve (again allowing for 0.03 population above the fixed limit). He concluded that, where there were major differences in the level of per capita consumption, the model cannot predict reliably the prevalence of heavy drinkers from per capita consumption alone. However, in general a substantial increase in overall consumption would be accompanied by an increase in the prevalence of heavy usage—it was difficult to find realistic examples where this had not occurred. The argument continued; Duffy (1980) began by noting that it had been suggested that the proportion of excess drinkers tends to be influenced by the square of the effect on the mean consumption (i.e. a modest alteration in average consumption in population appreciably influences the number of heavy users or the drinking of those in the heavy usage category). He disputed this suggestion and reiterated some of his claims about the poor fit in the empirical data, but did conclude that: (i) if one population has more excessive drinkers than another, it will usually have a higher per capita consumption; and (ii) that if the number of excessive drinkers decreases, then, other things being equal, so will the mean consumption.

The statistical debate about the validity of the Ledermann approach has led to a shift towards this 'softer' hypothesis with a conditional acceptance, even by his most vehement critics, of a relationship between overall consumption and the prevalence of heavy drinking.

From an empirical point of view, the evidence to support or refute the Ledermann approach appears to be contradictory. For example, a study in four Scottish towns (Plant and Pirie, 1979) found no clear relationship was evident between the proportion of drinkers or abstainers in any one town and the proportion of 'heavy drinkers'. However, the relative levels of self-reported average alcohol consumption in the four towns were closely related to rates of alcohol-related crimes, hospital admissions for alcoholism and alcoholic psychosis and rates of death from liver cirrhosis and suicide. These and other findings have led one of these authors to conclude (Plant, 1979) that:

'surveys indicate that as far as reported drinking habits go alcoholics fit into a continuum without apparently being a distinctive hard core group that would present a bi-modal curve'.

Plant (1979), however, goes on to suggest that no great generalization about the alcohol consumption curve has empirical validity.

It has been argued previously that one of the better methods of 'testing' the empirical validity of Ledermann's approach involved analysing changes in a population's alcohol consumption over time using longitudinal data. One such study has been carried out in England (Cartwright *et al.*, 1978a, 1978b). A population sample was interviewed in 1965 about drinking problems and habits and was followed up in 1974. The results showed that over the nine-year period, per capita consumption of alcohol increased by 47 per cent. The increase in consumption was not due to an increase in the prevalence of drinking or the frequency with which drinking occurred, but due to an increase in average daily consumption. The results also showed that the increase in mean consumption involved a redistribution of the drinking population into successively higher consumption categories. The 1974 data also showed an increase in alcohol problems and an analysis of variance showed that the increased prevalence of problems in 1974 was due to the population consuming more and this relationship held within demographic sub-groups. These results also showed that the level of alcohol problems varied according to age, sex and occupational status group for similar levels of consumption. Also, those who drank more on average per day were more likely to have high levels of drinking problems. Also of relevance was the finding that after allowing for both total consumption and frequency there was still a difference in the levels of problems reported. The authors suggest that this may be partially explained by individual vulnerability factors.

Now, this evidence appears to support the Ledermann model in the sense that as mean per capita consumption increased so did the level of heavy drinking and the level of alcohol problems. Cartwright *et al.* (1978b) suggest that an alternative explanation to Ledermann's is that the apparent 'fixed' relation between increased consumption and increased problems can be explained by the stability of the underlying drinking patterns. They state:

'Patterns of drinking behaviour are highly related to the demographic structure of a population and reinforced by strong cultural norms which dictate drinking styles. Thus, in a stable culture, drinking patterns are unlikely to change drastically in the short term.'

So whatever sparked off increases in consumption, the stability of underlying drinking practices meant that the population was affected uniformly. More studies of this kind need to be carried out to understand more fully the nature of the relationship between overall consumption and the prevalence of heavy drinking and the prevalence of alcohol-related problems.

Alcohol control policies in the UK

Bruun *et al.* (1975) have identified the following alcohol control measures: age limitations, type and frequency of outlets and hours of sale, alcohol content and type of beverage, marketing and profit seeking, and pricing and taxation. A further control policy involves the use of education.

A number of these measures have been adopted in the UK, but it is always difficult to judge whether they were adopted for public health reasons.

The minimum age for buying alcoholic beverages is 18 years in England and Wales, although children over 14 years of age can go into a bar but not buy or consume alcoholic drinks. How effectively this law is enforced is difficult to ascertain. The retail licensing laws in England and Wales are based on:

> 'the proposition that excisable liquor cannot be supplied or sold in retail quantities to the public without prior authority' (Davies, 1979).

There are four different types of licences: full on licence, restricted on licence, club licence, and off licence.

In England and Wales the licensing laws restrict the hours in which alcoholic beverages may be served or sold on licensed premises. On weekdays, the usual opening hours are 11 a.m.–3 p.m. and 5.30 p.m.–10.30 p.m. (in some places the hours are extended to 11 p.m.) and on Sundays, Good Friday and Christmas Day the hours are limited to 12 noon–2 p.m. and 7 p.m.–10.30 p.m. Compared with the rest of Europe, the United Kingdom has fewer permitted hours during which alcoholic beverages are available than in any of the other European countries; only Ireland, Norway and Sweden have nationally standardized restrictions in permitted hours for the sale and serving of alcoholic beverages (Davies, 1979). Scotland now has marginally longer permitted hours for the sale of alcoholic beverages than England and Wales.

During the early 1970s two government departmental committees, one for England and Wales under the chairmanship of Lord Erroll and one for Scotland under the chairmanship of Clayson, were appointed to examine the licensing laws. The Erroll Committee reported in 1972 and the Clayson Committee in 1973. Both these committees proposed relaxation of the licensing laws. The principle upon which such an approach is based is different to the more traditional approach where licensing laws were used as restrictions to purchase and consume in days when incomes were low. At the present time, when incomes are relatively high, according to Clayson (1977):

> 'The role of licensing laws has changed. Its role now is to mitigate the evils we all see by reducing the pressure to drink; by improving the quality of leisure; by discouraging drinking as an end in itself; and by encouraging moderate drinking as part of some other social activity.'

The Erroll Committee, amongst other recommendations, proposed to reduce the legal age for on-premises consumption from 18 to 17 years and, as an attempt to integrate drinking into the family, recommended that, where the establishment met certain prescribed standards and the licensee was willing, the grant of a children's certificate would allow the family to enter the premises for refreshment (HMSO, 1972). Both of these recommendations were rejected by the Government and the recommendations for liberalization were the focus of much criticism from a variety of different quarters (Robinson, 1974).

With regard to controls on industry's marketing and profit-seeking activities in relation to the manufacture and distribution of alcoholic beverages, the Advertising Standard's Association and the Independent Broadcasting Association require alcohol advertisements to conform with codes of practice which have been changed in recent years. However, this is purely a voluntary agreement between industry and those two bodies at present.

Governments could influence alcohol consumption through changes in taxation on alcoholic beverages and thus through manipulation of the price of alcoholic beverages. In the United Kingdom, regular adjustments to taxation on alcoholic beverages are made, although there is no evidence to suggest that these adjustments occur for reasons of public health or even to influence consumption. Taxation on alcohol is used purely as a source of revenue for the Government. Each type of alcoholic beverage has a different rate of tax. The taxes are excise duties but since the United Kingdom joined the EEC all alcoholic beverages have been subject to VAT.

The excise duty on beer is a basic rate at a certain strength plus a set amount for each additional degree of gravity. Brown (1978) reports the excise rate for beer to be £17.42 per barrel of 36 gallons, plus 58.08 pence for each additional degree. For spirits there is a set amount per proof gallon which is £27.013 per proof gallon (Brown, 1978). For wine the system is more complex. For light wines, under 10 per cent, the excise duty is £3.751 per gallon; for middle wines, 10 per cent to 15 per cent, the excise duty is £3.751 per gallon; but for wines 15 per cent to 18 per cent, it is £4.4165 per gallon (Brown, 1978).

The excise duty on spirits is three times higher than on beer per quantity of alcohol content and the tax on wine is one and a half times that on beer. However, since VAT has been introduced, the spirits : beer tax ratio has decreased but the beer : wine tax ratio has increased. The tax is particularly heavy on imported wine (Brown, 1978). One of the justifications for the higher rate of excise duty on spirits seems to be based on the theory that spirits are potentially more harmful from a physical, moral and social point of view.

The alcoholic content of beer in the UK is on average 3–7 per cent, although the range rises from 2.8 per cent to about 11 per cent. According to Brown (1978), it is estimated that about 90 per cent of all beer consumed is sold in pubs, clubs and restaurants. This is in contrast to spirits and wine, where 50 per cent of spirits and 30 per cent of wine are consumed in licensed premises. Brown (1978) suggests that, as preferred drink is beer and beer is more likely to be consumed in the public house, this pattern of drinking encourages moderation.

Between 1961 and 1977 the Government adjusted the excise duty on beer on eleven different occasions, raising it from £6.15 per barrel at 1030° to its present rate. Over the same period the Government adjusted the tax on spirits on thirteen different occasions, raising it from £11.6 per proof gallon in 1961 to its present level (Brewers' Society, 1979).

Between 1962 and 1979, the price of beer has kept pace with the RPI and only on three occasions during this period has it fallen below it (Brewers' Society, 1979). However, for wines and spirits the picture is different and, throughout this period, prices have consistently lagged behind the RPI.

Davies (1979) shows that the retail price of alcoholic beverages lagged behind increases in the per capita disposable incomes for the period 1971 to 1975, which suggested that the real price of alcoholic beverages had fallen relative to incomes and, in particular, the real price of wine and spirits. However, Davies reports (1979) that in 1976 the retail price of alcoholic beverages rose faster than per capita disposable incomes, making the real cost of alcoholic beverages more expensive. Davies is quick to point out that this was not due to any public health measure but an inadvertent result of economic circumstances.

Once again, this increase in price was a function of economic circumstances rather than due to concern about public health.

Availability of alcoholic beverages may have been controlled in the UK by regular adjustments to taxation and through control over permitted hours in which alcoholic beverages can be sold. These controls are more restrictive than are found in most other European countries and may account for the United Kingdom's relatively low level of alcoholic consumption and low level of alcoholism. However, throughout the period 1973 to 1975 in the UK the real price of some alcoholic beverages has fallen and this might partially account for the sharp increase in consumption since 1970.

As has been stated before, some of these measures may have been introduced for reasons other than for those of alcohol control. However, more recently there has been a series of recommendations from government committees about the prevention of alcoholism which have called for the tightening up of the present controls and the development of other measures specifically in the name of alcohol control. For example, the Advisory Committee on Alcoholism (DHSS, 1977a) recommended the following.

1. Health education designed to alert people to the dangers of alcohol and to discourage excessive drinking should be encouraged and expanded.

2. The presentation of alcohol to society, particularly in advertisements and the media, should be modified to produce a less one-sided picture of its effects.

3. Fiscal powers should be utilized to ensure that alcohol does not become cheaper in real terms.

4. Legal restrictions on the availability of alcohol should be enforced rigorously and should not be relaxed until there is sufficient evidence that to do so would not cause increased harm.

5. People who may be developing drinking problems should be encouraged to recognize these problems and to seek help.

At a similar time, the government consultative document, Prevention and Health (HMSO, 1977b), was published and, as with tobacco, presented a much less strong set of recommendations than those of the House of Commons Expenditure Committee on Prevention (HMSO, 1977a). Once again, as with tobacco, the emphasis was on teaching individuals to look after themselves. Whilst the consultative document emphasized the need to put more government money into health education, it stated:

'Each individual must be responsible for ensuring that his drinking does not lead to harm to his own health and well-being or to harm for others at home, at work or on the roads ... There is a need for a substantial change in social attitudes and more awareness of the dangers of alcohol increase.'

The consultative document rejected the Sub-committee's recommendation to support health education through revenue received from the sale of alcohol but accepted their recommendations that the media should be prepared to present a more balanced approach to alcohol.

The Expenditure Sub-committee also recommended that the price of alcoholic beverages should not fall in real terms to prices and incomes. The consultative document, whilst accepting the link between the price of alcohol and consumption, was more qualified in its conclusions. It states:

'However, the general implications for the government's fiscal, industrial, counter-inflation and social policies would have to be taken into account as would also international considerations.'

It goes on to emphasize the anti-social nature of such policies:

'It might be regarded as unreasonable to penalise the great majority of people who drink without harm in the hope of deterring the minority whose drinking does or might cause harm to themselves or others.'

Finally, the consultative document recommended that a consultative document specifically focusing on alcohol problems should be produced the following year. However, at the time of writing such a document has not been published.

In summary, the Government has yet to produce a comprehensive strategy for the prevention of alcoholism. As with tobacco, it has refrained from pursuing legal and fiscal policies specifically aimed at alcohol control and once again the Government's approach reflects its general approach to health policy, which is that it should be subordinate to other aspects of economic policy.

How effective are alcohol control measures?

The rationale on which many government alcohol control measures are based is that there is a strong association between the level of alcohol consumption in a country and the prevalence of 'heavy' drinking. Public health measures were aimed at reducing general consumption, so as to cut down the prevalence of heavy drinkers. Recent evidence has questioned the existence of such a relationship, at least in the form in which it was originally proposed. So, in the following section two different but interrelated questions need to be asked. First, do these control measures actually influence overall consumption? and, secondly, what impact do these control measures have on the incidence and the prevalence of heavy drinking and associated alcohol problems?

The following control measures will be considered: age limitations, type and frequency of outlet and hours for sale, marketing and profit seeking, monopoly and licensing systems, education, and price and taxation. However, some control measures vary according to beverage type, so beverage type will be considered within each control measure. Differential controls on different types of beverage are based on the assumption that certain types of alcoholic beverage are more likely to cause short- and long-term problems than others. The most common view is that beer is the least harmful and spirits the most harmful of alcoholic beverages. The evidence to support this proposition can be found in Swedish studies (Brown, 1978). These studies have specifically focused on the short-term problems associated with heavy drinking. Some of these studies have looked at the differences in blood alcohol level induced by ingestion of the same quantity of alcohol in different beverage types. Spirits give the highest blood alcohol value, followed by fortified wine, light wine and malt beverages. These studies (Brown, 1978) showed that it was the buffering effects of substances in beer and wine rather than the dilution effect which brought about these differences. This has obvious implications for accident rates. Brown (1978) also presents evidence which shows that subjective feelings of intoxication vary according to beverage type. Subjects were more likely to feel intoxicated after the consumption of whisky than they were after the consumption of wine. More objective evidence suggests that the intoxication effect of alcohol in spirits of 40% alcohol by volume is more than three times that in beer of 5% by volume.

The evidence certainly suggests a relationship between beverage type and drunkenness and beverage type and blood alcohol levels. This relationship supports the contention that spirits are more likely to produce short-term problems than wines or beers.

Differences in the long-term effects of alcohol consumption according to beverage type are more difficult to substantiate. For example, Brown (1978) concludes:

'There are sufficient examples in the literature, however, to at least suggest that long-term effects, as well as short-term effects, vary to some degree depending on the beverage consumed.'

On the other hand, Popham *et al.* (1975) suggest that there is no evidence to support an association between beverage type and liver cirrhosis. They compared countries with similar per drinker rates and examined the relationship between percentage contribution of spirits to total alcohol consumption and liver cirrhosis mortality. Little relationship was found and they conclude:

'that there is no "beverage of moderation" or for that matter a "beverage of excess". Any one of the three types of beverage may be used without a greater or lesser risk of becoming a pathological drinker. Conversely, a dependence on alcohol can be maintained as well on beer or wine as on spirits.'

The degree of differentiation in control measures in a country by beverage type appears to be a function of the preferred beverage type in a country (Brown, 1978). In countries where beer or wine predominate, all beverages are more likely to be treated alike than in those countries where the preferred type of beverage is wine or is mixed. Brown (1978) quantifies this difference and shows that in 'mixed' or 'spirits countries' on average there are 4.4 policy areas where fermented beverages receive preference over distilled beverages, but for 'wine and beer countries' the average is only 1.7 policy areas.

Age limitations
The case for the use of age limitations is that they should be used to postpone the age at which people can legitimately start to drink until as late as is possible. Evidence from research in Canada (Schmidt and Kornaczewski, 1975) showed a reduction in age limit, from 21 to 18 years, was accompanied by a substantial rise in the consumption level of the 18 to 20 age group. Further evidence to support this proposition comes from Smart (1977) who examined changes in alcoholic beverage sales after reductions in the legal drinking age in a number of different states in the US. Comparisons were made between changes in the sales of beers, wine and spirits in twenty-five states which lowered legal drinking ages and adjacent states where no change in the legal drinking age occurred. Most of the states which changed drinking ages had an increase in beer sales, whereas the unchanged ones did not. The increase in beer sales in the 'changed over states' as compared with the 'no change' states was 5.7 per cent. The differences for wine and spirits are not statistically significant.

Apart from increase in consumptions, other measures of 'alcohol' problems such as changes in the incidence of road accidents have been measured against changes in age limits for the drinking of alcohol. For example, Whitehead (1980a) in a review concluded that an increase in the availability of alcohol through a reduction in age limitations has been shown to result in a dramatic increase in alcohol-related problems that are associated with automobile collisions. On the other hand, it is argued that age limitations encourage secret drinking and therefore support the more 'unhealthy' approaches to the use of alcohol (Davies and Stacey, 1972). Bruun *et al.* (1975), in summary of the evidence on the value of age limitations as an alcohol control measure, state that:

> 'Findings suggest that age limits may well exercise a restraining influence and that lowering the legal drinking age may lead to an increase in consumption and alcohol problems if people begin to start drinking younger'

(See also Bourgeois and Barnes, 1980.)

Type and frequency of outlet and hours for sale
In considering the relationship between overall consumption and controls over availability, a methodological problem arises. Changes in availability may have arisen as a result of changes in drinking practices which were produced by social processes. Thus, changes in consumption may be due to changes in drinking practices, as controls of alcohol availability may be mirrors of the latter patterns (Bruun *et al.*, 1975).

In countries such as the UK, it has been assumed that hours of sale are effective ways of controlling problems associated with alcohol. The evidence to support this assumption is difficult to find. For example, a study (Popham *et al.*, 1975) carried out in Toronto found an association between tavern closing hours and patterns of arrest for drunkenness between 8.00 a.m. on Monday and 8.00 a.m. the following Sunday. However, a similar examination of the arrests for drunkenness between 8.00 a.m. on Sunday and 8.00 a.m. on Monday, when the taverns were closed, showed an identical pattern. The authors concluded that the hours of sale reflect the drinking habits of the community rather than vice versa.

The assumption that the more outlets there are for drinking the more people will drink, the higher the rate of consumption will be, and the higher the rate of drunkenness, is also difficult to substantiate. Popham et al. (1975) compared the incidence of alcohol problems with the number of outlets in the USA and England. They found no significant relationship in the predicted direction and in England the evidence suggested a slightly inverse relationship.

In spite of this evidence, which shows no relationship between specific controls on the availability of alcohol and the incidence and prevalence of alcohol problems, there is some evidence of a relationship when more general changes in availability occur. These general changes in alcohol availability include prohibition which occurred in the US, relaxation of previously stringent controls such as occurred in Finland, and strikes in the alcohol industry which occurred in Sweden and Finland. The Swedish strike in 1963 involved the cessation of distribution from the monopoly distribution centre to monopoly stores for three months. This led to the rationing of spirits. Spirit sales eventually fell markedly but wine sales remained constant and beer sales increased. Brown (1978) reports that drunkenness, industrial and road accidents, admission to hospital as a result of alcoholic effects, and the number of liver cirrhosis cases, all fell. The Finnish strike of 1972, too, involved the reduction in the availability of spirits because of a strike in the retail stores. In this case, wine and spirits were not available for domestic consumption but were available in restaurants. Beer was not affected (Brown, 1978). The results of the five-week strike show a marked decrease in the number of arrests for drunkenness but little change (only a slight drop) in overall consumption. Brown (1978) reports that one negative effect of the strike was the increase in the purchasing of distilling equipment and the consequent increase in the illicit production of spirits.

The impact of the strike—the reduction in drunkenness—clearly reflects the drinking practices of the Finns. The preferred beverage in Finland is spirits and the Finns tend to drink heavily at specific times, such as weekends. The Finns, however, do not drink very frequently and their patterns of drinking are borne out by their relatively high rate of alcohol poisoning compared with other Nordic countries (Brown, 1978).

Finland also saw a relaxation of its stringent alcohol control system with the introduction of the Medium Beer Act and the Alcohol Act of 1968. The Acts led to increases in the availability of spirits in rural areas and medium beer was allowed to be sold in food and grocery stores. This latter change was the most significant and, in addition, the minimum age for the off-premises consumption of medium beer was 18 years compared with 20 years for off-premises consumption of other alcoholic beverages (Brown, 1978). The changes were intended to modify the drinking practices of the Finns by encouraging a shift from spirits to beer. However, results have shown a significant increase in the overall consumption of alcohol. Contrary to expectations, the consumption of spirits has continued to rise and beer consumption, whilst initially rising markedly, has levelled off (Bruun *et al.*, 1975) and is now falling (Brown, 1978).

Monopoly and licensing systems
Countries can be differentiated according to whether they have a monopoly system controlled by the government or a licensing system with alcohol production and manufacture being in the hands of private enterprise.

In monopoly systems, the governments vary according to the extent of their control. For example, in France the State has a monopoly for only the purchase and sale of alcohol. However, there is a licensing system which distinguishes between beverage type. Licences involving the selling of less strong alcohol are easier to obtain than 'full' licences, so there are more outlets selling lighter alcoholic drinks (Brown, 1978).

In Finland and Sweden the State has a monopoly over almost the complete process of production, manufacture and distribution of alcohol. The object of the Swedish system is to cut down the harmful effects of alcohol. Brown (1978) lists the basic principles of the Swedish legislation. The emphasis is on discriminating against the sale of stronger drinks, which involves the reduction of the profit motive in the sales of these drinks and a differential system of taxation. The Finnish monopoly system also aims to reduce the harmful effects of alcohol and to cut out illicit production. Not all monopoly systems are organized predominantly to minimize the health and social problems created by alcohol. Some are mainly organized to maximize revenue for the State. Some authors (Popham *et al.*, 1975) have tried to compare the effects of the monopoly system with the licensing system.

Certainly, countries such as Norway do have a relatively low rate of deaths from cirrhosis of the liver compared with other European countries, but in 1974 their rates were no lower than those found in England and Wales, which has a licensing system (Davies, 1979).

Marketing and profit seeking

The consumption of alcoholic beverages has also been related to the expansionist activities of private enterprise such as profit seeking and marketing and distribution.

As has been shown, many countries, for example in Europe—France, West Germany and Switzerland and Austria (Davies, 1979)—have state alcohol monopolies which control the production and/or distribution of alcoholic beverages, although only in Norway, Sweden, Finland and Poland, out of the European countries, is the alcohol state monopoly specifically aimed at the removal of private economic interests from the production and sale of alcoholic beverages. Davies (1979) points out that only in Poland do these controls apply to all alcoholic beverages. He also points out that, even in state alcohol monopolies, there may be a conflict between economic interests and health interests.

According to Bruun *et al.* (1975), there is evidence of a drop in consumption in Sweden, Norway and Finland due to the use of controls on marketing and production. Belgium, Denmark and Sweden have no advertising of any kind on the broadcast media, but advertising of alcoholic beverages is allowed in other forms of media. In Norway, Finland and Czechoslovakia all advertising and promotions of alcoholic beverages are banned. The only control in the UK on marketing and profit seeking is a voluntary agreement on the content of advertising. As with tobacco, there is still uncertainty as to the relationship between advertising and total consumption of alcohol.

Wilkinson (1970) presents evidence on the effects of the 'Babycham' advertising campaign of 1959 which involved the brand owners spending a considerable amount of money promoting this sparkling alcoholic perry. The aim was to influence young women's drinking habits which, according to Wilkinson's anecdotal evidence, it did. Whether it increased drinking or merely changed habits is difficult to judge.

Bourgeois and Barnes (1980), in a brief review of advertising's effects on the consumption of alcohol and cigarettes, concluded:

> 'One thread runs through these studies—namely, that total advertising in a particular industry has not been shown to affect aggregate demand for the products of that industry. But if advertising cannot be shown to affect aggregate demand, why do manufacturers spend millions of dollars on advertising for their brands...'

They suggest that advertising affects brand sales alone, but this conclusion ignores the evidence from the Norweigian experience although in Norway other control measures such as education were also included in a more general programme. The uncertainty about the effect advertising has on the consumption of alcoholic beverages was the justification for a further study by Bourgeois and Barnes (1980) based on Canadian National Statistics.

They, quite rightly, acknowledged the vast range of factors that influence alcohol consumption and attempted to account for many of them in their multivariate analysis. The dependent variables were: per capita consumption of beer, per capita consumption of wine, per capita consumption of spirits and per capita consumption of total alcohol. The independent variables were divided into controllable marketing variables, semi-controllable and non-controllable non-marketing variables. The marketing variables were made up of: print advertising, broadcast advertising, price index, relative (to income) price index, tax index, number of liquor stores, provincial minimum drinking ages and introduction of the breathalyser. The other two types of variable contained a mixture of social, economic, demographic and cultural factors such as disposable income, religion, ethnicity, rate of unemployment, and type of housing.

Results from this study show that more variance was explained by the uncontrollable variables than is explained by the controllable marketing variables. According to Bourgeois and Barnes (1980), of the marketing variables, the level of liquor taxes and the minimum drinking age might be the best ways of reducing per capita consumption.

They also found interrelationships influencing the consumption of beer, wine and spirits—and action taken to reduce consumption in one led to an increase in consumption in another.

The results also showed that whilst there was no significant relationship between the level of print advertising for alcoholic beverages and total per capita consumption of absolute alcohol, a significant relationship was found between the level of print advertising for alcoholic products and per capita consumption of beer. Conversely, there was an inverse relationship between the level of print advertising of alcoholic products and per capita consumption of spirits. Whilst this is interesting in that it apparently indicates that advertising has different effects on drinking habits according to beverage type, it would have been useful to examine per capita consumption of beverage by the level of advertising of that beverage.

The evidence from Bourgeois and Barnes' study (1980) suggests that advertising might not be one of the more powerful influences on consumption, particularly for some types of beverage. However, in relation to the consumption of beer it was the most powerful of the marketing variables and thus may be one of the more practical measures for limiting the consumption of beer that policy makers have available to them.

Education through mass communication

Two mass education campaigns concerned with alcohol control have been carried out and evaluated in the United Kingdom in recent years. However, each campaign had different objectives.

The Health Education Council carried out a campaign in 1974 which was evaluated in the Tyne-Tees area. The campaign, lasting four to five weeks, aimed to create awareness and inform about the dangers of alcoholism through a multi-media campaign (see Gatherer *et al.*, 1979). Pre- and post-advertising interviews were carried out and a third interview was carried out three months later. Seven hundred and fifty street interviews were carried out at the three different stages with those aged between 16 and 45 years.

The results showed that whilst awareness of the campaign was high and there were significant changes in attitude amongst, particularly, the young in the 'right' direction, no long-term beneficial change in teenage drinking habits took place and both frequency and quantity of drinking were increasing. It seems that the campaign achieved its aim of informing people and changing attitudes amongst some groups. However, as has already been emphasized, this does not necessarily lead to a change in behaviour.

The second study (Plant *et al.*, 1979) involved the evaluation of a more ambitious campaign carried out in Scotland in 1976 which aimed to prompt individuals with a drink problem to seek help and to reduce alcohol consumption. Television commercial films were shown in Area A from months 1 to 8 inclusive of campaign and shown in Area B from months 3 to 8. There was also widespread newspaper coverage at the same time. Two surveys were carried out, the first one in month 3 when Area A had received two months exposure to the campaign and Area B had had no exposure. This was followed up by an interview in month 9 when Area A had received eight months exposure and Area B six months. Also, information was collected about clients referred to alcoholism treatment centres in the areas and an analysis was made of all letters sent to the Health Education Agency in response to the campaign. The results showed no general effect on the consumption of alcohol. Also, the television films appeared to have more penetration than the press. Referrals to one council on alcoholism increased by 65 per cent, but this may have been due to a local campaign. The Health Education Agency received on average sixty-seven letters a month in response mainly to the TV commercials.

In summary, the evidence from these two campaigns is that education through the mass media, although showing no significant impact on behaviour in the short term, appears to influence knowledge and sometimes attitudes. By itself it obviously would have a limiting impact on alcohol use but, in combination with other government alcohol control policies, it could help to provide the necessary climate for a change in alcohol consumption.

Price and taxation

Taxing alcohol and thereby increasing its price has been a practice adopted in many countries and the UK is no exception. Although, as has been shown, taxation on alcohol has been used principally for obtaining revenue rather than as a public health measure, the fall in the real price of alcoholic beverages in the UK during the first half of the 1970s further suggests that the annual adjustments to price have been inspired by motives other than those associated with public health.

The relationship between price and alcohol consumption is a complicated one and has received a large amount of attention from researchers. Bruun *et al.* (1975), in their review, concluded that the consumption of alcohol is affected by price level as well as availability. Their rigorous evaluation of the relationship between price and alcohol consumption can be summarized in the following way.

In general, Bruun *et al.* (1975) found that alcoholic beverages seem to behave in consumer markets like any other commodity. The variation in the demand for alcoholic beverages is associated with changes in price and changes in income. As the price of alcohol increases, so demand for alcohol decreases and, as consumer incomes increase, so then the demand for alcoholic beverages increases. So alcoholic beverages can be said to have a relatively high price and income elasticity as demand seems to react strongly to change in one or the other. However, the value or strength of both price and income elasticity of alcoholic beverages varies according to different regions and different periods, as it does between different types of alcoholic beverage. Elasticity values are also affected by the prices of other commodities and by income level and by prevailing alcohol control policies.

Consumer preferences are not homogeneous but vary between individuals and between social groups. Consumer preferences also change over time in response to changing lifestyles, changing marketing practices of the industry and changing control policies.

Further evidence of the association between the consumption of alcohol and the relative price is found in a study examining this association and the relationship to deaths from liver cirrhosis between 1928 and 1967 in Ontario, Canada (Popham *et al.*, 1975). Popham and his co-workers concluded:

> 'The role of relative price was examined in virtually every jurisdiction for which the relevant data were available, both regionally and, where possible, through time. Almost universally relative price was found to be very closely associated with indices of consumption and alcoholism.'

Popham *et al.* (1975), however, do suggest that the relative price of alcohol is not the only important variable responsible for differences in alcoholism prevalence. They suggest indigenous attitudes to alcohol and heavy drinking are also important and illustrate this by pointing to the low level of alcohol consumption in the Netherlands even though prices are relatively low. They account for this in terms of the population intolerance to drunkenness. On the other hand, they suggest that there appear to be no instances of a country having a high consumption with high prices.

One of the best examples which illustrates a relationship between price and consumption of alcohol came from Denmark around the time of the First World War (Neilson, 1965). Due to food shortage, the price of aquavit was raised about twelve-fold whilst that of beer was increased by only about 60 per cent. The alcohol consumption per capita decreased from 6.7 to 1.6 l of absolute alcohol within two years; it was due predominantly to diminished aquavit and only later an increase in beer consumption occurred. In parallel with this marked alteration in consumption, there was a dramatic decline in registered patients with delirium tremens and the death rate from chronic alcoholism dropped from 12 to 2 per 100 000 inhabitants.

Bruun *et al.* (1975) suggest that price reduction, either deliberately to control illicit trafficking or inadvertently through an increase in real incomes, may be harmful particularly because of the dependent nature of drinking alcohol. A temporary relaxation in price control may not be able to be countered by a subsequent increase in price. Control measures can be used to regulate prices of alcohol substitutes as well as their availability and thus make the substitution more attractive. Thus alcoholic beverages drunk with meals could be replaced by non-alcoholic beverages.

A study carried out in Canada (Johnson and Oksanen, 1974), which examined the social and economic determinants of alcohol consumption, showed that both price, which was deflated by the consumer price index, and disposable income were significantly associated with the demand for beer, wines and spirits. However, more important from a control point of view was that the price elasticity of spirits was greater than that of wine. Beer was least affected by price. This, according to Johnson and Oksanen (1974), suggests a need for a differential taxation system. The authors also found that social and cultural factors such as ethnicity, religion and educational level were also associated with consumption. Ethnicity was found to be highly significant in consumption for beer and wine; religion was found to be highly significant in spirits and wine, and level of education was significant in the consumption of spirits but nothing else. This evidence seems to support the proposals of Bruun *et al.* (1975) that for alcohol, control policies should always take into account the values and customs of the various cultural and social groups involved.

This point about the differential price elasticities of alcoholic beverages is important as many countries adopt taxation systems for discriminating against spirits and towards low-alcohol beers. Brown (1978) presents evidence on the relative weights of special taxes by alcoholic beverage within twenty different countries. With the exception of Japan, the weight of taxation is always heavier on distilled products than on beer. Brown quantifies these differences and shows that the mean rate of tax on spirits is 4.5 times higher than that on beer. The average tax on beer is a little higher than that on table wine as many countries do not levy special taxes on wine.

The greater price elasticity of spirits compared with other alcoholic beverages means that governments can apply differential taxation systems without losing revenue because of large price increases. However, if there are no long-term differences in harmful effects according to alcoholic beverage (Popham *et al.*, 1975), then the government may be in a more difficult situation in that it would need to boost the price of beer to such a degree that it may begin to lose a substantial part of its revenue. Thus, governments favour differential taxation of spirits even though it may only serve as a 'social control' measure for reducing drunkenness. Brown (1978) presents further evidence which supports the weak nature of price elasticity for beer. Brown (1978) shows that the weight of taxation, calculated as a percentage of the retail price of beer in a country, bears no relation to the amount of beer consumed. She accounts for this pattern in terms of the dominance of the indigenous populations' traditional drinking practices and preference.

Further evidence on the relationship between the consumption of beer and changes in taxation are shown in Fig. 5.7, which compares the consumption of beer in the UK over the period 1925 to 1978 with changes in taxation on beer. There were three periods in which there was a very rapid rise in taxation—the early 1940s, the early 1960s and the late 1970s. These changes did not appear to be related directly to variation in beer consumption—in particular, depression of beer consumption. Ball (1977), in his review of statistical estimates of the demand for beer, also found a low price elasticity. Data on income or expenditure elasticity showed consistent results with low positive figures for short runs, but one study suggested that, in the long run, income elasticities might be high.

The Finnish Government, as has been shown, attempted to shift the proportion of the population drinking strong alcoholic beverages such as spirits to lower alcoholic beverages such as medium beer. A number of measures were used and one of these was the differential pricing (and taxation) borne more heavily by stronger alcoholic beverages. The Finnish Government hoped for a drop in alcohol consumption with beer accounting for 50 per cent of the alcohol consumed (Brown, 1978). This percentage was achieved, although since then beer has been losing its share of the market, mainly to spirits.

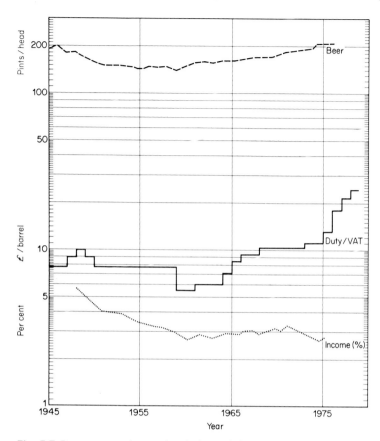

Fig. 5.7 Beer consumption per head of population, percentage of personal income spent on beer, and Excise duty/VAT, UK 1945–78. (Source: Brewers' Society, 1979.)

Summary

Compared with most other European countries, the United Kingdom has a relatively low level of total consumption of alcohol and a low level of heavy drinking. However, over the last decade the UK has witnessed one of the largest increases in alcohol consumption in Europe. The availability of alcohol in terms of the number of permitted hours of drinking in licensed premises and legal age limits is more limited in the UK than in most other European countries. However, there have been no direct restrictions on the manufacture of alcoholic beverages and the real prices of alcoholic beverages have fallen during some periods, even though alcoholic beverages are more heavily taxed in the UK than in most other European countries. The taxation system in the UK discriminates against spirits and in favour of beer. The philosophy behind this system seems to be primarily economic in that it is the most lucrative means of obtaining revenue without risking a drop in consumption.

The two theories of prevention which support the role of government in alcohol control—the integration theory and the Ledermann model—both appear to be incomplete explanations of problems of heavy consumption at the present time (Whitehead, 1980b). Changes in price through taxation appears to be one of the genuine measures of influencing consumption although it has different effects according to beverage type. More evidence of the long-term effects of price control on consumption and on alcohol problems is needed. Further evidence is also required on the relationship between price, consumption and the country's traditional drinking practices. General controls over availability seem to have the effect of controlling drunkenness and associated problems, although once again this effect may be a function of indigenous drinking habits. Further evidence is needed on their long-term impact on consumption and on alcohol problems.

The apparent failure of the UK Government to develop a more comprehensive strategy for alcohol control may be due to:

(i) the lack of convincing evidence to support the effectiveness of alcohol control policies;

(ii) the fact that alcohol problems, in terms of physical harm, appear to be relatively low compared with other countries in Europe.

Recent government reports, however, recommended the reinforcement of present controls because of increasing concern about acute alcohol problems. However, the lack of a coherent policy once again may also reflect the costs of these policies to the Government in terms of a loss of revenue, alienation of a segment of industry, and alienation of a segment of the voting public who drink for pleasure without any harmful effects.

Bruun et al. (1975) identify other costs, such as the use of alternative toxic substances if alcohol is severely controlled. The dose–response relationship between smoking and ill-health implies that long-term public health policy should aim at reducing the prevalence of smoking to as low a level as is possible. In the case of alcohol, it is the heavy drinkers who are at most risk of ill-health and it is to them that the public health policy should be directed.

Certainly, if the Government does adopt more decisive public health measures to reduce total consumption of alcohol, it must ensure that social drinkers are not penalized.

Constituents of food and diet and cancer: policies for prevention

Introduction

In Chapter 3 the evidence suggested that food, food additives and diet may be potential sources of carcinogens. The wide variety of different substances involved which may generate a wide variety of different effects means that some kind of classification is necessary. In this particular context, the classification will be made in terms of implications for prevention and it will be based on the premise that controlling artificial inputs to food and diet is, at least in theory, more straightforward than controlling natural constituents or contaminants. However, as Jukes (1977) points out, the distinction between an additive (artificial) and non-additive is conceptually incorrect. He states, when discussing the value of the Delaney amendment in the US:

'Its existence has focussed attention on certain food additives, while "non-additive" carcinogenic substances in food may be ignored or given tolerances.

There is no rational basis for drawing regulatory distinctions between various carcinogens on the basis of whether they are natural or man-made or present advertently or inadvertently.'

He argues for a more comprehensive appraisal of carcinogens and illustrates this by pointing to the need to assess the relative importance in terms of carcinogenic risk of such natural substances as saturated fats or natural contaminants such as aflatoxin B compared with artificial additives such as saccharin.

Certainly, Jukes is right in the sense that over-exaggeration of the relative importance of artificial additives may be unscientific and present a misleading picture. He is correct also in arguing that a regulatory distinction between additive and non-additive may be conceptually irrational. However, from the point of view of prevention policy, different policies may be needed for controlling, for example, nitrite used as a preservative in meat and nitrite produced through the conversion of nitrates that naturally occur in vegetables, water and soil by human saliva. A recent government report (MAFF, 1978a) suggested that the major source of nitrate in the diet of the average person is vegetables which account for 40–50 per cent of the average person's weekly intake. The level of nitrate in vegetables might be controlled through the regulation of nitrogen fertilizer used in agriculture or through changes in diet, whereas nitrite used as a preservative might be controlled by the regulation of food manufacture. So the classification used here will be based on implications for policy. The classification is 'two-fold'.

(i) Naturally occurring carcinogens which include:
  (a) constituents, e.g. nitrosamines;
  (b) contaminants, e.g. aflatoxins.
(ii) Additives introduced during the manufacture and processing of a product, e.g. cyclamates.

The other dimension which is not accounted for in this classification is carcinogens which are associated with different forms of diet. In this case, the food substances themselves or the combination of substances may put the individual at a higher risk of certain types of cancer, such as the proposed relationship between cancer of the colon and high-fat and low-fibre diets. Dietary 'imbalances' therefore have further implications for policy which are different to the two described in the above.

Food consumption in Britain

In this section, changes in dietary habits and food production and distribution techniques in Britain will be discussed in terms of their implications for risks of different forms of cancer.

With regard to the nature of food production, the food industry, like the alcohol and tobacco industries, is predominantly concerned with economic as opposed to public health concerns. Food, unlike tobacco and alcohol, is a basic need in the sense that it is essential for the long-term maintenance of human life. However, with the Industrial Revolution there developed a large consumer market, particularly in urban areas; this generated the need for mass production and thus the beginnings of the food industry. With the increasing mass production and distribution of food, food itself became a market commodity.

As a result of this change, levels of malnutrition have decreased markedly and there now exists an attractive and varied diet for a large proportion of consumers. However, this expansion of the food industry also has had some deleterious effects.

Doyal (1979) points to a number of different aspects of present-day food production and manufacture which may increase the consumers' exposure to harmful agents. The increasing use of chemicals in agriculture such as in fertilizers, insecticides, herbicides and fungicides, not only has made the industry less labour intensive and provided further market outlets for the chemical industry, but has meant that the food product which finally reaches the consumer may contain additives which may contaminate. Doyal (1979) also highlights the dramatic increase in food processing in the UK since the Second World War. She argues that, if the product has to be marketed nationwide, it must be identical wherever it is sold in terms of taste and quality and it must be able to withstand travel and have a long shelf life. To meet these needs, artificial flavourings and preservatives are added to food products. Some of these additives may be a health risk.

Doyal (1979) identifies another function of artificial flavourings and additives. She argues that the food manufacturer's need to create a new product to expand demand has also led to the increasing use of flavourings and additives.

In relation to cancer, as has been suggested, the importance of artificial additives compared with natural constituents and contaminants has yet to be appraised. However, the increasing use of additives may have created an additional contribution to carcinogenic risk, although their benefits in terms of reducing natural hazards in food, and reducing wastage, may outweigh the costs (Frazer, 1977).

Truswell (1979) has identified the following dietary recommendations for cancer prevention. Cancer of the oesophagus—less alcohol, but no recommendation for reduction in consumption of a specific type of beverage; breast cancer—less fat, less obesity, and slower growth in childhood; cancer of the colon—less fat, less grilled meat, more fibre (which type?); cancer of the rectum—less stout (beer); cancer of the endometrium—less obesity and less fat; cancer of the stomach—less nitrate or salt, less fermented foods, more refrigerated foods, more salad, fresh fruit, milk; cancer of the liver—avoidance of mouldy foods (aflatoxins); cancer of the lung—adequate vitamin A.

Changes in the British diet over the last 100 years have been significant (Oddy and Miller, 1976). Perhaps the most marked trends have been a decline in the volume of fibre consumed and an increase in the consumption of refined carbohydrates (mainly sugar) and fat, each of which has been implicated in the aetiology of various different cancer sites (Doyal, 1979). Dietary patterns are primarily functions of social, cultural and economic considerations; changes can be accounted for in terms of the change in social structure and population growth (Elton, 1976). However, within British society, such changes influence different social groups in different ways. Doyal (1979) shows that the diets of poorer groups are much higher in sugar intake, white bread and potatoes but lower in brown bread intake and fruit intake than more affluent groups. For Doyal (1979), this suggests that these changes in dietary habits, that have occurred over the last 100 years, have affected the poorer groups disproportionately. However, the 'diseases of affluence', such as coronary heart disease, have also been associated with certain lifestyles and dietary patterns which include increases in the consumption of fats.

The most rapid change in eating habits in the UK has occurred during the post-Second World War period (Barker, 1978). In terms of packaging and storage of food, frozen foods have replaced tinned, pickled and fresh foods.

The increase in 'instant' foods has cut down the time spent preparing and cooking food. In addition, the range of foods available has expanded markedly, especially the increasing availability of foreign and continental-style foods either for consumption at home or in restaurants.

The reasons for such a rapid expansion in eating habits are complex. Factors such as changes in disposable incomes, the relative prices of fresh food compared with packaged food (Winegarten, 1978), the increasing geographical mobility of the consumer, the increasing complexity of lifestyles in post-industrial societies, the availability of a wider range of food products, plus the increasing sophistication of the food industry's promotion practices, all must play a part in influencing consumer tastes.

Apart from the change in the composition of diets indicated previously, it is difficult to judge whether these changes in eating practices have increased or reduced the consumer's exposure to hazards which are potentially carcinogenic. For example, the methods of storing and containing foods may be more hygienic and as such have reduced the risk of contamination, but the actual form of container may in itself be a health risk. For example, in the United States the use of acrylonitrile plastic for the bottling of beverages was banned due to the risk of carcinogenicity after these bottles had been marketed for over a year (see. Epstein, 1979).

Government policy for food and diet in the UK

Control of food constituents, contaminants and additives

The early 1950s saw the beginnings of the development in the United Kingdom of a complicated government apparatus designed to control food constituents, contaminants and additives. The most significant legislation was the Food and Drugs Act of 1955. The basic principles of this legislation were the protection of health and the prevention of consumer exploitation (Yellowlees, 1976). Section I prohibits the addition of any substance to food, the use of any substance as an ingredient in the preparation of food, the abstraction of any constituent from food, or the subjection of food to any other process or treatment, so as to render the food injurious to health. Section 2 prohibits the sale of any food which is not of the nature, substance and quality of the food demanded by the purchaser and Section 6 prohibits the use of a label or advertisement which falsely describes a food or misleads as to its nature, substance or quality, including its nutrition or dietary value. Section 8 prohibits the sale of food unfit for human consumption.

In the areas which each of these different sections cover, a series of regulations and acts has been passed over the last twenty-five years. The Act gives ministers the powers to make regulations covering:
   (i)   the composition of food, including claims for benefits or qualities of food;
   (ii) treatments or processes; and
   (iii) hygiene.

The Minister of Agriculture, Fisheries and Food takes the lead in making regulations dealing with composition and labelling, whilst the Secretary of State for Social Services takes the lead where the subject matter is hygiene (Giles, 1976).

Since 1955 the Act has been supplemented by a number of minor Acts which cover any gaps—Lead in Food Regulations (1959) Act and the Arsenic in Food Regulations (1961)—which lay down the maximum levels of lead and arsenic allowed in food. The Imported Food Regulations (1968) Act prohibits the import of food injurious to health. More recently, the Materials and Articles in Contact with Food Regulation Act (1978) has been passed which concentrates on controlling dangerous constituents of food packaging and other materials.

Several government committees have been set up in an advisory capacity to advise government departments on various aspects of food policy. The Food Standards Committee and the Food Additives and Contaminants Committee (FACC) advise principally the Ministry of Agriculture, Fisheries and Food. The terms of reference of the Food Standards Committee are:

> 'To advise the Minister of Agriculture, Fisheries and Food, the Secretary of State for Social Services, the Secretary of State for Social Services, the Secretary of State for Scotland and the Secretary of State for Northern Ireland on the composition, description labelling and advertising of food with particular reference to the exercise of powers conferred on Ministers by Sections 4, 5 and 7 of the Food and Drugs Act and the corresponding provisions in enactments relating to Scotland and Northern Ireland' (Ward, 1976).

This Committee is an independent body and was founded in 1947. Of more interest is the Committee on Food Additives and Contaminants which was set up in 1964. Its terms of reference are as follows:

> 'To advise the Minister of Agriculture, Fisheries and Food, the Secretary of State for Social Services, the Secretary of State for Scotland, and as respects Northern Ireland, the Head of the Department of Health and Social Services, on matters referred to them by Ministers in relation to food contaminants, additives, and similar substances which are, or may be, present in food or used in its preparation, with particular reference to the exercise of powers conferred on Ministers by Sections 4, 5 and 7 of the Food and Drugs Act 1955 and corresponding provisions in enactments relating to Scotland and Northern Ireland' (Weedon, 1976).

Weedon (1976) states that the Committee normally deals with chemical contaminants such as lead and arsenic and defines an additive as:

> 'a substance which is not natural to a food but which is added to it represents in essence what is generally understood by an additive'.

The Chairman states (Weedon, 1976) the role of the Committee as far as contaminants are concerned:

> 'is to encourage good agriculture, manufacturing and handling techniques so as to eliminate contamination of food as far as possible, or to reduce to a minimum the quantities that are unavoidable by setting limits as low as practicable'.

In the case of additives, Weedon (1976) states that regulation occurs through statutory permitted lists. The manufacturer has to satisfy the FACC on these counts:

(i) there is a real technological need for the additive and that this need could not be met by a substance which has already been permitted, or by use of different production techniques which would obviate the need for it;

(ii) that the additive is not a health hazard;

(iii) that details for defining the purity standards of the substance for use in food are available.

Goldenberg (1977) describes the series of consultations which are involved in this process of assessment of 'need' for a new additive. These consultations involve discussions with (i) consumer organizations, (ii) enforcement authorities, (iii) representations from individual firms, (iv) assessment by research associations, and (v) industrial food chemists and technologists.

So the emphasis is on the manufacturer providing proof of a technological need for the additive and proof of its safety before it is placed on the permitted list. These lists are reviewed every five years and, according to Roe (1973), on each review substances are classified into six different groups according to the nature of the evidence which identifies potential risk of toxicity.

The first group contains additives where the evidence suggests acceptability for use in food. The second group contains additives where evidence suggests provisional acceptability but further information is necessary and the position should be reviewed. Two groups contain additives which are possibly and probably toxic and it is recommended that they are not to be allowed in food. The final two groups contain additives which either cannot be evaluated as the data are inadequate or no information on toxicity is available at all.

According to Goldenberg (1977), some classes of additives are not controlled by the permitted list and are subject to the general provisions of the Act which states that it is illegal to use a substance which renders food injurious to health or to sell food which is unfit for human consumption. It is not clear how naturally occurring constituents such as nitrosamines would be controlled by the Act. Additives which were originally permitted but have been withdrawn from the permitted lists include brominated vegetable oils, various types of colouring agent, and cyclamates.

Roe (1973) also points out the nature of the evidence used to assess carcinogenicity. He states that the evidence used should be based on:

'Long-term feeding tests at several dose levels on two species of animal with adequate survival and complete histopathological evaluation is normally required.'

Roe states that a significant excess of malignant neoplasms in a test group as compared to a negative control group would lead to the additive not being permitted for use in food, irrespective of all other considerations. Roe (1973) states that in cases where no human data are available:

'It is normal to require evidence of no toxic effect in animals of levels of incorporation in food 100 times higher than those proposed for man. This factor may be reduced to 10 where satisfactory human data are available.'

The practical problem, when assessing the risks of permitting many additives in food, is primarily the lack of hard human data. In many cases, as Roe suggests, permitted tolerance levels have to be extrapolated from animal studies. For example, one additive that was banned by the Ministry of Agriculture, Fisheries and Food was the sweetener cyclamates in 1969. The FACC recommended the ban which came into force on 1st January 1970. The ban came as a result of a report from the US Food and Drugs Administration where cyclamates had already been banned. There was considerable controversy about the ban as the evidence on which the ban was based was on animal studies and there was no evidence to say that cyclamates can cause cancer in man.

Cyclamates were permitted in the UK in 1964 in soft drinks and sweetening tablets. They were used as non-calorie artificial sweeteners. They could be used particularly by those who were dieting as a slimming aid, or by diabetics and people suffering from obesity as an alternative to saccharin. Compared with the US and Canada where there were no controls over its use in most foods, the use of cyclamates was much more restricted in the UK. The FACC had produced reports on cyclamates on a number of occasions prior to 1968 but there were no suggestions that the evidence warranted a ban. The ban on cyclamates in the UK and in other countries was based on evidence from animal studies carried out in the US. The results from these studies were as follows:

'Male rats fed a 10 : 1 cyclamate–saccharin mixture for 105 weeks developed bladder tumours, some of which were malignant at the highest dose level tested—i.e. 2500 mg/kg body weight. Subsequent experiments confirmed the presence of this activity in rats for cyclamate alone at dose levels as low as 400 mg/kg body weight' (DHSS, 1970).

Considerable problems were involved in the interpretation of these results, particularly because of the species-specific responses of the bladder to a variety of chemical agents. As the DHSS commented (1970):

'None of the known human bladder carcinogens acts in a like manner on the rat bladder.'

According to the same report, the decision to ban was based on incomplete evidence. The report states (DHSS, 1970):

'Clearly prudence has to be exercised where human health is concerned but it is frequently impossible to back up a final decision by scientifically unassailable arguments. As cyclamates are not an essential food additive it was considered wrong to persist with their use while alternative artificial sweeteners—e.g. saccharins—are available.'

The justification for an immediate ban rather than procrastination was on the grounds of the long incubation period of malignant disease after exposure of man to some carcinogens and the lessons learnt from the cigarette and naphthylamine (DHSS, 1970). It appears that when evidence from animal studies creates reasonable doubt then action is necessary.

Stronger evidence may have been necessary to support the ban if saccharin had not been available. Certainly, the soft drinks industry, amongst others, may have put up stronger opposition if it had not been available. The failure to ban saccharin in the United States was due in part to the strength of the industry lobby. The implications of this are that much firmer scientific evidence on relative risk is needed from both animal and human studies which can be used as a basis for the policy decision. At present, the inadequacy of much evidence means that decisions can be heavily influenced by economic and political interests. Certainly, social and economic factors should be taken into account when assessing the costs and benefits of a policy decision, but these factors have to be taken into account after the scientific evidence on the potential health hazard is evaluated.

More recently, the FACC have been considering the use of nitrites and nitrates in cured meats and cheese (1978). The foods to which nitrates and/or nitrites can be added in restricted quantity are controlled by the Preservatives in Food Regulations (1975). Once again, the evidence on the carcinogenic nature of nitrites is derived from animal studies. One of the functions of nitrite is to prevent botulism (Culliton and Waterfall, 1978); it is necessary therefore to weigh up the costs and benefits of banning it. One of the recommendations of the British FACC in its white paper on the use of nitrites and nitrates in cured meats and cheese was as follows:

'Every effort should continue to be made to eliminate the use of nitrate and reduce nitrite levels as soon as practicable and with this in mind the position should be reviewed no later than two years from the date of publication of this Report' (Food and Contaminants Committee, 1978).

Over the last five years the Ministry of Agriculture, Fisheries and Food has begun to take increasing interest in the problem of food contamination and a steering group has been set up specifically to look at this topic (MAFF, 1978b). As a result of this interest, a working party on vinyl chloride content of food packaging and its dangers for food consumption was set up and produced a report in 1978 (MAFF, 1978a). The main concern was with the amount of vinyl chloride used in PVC food containers. This report showed that PVC was used in food for bottling mainly liquid foods, in rigid film (mainly tubs), flexible film, bottle closure liners, lacquered foods and heat aluminium foil. The results of the survey indicated that the maximum likely intake per person of vinyl chloride from foods packaged in PVC is very small (May 1976—0.1 μg/day). But perhaps the most interesting result was the significant reductions in the amount of vinyl chloride used in PVC containers due to changes in manufacturing and processing methods. Between April 1974 and February 1977 the proportion of PVC bottles containing less that 1 mg/kg of vinyl chloride changed from 0 per cent to 100 per cent. It must be emphasized that this was as a result of co-operation on a voluntary basis between industry and the Government.

A similar type of report was carried out on vinylidene chloride levels in food contact materials and in foods (MAFF, 1980). Vinylidene chloride (VDC) is used mainly in food packaging, such as in films used to vacuum package poultry and meats and as a coating on a variety of traditional packaging materials. The Survey found that the levels of VDC found in food were restricted to certain types of food only and the levels of VDC detected were very low. The maximum possible (overestimate) daily intake of VDC per capita from food was estimated at no more than 1 mg/day.

Other government advisory committees exist to provide the Government with expertise on the more medical aspects of food policy. These are the Committees on Medical Aspects of Food Policy, on Mutagenesis, on Toxicity and on Carcinogenesis. The latter Committee's terms of reference are as follows:

'(1) To assess and advise on the carcinogenetic risk to man of substances which are:
   (a) used or proposed to be used as food additives, or used in such a way that they might contaminate food through their use or natural occurrence in

agriculture, including horticulture and veterinary practice, or in the distribution, storage, preparation or packaging of food;

(b) used or proposed to be used, or manufactured or produced in industry, agriculture, food storage or any other work place;

(c) used or proposed to be used as household goods or toilet goods and preparations;

(d) used or proposed to be used as drugs, when advice is requested by the Medicine Commission, Section 4 Committees or the Licensing Authority (in accordance with the Medicines Act);

(e) used or proposed to be used or disposed of in such a way as to result in pollution of the environment.

(2) To advise on important general principles or new scientific discoveries in connection with carcinogenic risks, to co-ordinate with other bodies concerned with the assessment of carcinogenic risks and to present recommendations for carcinogenicity testing.'

The activities of the above advisory committee are not published so it is difficult to know how they do their work. This is an example of a general problem in this area where information on the activities of some government committees is not publicly available. In the United States, in contrast, the 1973 amendments to the 1967 Freedom of Information Acts make it possible for concerned citizens to obtain copies of documents on the basis of which agencies make decisions and regulatory policies (Epstein, 1979).

The justification for keeping the information, which these advisory committees use to make their decisions about what constitutes a risk and what does not, secret is probably that making the information publicly available might lead to the creation of a number of unwarranted health 'scares' which may have a harmful impact. It might be argued that these 'scares' would be generated by lay people who do not have the expertise to evaluate the scientific evidence. Thus, not publishing these materials is justified on the grounds that it would cause more harm than good.

On the other hand, it may be possible to present the evidence in a manner which is comprehensible to the majority of people. In addition, publication of the work of the committee which would involve declaration of the topic being studied, the information being reviewed, the weight given for various positive/negative results obtained and the overall judgement made about the degree of risk to humans from the agent involved, would mean that these procedures could be openly evaluated by others in the scientific community. This could lead to further information being provided by outside sources which may have been misjudged or ignored by the committee. Also, information from experts not represented on the committee may also be of some use. Publication of procedures and decisions would also place the committees above any accusation that might suggest certain interests are being protected through secrecy.

In summary, the legislation in the UK gives government departments powers to ban additives that are injurious to health and contaminants, both intentional and unintentional (such as pesticide residue), and natural constituents which render them unfit for human consumption. The problem here is in the definition 'injurious to health' and 'unfit for human consumption'. Certainly, some substances have levels of intake which are not dangerous to humans. It is also unclear if government committees are concerned or would be concerned with natural constituents in food which are potentially carcinogenic and how they would go about regulating their use. Although the recent government committee on food contamination (MAFF, 1978b) has discussed the use of total diet studies which monitor average intake of food, it gives no indication of the range of contaminant intakes in the population as a whole. For Truswell *et al.* (1978), in a review of evidence from a Swedish conference on food and cancer, suggested that:

'Of the potential sources of harm in foods the largest by far are microbiological contamination and, next, nutritional imbalance. Risks from environmental contamination are about 1000 times less and risk from pesticide residues and food additives can be estimated as about a further 100 times smaller again.'

They suggest that naturally occurring compounds in food are far more important as potential agents of toxicity than intentional additives.

One obvious problem with focusing on natural constituents and contaminants is the difficulty of obtaining scientific data on their harmfulness. Also, unlike additives where permitted lists provide regulation, in the case of natural contaminants and constituents it may be a matter of trying to change practices in agriculture and husbandry or even to change domestic practices for keeping, preparing and cooking food.

Dietary imbalance

Only in recent years has the UK Government attempted to develop a comprehensive dietary policy. In the discussion booklet on Eating for Health (DHSS, 1978) much of the emphasis was on the relation between diet and coronary heart disease; mention was made of the possible association between low-fibre diets and cancer of the large bowel and diverticulitis.

Once again, when laying out their dietary recommendations, emphasis is placed on the individual's responsibility for maintaining a balanced diet. No mention is made of policies on food production and processing or establishing dietary goals to which food or the agricultural industries could adhere. There is no mention of the difference in diets between different groups due to social and economic inequalities, nor any indication of how this could be rectified. Emphasis is placed on individuals cutting down on fats and sweet foods and eating a diet consisting of a mixture of foods from: cereals, milk and dairy foods, fruit and vegetables, fat and oils, meat, fish, and non-dairy fats and oils. Special mention is made of the problem of obesity and also the need to eat more bread, fish, fruit and vegetables; these might replace fatty and sweet foods.

A number of these recommendations have implications for cancer, but cancer was just one of many diseases for which these dietary principles were designed. One major difficulty is the development of a general set of dietary principles which take into account the necessary details for those at high risk of specific diseases. This is of particular relevance for cancer as different dietary imbalances may be associated with different cancer sites.

In summary, it is evident that the Government's role in attempting to influence food choice is through propaganda and control over standards. Wheeler (1978) clearly identified the role the British Government has taken in influencing food choice. She states:

'Government may intervene to subsidise a certain sector of agriculture, or to stabilise food prices against sudden fluctuations; but these are economic manipulations, carried out irrespective of any nutritional considerations . . .'

She goes on:

'Government food price policies do not at present include any bias towards "good" and away from "bad" food, unless we argue that the tax on alcohol represents a judgment about the balance between the social costs and benefits of its consumption.'

Wheeler acknowledges the presence of some legislative controls but says they are passive rather than innovative. They do not attempt to change dietary habits. She states:

'There is legislation for reinforcing the nutrient content of some foods (flour and salt for example) and for clean, non-contaminated food without noxious additives. But this "health and hygiene" legislation is all designed to maintain good standards in the foods which we already like and choose to eat.'

As Wheeler (1978) argues, in contrast to the aggressive attitude of food producers, the Government has taken a passive position on influencing food choice. Wheeler also questions whether the Government has the legislative apparatus to influence food and agricultural policy. One problem with dietary policy, as with other aspects of food policy, is the lack of scientific data upon which rational decisions can be made. Foster (1973) argues that there is a need for more research funds to be injected into the area of food safety which would attract many more scientists. One way of attempting to change beliefs and practices is through education but, as yet, in this country there is no evidence to assess the relative value of (i) mass communication, (ii) group education, (iii) individual instruction with regard to changing dietary practices.

Alternative government policies for the control of food and diet in relation to cancer prevention

Control of food constituents, contaminants and additives

In the United States, the Food and Drug Administration (FDA) is responsible for the control of food and animal feed additives, cosmetics and drugs. Under an Act of 1938, the FDA has the power to prohibit the sale of food which contains natural substances or additives which are potentially harmful to health. An anti-cancer clause, commonly called the Delaney Amendment, was subsequently attached to the 1938 Act. This clause states that:

'No additive shall be claimed to be safe if it is found to induce cancer when ingested by man or animal, or if it is found after tests which are appropriate for the evaluation of safety of food additives to induce cancer in man or animal.'

This clause has been invoked on several occasions and the powers of the FDA under the Delaney Amendment were actually thwarted in the case involving the intention to ban saccharin (Epstein, 1979). Despite its infrequent use, the Delaney Amendment has come under fire from a number of different quarters (see Hutt (1979) for detailed discussion). Jukes (1979) suggests that the legislation ignores both the natural constituents and contaminants and places an exaggerated emphasis on 'additives'. Jukes also suggests that the clause does not recognize a no-effect level of a carcinogen and suggests that there must be a threshold level for carcinogens. Roe (1973), in a more detailed discussion of the issue, outlines the assumptions upon which the Delaney Amendment is based. Roe (1973) states:

'Nobody knows whether there is a threshold dose for any carcinogen below which it produces no effect. However, it is widely assumed that the effect of a carcinogen is irreversible and that the effects of a series of exposures to a carcinogen are cumulative.'

Roe (1973) then suggests that the assumptions are unrealistic. He states:

'This regulation would make good sense (1) if it were possible to distinguish absolutely between carcinogens and non-carcinogens by means of animal tests, (2) if it were possible to devise a diet that was free of naturally occurring carcinogens, and (3) if the effects of carcinogens were really irreversible.'

An additional problem, as has been shown in the case of the banning of cyclamates, is the validity of extrapolating from animal studies to humans (see Foster, 1973).

For Roe (1973), the answer lies with the assessment of relative safety and risk:

'Commonsense as well as data from animal studies should be used to devise a diet for humans that carries the least overall carcinogenic risk from all sources— food constituents as well as additives and contaminants.'

In the case of natural constituents or natural contaminants, some of the problems of control are more difficult. A good example of the various different regulatory problems involved can be found through examination of attempts to control the natural contaminant aflatoxin. Linsell (1979) has outlined the various stages which are necessary in the investigation of a dietary carcinogen. These are as follows:

(i) identification as carcinogen—through animal studies of toxicity, carcinogenicity and mutagenicity;

(ii) identification of human exposure—dietary availability demonstrated;

(iii) association with specific human tumour—correlation studies;

(iv) intervention programmes:
  (a) monitor exposure and trends of incidence,
  (b) prevent contamination;

(v) eradication of the cancer—primary prevention.

Whilst Linsell (1979) does go through each of the above stages in his account of how aflatoxin was identified as a human carcinogenic agent, it is on the fifth stage that the following discussion will focus. There are two types of decision which involve the control of aflatoxin. These are, according to Linsell:

(i) regulations to prevent contaminated foods reaching the markets of industrialized countries where food supplies are centralized—these foods can either be directly exported or exported in the form of animal feeds;

(ii) primary prevention for developing countries where populations live off the food that they grow themselves.

Much more progress has been made in the control of contaminated goods reaching developed countries. Before this is discussed, it is necessary to identify a problem which has implications for both types of decisions. Restrictions on the production of foods such as peanuts in some developing countries has serious economic implications. Some of these foods not only are the staple diet for the indigenous population, and provide important sources of protein, but provide important sources of revenue when they are exported directly or in the form of animal feed. In countries such as The Gambia, Nigeria and Senegal, the estimated percentage of the population involved in the groundnut industry in each country is > 60 per cent, 35–40 per cent and 70 per cent, respectively (Linsell, 1979).

With regard to the control of contaminated foods reaching industrialized countries, Linsell (1979) suggests that the most significant controls are on imports rather than through domestic production. For example, in the UK the port health authorities have been monitoring aflatoxin in groundnuts since the 1960s and, in 1973, 13 per cent of all groundnut imports were found to contain aflatoxin in amounts exceeding 0.05 mg/kg and were not used for direct human consumption (MAFF, 1978b). Linsell (1979) shows the wide choice in tolerance levels accepted by different countries and some have insisted on a zero level. He states that the zero limit for food is usually 5 mg/kg and 10–100 mg/kg for feeds. The EEC tolerance limits for aflatoxin B in animal feed is not more than 50 mg/kg for any type of feed to any type of farm animal. As Linsell (1979) points out, this involved the lowering of maximum limits in some countries which may have considerable economic implications for exporters to EEC countries. The effectiveness of these controls can only be assessed by careful monitoring.

The second form of control, that is the control over the production of these foods so as to reduce the risk of exposure to the indigenous population, has made little headway. According to Linsell (1979), this may constitute the greater risk and, although methods for improving husbandry and agricultural practices do exist, they need to be implemented.

The example of aflatoxin not only illustrates the various types of regulatory procedure needed for the control of natural contaminants but also emphasizes the necessity to examine the social and economic consequences of policy decisions. In the case of aflatoxin, restrictions on the use of food substances by the indigenous populations may not only be difficult to implement but may constitute a health risk in that they may involve depriving the population of an important constituent of its diet. In addition, such restrictions may also involve depriving the economy of a large source of revenue which could in itself provide the funds for supporting public health programmes.

Dietary policies for cancer prevention
Several countries, in particular Sweden, Finland and the US, have attempted to develop more comprehensive and rigorous sets of guidelines for a dietary policy. In the last few years the US Government has produced a set of dietary goals (1977) which have recently been amended (1978). They are as follows:

(i) to avoid overweight, consume only as much energy (calories) as expended; if overweight, decrease energy intake and increase energy expenditure;

(ii) to increase the consumption of complex carbohydrates and 'naturally occurring' sugars from about 28 per cent of energy intake to about 48 per cent of energy intake;

(iii) to reduce the consumption of refined and processed sugars by about 45 per cent to account for about 10 per cent of total energy intake;

(iv) to reduce overall fat consumption from approximately 40 per cent to about 30 per cent of energy intake;

(v) to reduce saturated fat consumption to account for about 10 per cent of total energy intake; and balance that with poly-unsaturated and mono-unsaturated fats, which should account for about 10 per cent of energy intake each;

(vi) to reduce cholesterol consumption to about 300 mg a day;

(vii) to limit the intake of sodium by reducing the intake of salt to about 5 g a day.

Wheeler (1978) reports that the McGovern Committee also recommended a more aggressive government position through:

'(i) government funding of education programmes related to dietary goals;

(ii) requiring labelling of foods in terms of fat, sugar cholesterol, salt and energy content;

(iii) setting up of a joint agriculture health committee to consider the implications for agricultural policy of subjects of concern in nutrition and health.'

The problem, once again, with these dietary goals is the lack of evidence to support them. Wheeler (1978) argues that the evidence supports only goal (vi) in terms of possible benefit to some people. Simopoulos (1979), too, questions the scientific basis of the Dietary Goals. He suggests that the concept of universal dietary goals is a mistaken one and what is needed are specific dietary guidelines aimed at specific groups.

It is evident then that before dietary goals are formulated by governments, there is a need for more research evidence to be collected and collated. This evidence can be used as a basis for policy formation. However, attempts to formulate a more comprehensive food and nutrition policy aimed at influencing both the practices of the food industry and the dietary practices of the general public form a more rational approach to prevention than merely supporting *ad hoc* propaganda aimed at informing individuals about 'health' diets.

Summary

There exists in the UK a complicated machinery aimed at controlling the use of additives and contaminants in food. The effectiveness of this machinery is difficult to assess. The system of regulation is through permitted lists and each new additive has to justify being placed on the list on a number of different counts. The lists are reviewed five-yearly. Cyclamate is an example of an additive which was banned in the UK but this decision was seen to be controversial as it was said to be based on inadequate evidence. The lack of hard animal and human data in this area, and in the area of dietary control, imposes serious difficulties in the interpretation of data and the evaluation of their implications for policy. This lack of hard human data has meant that regulations in the US which contain an anti-cancer clause have had to base their decisions on animal data. Thus, this form of legislation has come under increasing attack over the correctness of decisions. In addition, the notion of complete safety which this legislation appears to support has been criticized for being impractical and unrealistic.

No coherent government policy for diet has been developed by the UK Government. This may be due to the lack of adequate scientific information, although it may also be due to the emphasis on the idea in governmental philosophy that the responsibility for health lies with the individual.

Evidence for effective methods of influencing dietary practices are difficult to find. Further research is needed to evaluate the importance of government fiscal policy, controls over availability and different types of education campaign in influencing dietary practices. Evidence is also needed on the efficacy of national dietary goals as opposed to dietary programmes aimed at specific at-risk groups and at the prevention of specific illnesses.

Medicines and cancer: policies for prevention

Government control of medicines in the UK

No legal controls or sanctions on medicines existed in the United Kingdom until 1968. Before that time there was no legal restriction apart from those listed under the Therapeutic Substances Act on what drugs or medicines were used and any medicine, irrespective of how dangerous or how inadequately tested it was, could be marketed. However, as a result of the thalidomide disaster, and its eventual withdrawal from the UK market in 1961 (see Sjostrom and Nilsson, 1972), more concern was expressed about the need to institute controls over the marketing of drugs.

As a result, in 1963 the Committee on Safety of Drugs was set up and its functions were basically threefold. They were to:

(i)   advise whether a new drug should be submitted for clinical trials;
(ii) advise whether a new drug should be released for marketing;
(iii) carry out studies of adverse reactions to drugs in general use.

This was essentially an advisory committee and the pharmaceutical industry was not legally obliged to submit its drugs for pre-market approval. This advisory committee was eventually taken over by the Committee on the Safety of Medicines which was set up in 1971 by the Medicines Commission under the 1968 Medicines Act (HMSO, 1979b). This Act had been introduced by the Government to secure better controls over the safety, quality and efficacy of medicinal products for human and veterinary use, the circumstances in which they are sold or supplied, their labelling and description, and their sales promotion. Under the 1968 Act, all persons wishing to market medicines have to hold a product licence, the grant of which is determined primarily by reference to the criteria of safety, efficacy and quality. The Medicines Commission set up the Committee on the Safety of Medicines to advise on safety, efficacy and quality of medicinal products for human use for which licences or certificates are sought under Part II of the Act. From 1st September 1971, no new medicinal product could be marketed without a product licence and no clinical trial could be initiated without a clinical trial certificate.

For medicines which are already on the market, and have either passed through the product licensing system or through previous machinery before 1st September 1971, irrespective of safety, quality, efficacy, there is what is called 'an adverse reaction reporting system'. This system, initiated by the Committee on Safety of Drugs and carried on by the Committee on Safety of Medicines, is a voluntary reporting system. Doctors are asked to report any abnormal or serious event following the use of a drug and to report all but trivial events with recently introduced drugs (Inman and Vessey, 1978). In addition, reports are received from drug companies, from copies of death certificates received from OPCS, and from papers sent to the Committee before publication.

Inman and Vessey (1978), in their account of the adverse monitoring system, identify a number of weaknesses. They argue that the major weakness is the under-reporting of adverse reactions. Failure to report may be due to a high threshold of suspicion by prescribers or may be due to unwillingness to make a report even though an adverse reaction has been identified. Inman and Vessey (1978) suggest that some of the reasons for the occurrence of the latter type of behaviour may be due to ignorance about the Committee's requirements, fear of involvement in litigation or in investigation of prescribing practice, a feeling of guilt for having harmed a patient, and a mistaken belief that only safe drugs are passed for marketing. Inman and Vessey (1978) also identify two other weaknesses in this voluntary reporting system. They argue that the data are inadequate for total exposure to a given drug. The second weakness is:

'the fact that only temporally-related and pharmacologically reasonable adverse effects tend to be reported'.

Examples of medicines which have not been allowed on the market or have been taken off the market for reasons of risk of carcinogenicity are difficult to find. One example is the carcinogenicity tests which were carried out on oral contraceptives. In 1964, the Committee on Safety of Drugs examined this issue and decided that long-term studies of toxic effects of oral contraceptives and their active constituents were to be examined. Results of the long-term animal studies were considered by the Committee on Safety of Medicines in 1972 and they concluded:

'Although carcinogenic effects can be produced when some of these preparations are used in high doses throughout the life span in certain strains of rat and mouse, this evidence should not be interpreted as constituting a carcinogenic hazard to women when these preparations are used as oral contraceptives' (DHSS, 1973).

The Committee stated that they intended to keep a close watch on all contraceptives in clinical use.

When considering the efficacy and safety of drugs, there is the obvious issue of weighing up the therapeutic costs against therapeutic benefits. Sometimes these decisions are made without the help of the government machinery and drugs are voluntarily taken off the market by drug companies as a result of either pressure put on them by the medical profession or through information published in medical journals. Sometimes doctors are not satisfied with drugs and choose not to use them or prescribe them.

The effectiveness of the present system of product licensing and adverse reaction system is difficult to evaluate. However, according to Inman and Vessey (1978), the present adverse reaction reporting system and its alternative, a more intensive type of monitoring system, may not be very reliable ways of identifying the carcinogenic, mutagenic or tetragenic effects of drugs. This may involve long-term and detailed monitoring for events which may often be rare. Inman and Vessey (1978) suggest the answer might be a more improved method of medical record linkage. Alternatively, they argue that some method must be devised for bridging the gap between clinical trials and widespread marketing of a new drug. One novel suggestion that Inman and Vessey (1978) make is for a 'recorded drug' system. These new drugs could be used by any doctor for any of his patients where the need arises, but the doctor has to submit follow-up reports at appropriate intervals. These reports would be collected and evaluated until the drug was ready for general release.

Summary
Medicines are controlled in the UK by the statutory requirement to have a licence before marketing. This licence is authorized by the government department on the basis of evidence received from its expert committees. Product licences are given on the basis of their fulfilling the requirements of an evaluation which focuses on the safety, efficacy and quality of the substance.

There also exists an adverse reaction monitoring system which operates on a voluntary basis and is a system for monitoring drugs that have been marketed.

The value of such a system has been questioned, particularly in terms of its reliability for collecting information on the carcinogenic effects of drugs.

Government control of medicines in other countries

The USA appears to be the leading nation when it comes to the control and legislation of the manufacture of medicines. The 1938 Food, Drug and Cosmetic Act provided the first government controls of medicines in the world over the safety of medicines. These controls included: controls over the advertising of drugs and the need to present information on side-effects and effectiveness; controls in drug manufacture and the requirement to present evidence for the effectiveness and safety of new drugs.

The power to licence drugs and medicines rests with civil servants in the USA. This system has been criticized because it leads to over-caution and it is claimed that many perfectly good drugs do not reach the marketplace (Dunlop, 1973). Even if these criticisms are correct in identifying the FDA civil servants' propensity to adopt decisions which are over-cautious about the adverse effects of drugs, this system proved invaluable in the case of thalidomide. The FDA's civil servants withstood considerable pressure from the drug companies and postponed the introduction of thalidomide to the US market.

The thalidomide case also identified a further problem which is still to be rectified. This problem involves the lack of uniformity amongst countries through-out the world over the controls of medicines and drugs. Thus, it is possible for a drug to be banned in some countries on the grounds that it is dangerous and still be marketed in other countries where regulatory controls are not as stringent or scientific information is not available (Sjostrom and Nilsson, 1972).

Conclusions

Governments have three different policy options for the control of environmental agents and consumer products. They can either:
   (i) ban the hazard or hazardous substance completely;
   (ii) restrict the dose of the substance or limit the exposure to the substance;

(iii) educate or equip the population at risk to be able to cope with the hazard safely.

Over the last thirty years, legislation has developed in the United Kingdom which has made it possible for the Government to ban medicines and food and food additives which are a carcinogenic risk. There are various gaps and loopholes in this legislation which have been outlined and, unlike in the US, no legislation with a specific anti-cancer clause has been developed. The advantages and disadvantages of such anti-cancer legislation have also been discussed. There are some classes of substance, such as tobacco and alcohol, where there is evidence of carcinogenic risk but no government regulations exist which could ban them if required. However, it might be possible, when the legal niceties of individual cases are taken into account, for tobacco to be described as a drug and included under the Medicines Act and alcohol to be described as a food and included under the Food Acts. However, what is more likely is that specific legislation should be developed for the control of each of these different substances.

Despite the presence of legal controls for medicines and food products, the first option—the banning of a hazard or hazardous substance—has seldom been taken. Why has this been the case? A related question is why has so little been done about developing legislation to control substances such as tobacco?

This review has thrown light on a number of factors which might explain the approach adopted in the United Kingdom. The following will attempt to describe briefly the most important of these factors.

1. There is a lack of good scientific animal and human data on the potential carcinogenic risks of certain substances which is a prerequisite for policy. A good example of this is found in the area of food contaminants and additives.

2. There is a lack of good scientific data on the efficacy of different policies for control. The case of alcohol illustrates this clearly with the difficulties involved in assessing how far controls over overall alcohol consumption in a society will influence the prevalence of heavy drinking.

3. Government decisions about control are clearly influenced by political, economic and social considerations. An example of this is the Government's unwillingness to control the production of tobacco, which might involve alienating the tobacco industry and, more importantly, cut down a valuable source of revenue for the Government.

4. Policies of non-intervention and intervention are clearly influenced by the ideological positions of individual governments. The emphasis on voluntary agreements between governments and industry on a number of issues highlights the essentially predominantly non-interventionist position of British governments.

5. The lack of a coherent government policy for cancer control in the UK reflects the low priority that the UK Government has traditionally placed on prevention. More recently, government statements on prevention have been made, although with the emphasis on individual rather than government responsibility for action.

More research is needed, therefore, to identify the carcinogenic risks of substances as well as on the relative value of different policy options. This information should be the basis for policy decisions about cancer control. Health and economic policy are clearly interlinked but it must be emphasized that if a government is genuinely interested in the prevention of ill-health, be it cancer or any other illness, then it must face the economic and political costs which such a policy might bring. Clearly, contemporary government policies for prevention of illness are severely constrained by the Government's commitment to economic aims which are not compatible with the promotion of health (Renaud, 1978). A positive prevention policy for cancer would involve the Government becoming directly involved in regulating the environmental, economic and social forces that may play a part in the production of ill-health.

References

Atkinson, A. B. and Skegg, J. L. (1974). *British Journal of Preventive and Social Medicine* **28**, 45.
Atkinson, A. B. and Townsend, J. L. (1977). *Lancet* **ii**, 492.
Ball, J. (1977). *Effective Changes in Income and Price on Demand for Beer*. Economic Development Committee for the Food and Drink Manufacturing Industry, London.
Barker, T. C. (1978). In *Diet of Man: Needs and Wants*, pp. 163–86. Ed. by J. Yudkin. Applied Science Publishers, London.
Bjartveit, K. (1977). *Health Education Journal* **36**, 3.
Bourgeois, J. and Barnes, J. (1980). *Journal of Advertising Research* **19**(4), 19.
Brenner, M. H. (1972). *American Journal of Public Health* **65**, 1279.
Brewers' Society (1979). *U.K. Statistical Handbook*. Brewers' Society, London.
Brewers' Society (1980). *U.K. Statistical Handbook*. Brewers' Society, London.
British Medical Journal (1979). Editorial, **2**, 1610.
Brown, E. R. and Margo, E. G. (1978). *International Journal of Health Services* **8**(1), 3.
Brown, M. M. (1978). *Alcohol Taxation and Control Policies, International Survey*, Vol. 1. Brewers' Association of Canada.
Bruun, K., Edwards, G., Lumis, M. *et al.* (1975). *The Finnish Foundation for Alcohol Studies* **25**, Finland.
Capell, P. J. (1978). *Health Trends* **10**, 49.
Cartwright, A. K. J., Shaw, S. J. and Spratley, T. A. (1978a). *British Journal of Addiction* **73**, 237.
Cartwright, A. K. J., Shaw, S. J. and Spratley, T. A. (1978b). *British Journal of Addiction* **73**, 247.
Central Statistical Office (1979). *Social Trends*. HMSO London.
Chilvers, C. (1980). Personal communication. Division of Epidemiology, Institute of Cancer Research, London.
Clayson, C. (1977). In *Alcoholism*, pp. 78–87. Ed. by G. Edwards and M. Grant. Croom Helm, London.
Crawford, R. (1977). *International Journal of Health Services* **7**, 663.
Culliton, B. J. and Waterfall, W. K. (1978). *British Medical Journal* **2**, 1613.
Cust, G. (1979). In *A Preventive Medicine Viewpoint in Health Education: Perspectives and Choices*, pp. 64–92. Ed. by I. Sutherland. George Allen & Unwin, London.
Davies, J. and Stacey, B. (1972). *Teenagers and Alcohol: a developmental study in Glasgow*, Vol. 2. HMSO, London.
Davies, P. L. (1977). *The Ledermann Curve, Papers of a Conference*. Ed. by P. L. Davies. Alcohol Education Centre, London.
Davies, P. (1979). *British Journal on Alcohol and Alcoholism* **14**(4), 208.
Davis, A. G. (1979). *Social Science and Medicine* **13A**, 129.
Dean, M. (1980). *Guardian* 4th January.
DHSS (1970). *On the State of the Public Health*. HMSO, London.
DHSS (1973). *On the State of the Public Health*. HMSO, London.
DHSS (1976). *Prevention and Health: Everybody's business—a reassessment of public and personal health*. HMSO, London.
DHSS (1977a). *Advisory Committee on Alcoholism: Report on Prevention*. HMSO, London.
DHSS (1977b). *Smoking and Professional People*. HMSO, London.
DHSS (1978). *Eating for Health, Prevention and Health*. HMSO, London.
Dight, S. (1976). *Scottish Drinking Habits*. OPCS, HMSO, London.
Doyal, L. (1979). *The Political Economy of Health*. Pluto Press, London.
Draper, P., Best, G. and Dennis, J. (1977). *Royal Society of Health Journal* **97**, 3, 121.

Draper, P., Dennis, J., Griffiths, J. and Popay, J. (1979). *Lancet* ii, 425.

Draper, P., Griffiths, J., Dennis, J. and Popay, J. (1980). *British Medical Journal* 2, 493.

Duffy, J. (1977a). *International Journal of Epidemiology* 6(4), 375.

Duffy, J. (1977b). In *The Ledermann Curve*, pp. 11–24. Ed. by D. L. Davies. Alcohol Education Centre, London.

Duffy, J. (1980). *British Journal of Addiction* 75, 147.

Duffy, J. and Cohen, C. R. (1978). *British Journal of Addiction* 73, 259.

Dunlop, D. (1973). *Medicines in Our Time*. National Provincial Hospital Trust, London.

Eiser, R., Sutton, S. R. and Wober, M. (1978a). *British Journal of Addiction* 73(2), 215.

Eiser, R., Sutton, S. R. and Wober, M. (1978b). *British Journal of Addiction* 73(3), 291.

Elo, O. (1979). In *Carcinogenic Risks: Strategies for Intervention*, pp. 21–40. Ed. by W. Davis and C. Rosenfield. International Agency for Research on Cancer, Lyon.

Elton, G. A. H. (1976). In *Ministry of Agriculture, Fisheries and Food—Food Quality and Safety: a Century of Progress*, pp. 82–104. HMSO, London.

Epstein, S. S. (1979). *The Politics of Cancer*. Anchor Books, New York.

Ferguson, P. (1976). *Marketing* 22, 22.

Food and Contaminants Committee (1978). *Report on the Review of Nitrites and Nitrates in Cured Meats and Cheese*. HMSO, London.

Foster, E. M. (1973). *Journal of the American Veterinary Medical Association* 163(9), 1056.

Frazer, A. (1977). In *Why Additives?—The Safety of Foods*, pp. viii–xvi. Ed. by British Nutrition Foundation. Forbes Publications, London.

Friedman, K. M. (1975). *Public Policy and the Smoking–Health Controversy*. Lexington Books, New York.

Gatherer, A., Parfit, J., Porter, E. and Vessey, M. (1979). *Is Health Education Effective?* Health Education Council Monograph Series, No. 2, p. 78.

Giles, R. F. (1976). In *Ministry of Agriculture, Fisheries and Food—Food Quality and Safety: a Century of Progress*, pp. 4–21. HMSO, London.

Goldenberg, N. (1977). In *Why Additives?—The Safety of Foods*, pp. 59–69. Ed. by British Nutrition Foundation. Forbes Publications, London.

Gray, N. (1977). *Lung Cancer Prevention*. Union Internationale Contre le Cancer, Geneva.

Hamilton, J. L. (1972). *Review of Economics and Statistics* 5(4), 401.

HMSO (1972). *Report of the Departmental Committee on Liquor Licensing*. The Erroll Report, London.

HMSO (1977a). *Expenditure Committee—Session 1976/77*.

HMSO (1977b). *Prevention and Health*. Department of Health and Social Security, Department of Education and Science, Scottish Office and Welsh Office.

HMSO (1979a). *Developments in Tobacco Products and the Possibility of 'Lower-Risk' Cigarettes*. Second Report of the Independent Scientific Committee of Smoking and Health.

HMSO (1979b). *Medicines Act 1968*, Chapter 67 (reprinted).

HMSO (1979c). *Royal Commission on the NHS*.

Hutt, D. B. (1979). In *Regulatory Aspects of Carcinogenesis and Food Additives: The Delaney Clause*, pp. 9–25. Ed. by F. Coulston. Academic Press, New York.

Inman, W. H. W. and Vessey, M. P. (1978). In *Recent Advances in Community Medicine*, pp. 215–30. Ed. by A. E. Bennett. Churchill Livingstone, Edinburgh, London and New York.

Jarvis, M. and Russell, M. A. H. (1980). *British Medical Journal* 1, 994.

Johnson, J. and Oksanen, S. (1974). *Applied Economics* 6, 293.

Jukes, T. H. (1977). *New England Journal of Medicine* 297(8), 427.

Jukes, T. H. (1979). *Journal of the American Medical Association* 241(6), 617.

Kirkwood, R. (1980). *A defence of cigarette advertising*. *Financial Times*, 29th May, 5.

Lancet (1979). Editorial *Silent Prevention*, i, 705.

Lancet (1980). Editorial, ii, 567.

Ledermann, S. (1956). In *Alcohol, Alcoholism, Alcoholisation*. Données scientifiques de caractère physiologique, économique et social, Institut National d'Études Démographiques, Travaux et Documents, Cahier No. 29, Presse Universitaires de France.

Lee, P. N. (1976). *Statistics of Smoking in the U.K.*, 7th edn. TRC, Research Paper, London.

Linsell, C. A. (1979). In *Carcinogenic Risks: Strategies for Intervention*, pp. 111–20. International Agency for Research on Cancer, Scientific Publications, No. 25, Volume 74.

Lint, J. (1977). In *The Lederman Curve*, pp. 1–10. Ed. by D. L. Davies. Alcohol Education Centre, London.

Lint, J. (1978). *British Journal of Addiction* 73, 265.

Lint, J. and Schmidt, W. (1968). *Quarterly Journal of Studies in Alcohol* **29**, 968.
Lint, J. and Schmidt, W. (1971). *British Journal of Addiction* **66**, 97.
McCron, R. and Budd, J. (1979). In *Health Education: Perspectives and Choices*, pp. 199–216. Ed. by I. Sutherland. George Allen & Unwin, London.
Macfarlane, A., Bland, M., Chalmers, I. *et al.* (1978). *International Journal of Health Services* **8**(2), 387.
McGuiness, T. and Cowling, K. (1975). *European Economic Review* **6**(3), 311.
McKeown, T. (1979). *The Role of Medicine*, Part 2: *Determinants of Health*. Blackwell, Oxford.
McKinlay, J. A. (1974). *A case for refocusing upstream the political economy of illness*. Unpublished paper, Boston University.
MAFF (1978a). *Survey of vinyl chloride content of polyvinyl chloride for food contact and of foods*. HMSO, London.
MAFF (1978b). *The surveillance of food contamination in the U.K.* HMSO, London.
MAFF (1980). *Survey of vinylidene chloride levels in food contact materials*. HMSO, London.
Manis, J. G. (1976). *Analyzing Social Problems*. Praeger Publishers, New York.
Miller, G. H. and Agnew, N. (1974). *Quarterly Journal of Studies in Alcohol* **35**, 877.
Muller, M. (1978). *Tomorrow's Epidemic: Tobacco and the Third World*. War on Want, London.
National Consumer Council (1979). *Inexpensive Cigarettes. Financial Times*, 22nd March.
Neilson (1965). In Bruun, K. *et al.* (1975). *The Finnish Foundation for Alcohol Studies* **25**, Finland.
Oddy, D. J. and Miller, D. S. (1976). *The Making of the Modern British Diet*. Croom Helm, London.
OPCS (1972). *General Household Survey Report*. HMSO, London.
OPCS (1977). *Population Trends* **7**, 18.
OPCS (1978). *General Household Survey Report*. HMSO, London.
OPCS (1979). *Cigarette Smoking, General Household Survey 1978*, Ref. GHS.
Orrego, H., Blake, J. E., Blendis, L. M., Kapur, B. M. and Israel, Y. (1979). *Lancet* **ii**, 1354.
Pernanen, K. (1974). In *Research Advances in Alcohol and Drug Problems*, Vol. 1, pp. 355–74. Ed. by R. J. Gibbins, Y. Israel, H. Kalaut, R. E. Popham, W. Schmidt and R. G. Smart. John Wiley, London.
Peto, J. (1974). *British Journal of Preventive and Social Medicine* **28**, 241.
Peto, J. (1976). *Lancet* **i**, 301.
Plant, M. A. (1979). *British Journal on Alcohol and Alcoholism* **14**(3), 132.
Plant, M. A. and Pirie, F. (1979). *Social Psychiatry* **14**, 65.
Plant, M. A., Pirie, F. and Kreitman, N. (1979). *Social Psychiatry* **14**, 11.
Popham, R. E., Schmidt, W. and de Lint, J. (1975). *British Journal of Addiction* **70**, 125.
Renaud, M. (1978). In *The Cultural Crisis of Modern Medicine*, pp. 101–22. Ed. by J. Ehrenreich. Monthly Review Press, New York and London.
Research Bureau Ltd. (1972). *Anti-smoking T.V. campaign: report of H.E.C. campaign* (mimeo).
Research Services Ltd. (1972). *Anti-smoking advertising: report of H.E.C.'s campaign* (mimeo).
Research Surveys of G.B. Ltd. (1974, 1975, 1976). *H.E.C.'s tar and nicotine advertising campaign* (mimeo).
Research Surveys of G.B. Ltd. (1976). *H.E.C.'s adolescent anti-smoking campaign* (mimeo).
Research Surveys of G.B. Ltd. (1977). *H.E.C.'s anti-smoking campaign* (mimeo).
Robinson, D. (1974). *British Journal of Addiction* **69**, 99.
Robinson, D. (1976). *From Drinking to Alcoholism. A Sociological Commentary*. John Wiley, London.
Robinson, D. (1977). In *Alcoholism*, pp. 60–77. Ed. by G. Edwards and M. Grant. Croom Helm, London.
Roe, F. J. C. (1973). *Proceedings of the Royal Society of Medicine* **66**, 23.
Royal College of Physicians (1962). *Smoking and Health*. Pitman Press, London.
Royal College of Physicians (1971). *Smoking and Health Now*. Pitman Press, London.
Royal College of Physicians (1977). *Smoking or Health—Third Report*. Pitman Press, London.
Royal College of Psychiatrists (1979). *Alcohol and Alcoholism*. Tavistock, London.
Russell, M. A. H. (1971). *British Journal of Addiction* **66**, 157.
Russell, M. A. H. (1973). *British Journal of Preventive and Social Medicine* **27**, 1.
Russell, M. A. H. (1974). *Lancet* **i**, 254.
Russell, M. A. H. (1976). *British Medical Journal* **1**, 1430.
Russell, M. A. H., Cole, P. V. and Brown, E. (1973). *Lancet* **i**, 576.

Russell, M. A. H. and Feyerabend, C. (1975). *Lancet* **i**, 179.

Russell, M. A. H., Jarvis, M., Iyer, R. and Feyerabend, C. (1980). *British Medical Journal* **1**, 972.

Russell, M. A. H., Wilson, C., Patel, V. A., Cole, P. V. and Feyerabend, C. (1973). *British Medical Journal* **4**, 512.

Schmalensee, R. (1972). *The Economics of Advertising*. North Holland, Amsterdam.

Schmidt, W. (1977). In *Alcoholism*, pp. 15–47. Ed. by G. Edwards and M. Grant. Croom Helm, London.

Schmidt, W. and Kornaczewski, A. (1975). *The Effect of Lowering the Legal Drinking Age in Ontario on Alcohol-related Motor Vehicle Accidents*. Proceedings of the Sixth International Conference on Alcohol, Drugs and Traffic Safety. Addiction Research Foundation, Toronto.

Simopoulos, A. P. (1979). *Journal of the American Diet Association* **74**(5), 599.

Single, E. and Giesbrecht, N. (1979). *British Journal of Addiction* **74**, 165.

Sjostrom, H. and Nilsson, R. (1972). *Thalidomide and the Power of the Drug Companies*. A Penguin Special, Penguin, London.

Skog, O. J. (1977). In *The Lederman Curve*, pp. 25–43. Ed. by D. L. Davies. The Alcohol Education Centre, London.

Skog, O. J. (1980). *British Journal of Addiction* **75**, 133.

Smart, R. G. (1977). *American Journal of Drug and Alcohol Abuse* **4**(i), 101.

TACADE/ASH (1977). *T.A.C.A.D.E./A.S.H. fact sheets*.

Todd, G. F. C. (1975). *Changes in smoking patterns in the U.K.* TRC Occasional Paper **1**, 7.

Truswell, A. S. (1979). *Nutrition and Cancer* **1**(3), 96.

Truswell, A. S., Asp, N., James, P. T. and MacMahon, B. (1978). *Nutrition Reviews* **36**(10), 313.

Tuckett, D. (1979). In *Health Education, Perspectives and Choices*, pp. 39–63. Ed. by I. Sutherland. George Allen & Unwin, London.

Turner, J. (1980). *New Society*, 19th June, 287.

Vuylsteek, K. *et al.* (1977). *Evaluation in a rural population of a T.V. programme on smoking and health*. Department of Hygiene and Social Medicine, University of Ghent, Belgium.

Ward, A. G. (1976). In *Ministry of Agriculture, Fisheries and Food—Food Quality and Safety: a Century of Progress*, pp. 22–41. HMSO, London.

Warner, V. E. (1977). *American Journal of Public Health* **67**, 643.

Weedon, B. C. L. (1976). In *Ministry of Agriculture, Fisheries and Food—Food Quality and Safety: a Century of Progress*, pp. 42–61. HMSO, London.

Wheeler, E. F. (1978). *Journal of Human Nutrition* **32**, 325.

Whitehead, P. C. (1980a). In *Alcohol Problems: Reviews, Research and Recommendations*, pp. 217–26. Ed. by D. Robinson. Macmillan, London.

Whitehead, P. C. (1980b). In *Alcohol Problems: Reviews, Research and Recommendations*, pp. 232–40. Ed. by D. Robinson. Macmillan, London.

Wilkinson, R. (1970). *The Prevention of Drinking Problems, Legal Controls and Cultural Influences*. Oxford University Press, New York.

Winegarten, A. (1978). In *Diet of Man: Needs and Wants*, pp. 317–50. Ed. by J. Yudkin. Applied Science Publishers, London.

Yellowlees, H. (1976). In *Ministry of Agriculture, Fisheries and Food—Food Quality and Safety: a Century of Progress*, pp. 62–81. HMSO, London.

6

The prevention of industrial cancer

Joan M. Davies

Introduction

Scope and outline

This chapter deals with various aspects of the prevention of cancer caused by industry. It is concerned mainly with occupational cancer—i.e. cancer caused by exposure to carcinogens at work—but in so far as occupational carcinogens may also affect users or may create neighbourhood hazards, much of it also applies to

Table 6.1 Industrial cancer: relevant groups

Medical and research bodies
    University departments of occupational medicine etc.
    Institutes for medical and related research
    The Royal Society of Medicine and other learned societies
    Funding bodies, including the Medical Research Council (MRC) and Cancer Research Campaign (CRC)

International agencies
    The World Health Organization (WHO), including the International Agency for Research on Cancer (IARC)
    The International Labour Organization (ILO)
    The International Atomic Energy Agency and the International Commission on Radiological Protection (ICRP)

Legislative and enforcement agencies
    The European Economic Community (EEC)
    The British Government (Parliament and ministers)
    The Health and Safety Commission (HSC)
    The Health and Safety Executive (HSE)
    The Department of Health and Social Security (DHSS)
    Coroners' courts and law courts

Representatives of both sides of industry
    Employers' associations
    Large individual firms
    The Trades Union Congress (TUC)
    Individual trade unions

Pressure groups
    Small groups concerned with local issues
    The Cancer Prevention Society
    The Society for the Prevention of Asbestos-Induced Diseases
    Friends of the Earth and other environmental protection groups

these risks; in general the issues are similar. Some carcinogenic products affect users without apparently involving a risk for the workers making them; for the most part these are products which are ingested by users, such as drugs. The industrial product which causes more cancer deaths than any other (the cigarette) is dealt with elsewhere in this book; it does not cause occupational cancer, although its use appears to enhance the effect of exposure to occupational lung carcinogens.

After a brief historical account of the growth of the recognition of occupational cancer, this introduction considers prevailing views on how much cancer today is in fact occupational. The second and main part of this chapter is concerned with the mechanisms of industrial cancer prevention: the identification of carcinogens, the enactment of legislation to prohibit or control them, and the enforcement of this legislation. It deals mainly with the UK, but developments in the USA are also described because of their implications for other countries.

In 1974, Munn remarked that 'In the entire history of occupational medicine there can be few industrial hazards that have aroused greater emotion or more muddled thinking than chemically induced cancer.' This emotion and muddled thinking has not dimished—rather the contrary—and the third section of the chapter attempts to convey some of the attitudes of the various participants in the process of attempting prevention. It is convenient here at the outset to present a list of the main bodies concerned, with the abbreviations subsequently used for many of them. The list is given in Table 6.1; it makes no claim to be exhaustive, and the categories are not mutually exclusive: bodies are listed under their main function heading. Markedly different attitudes may be found among employers, trade unions, government bodies (especially the Health and Safety Executive), research workers and pressure groups.

An historical view

In the whole field of the prevention of industrial cancer, we are in the midst of a transition—even a revolution. Although it may seem to us today that attitudes shift slowly and that enacting new legislation is a most lengthy process, present changes are rapid and radical compared with the slow progress of past decades. This applies to most aspects of the scene, be it ascertainment of carcinogens, preventive legislation, or the active participation of trade unions and pressure groups on a hitherto unprecedented scale. In no small way, these developments reflect an increased public concern with all aspects of health and the safety of the environment, as well as the development of relevant sciences, including epidemiology. They also reflect a notable change in the attitude of the workforce, expressed succinctly in a remark by the Chairman of the Hebden Bridge Asbestos Action Group, cited in *Safety* (issue of October 1979): 'In my early days people used to get round health problems by saying "It's an occupational hazard", we should no longer accept that there are such things as occupational hazards.'

But equally responsible for the revolution has been the steadily growing number of different industrial cancers which have come to light. The principal well-proven industrial cancers are listed in Table 6.2 in three groups; note that the references given for the third group do not necessarily relate to the earliest paper concerning a risk. In the early 1930s, Sir Thomas Legge (1934) listed only three groupings of workers as liable to occupational cancer affecting the skin, scrotum,

Table 6.2 Occupational cancers widely recognized at different dates

As listed by Legge (1934) in about 1932	
Workers making synthetic dyestuffs	Bladder cancer
Workers exposed to tar, pitch and certain oils	Skin cancer, scrotal cancer
Workers exposed to x-rays or radioactive substances	Skin cancer, bone cancer, lung cancer
Added by Hunter (1959)	
Gasworkers	Lung cancer
Asbestos workers	Lung cancer
Arsenic workers	Skin cancer, lung cancer
Bichromates manufacturing workers	Lung cancer
Nickel manufacturing workers	Respiratory tract cancer
Workers exposed to benzene	Leukaemia
Workers exposed to ionizing radiation or radioactive substances	Leukaemia
Added by 1980	
Rubber and cable factory workers	Bladder cancer (Case and Hosker, 1954; Davies, 1965); lung and stomach cancer (Health and Safety Executive, 1980)
Gasworkers	Bladder cancer (Doll et al., 1965)
Coal-miners	Stomach cancer (Stocks, 1962; Rockette, 1977)
Asbestos workers	Mesothelioma, gastrointestinal cancer (International Agency for Research on Cancer, 1973)
Woodworkers	Nasal sinus cancer (Acheson et al., 1968)
Boot and shoe (leather) workers	Nasal sinus cancer (Acheson et al., 1970)
Makers of zinc chromate pigments	Lung cancer (Davies, 1979)
Workers making mustard gas	Lung cancer (Wada et al., 1962)
Professional chemists	Hodgkin's disease (Olin, 1978)
Coke oven workers	Lung cancer, kidney cancer (Redmond et al., 1972)
Workers in beryllium production	Lung cancer, (Wagoner et al., 1980)
Workers exposed to bis (chloromethyl) ether (BCME) or chloromethyl methyl ether (CMME)	Lung cancer (Figueroa et al., 1973)
Workers exposed to vinyl chloride monomer (VCM)	Liver angiosarcoma (British Medical Journal, 1974)

bladder, lung and bone. Only the skin cancers appeared numerous, and up to the end of 1931 only twenty-three fatal cases of bladder cancer arising in synthetic dye manufacture had been reported to the Government's Factory Department. Legge cites at least seven cases of bone sarcoma from 1924–31, but the lung cancers to which he refers had occurred in Germany, not in England. Thus at that date, occupational cancer would have been a cause for concern, but the problem would have appeared well defined and, as a cause of death, industrial cancer would have seemed numerically insignificant.

When Hunter published *Health in Industry* in 1959, his list of occupational cancers was longer: even though the bladder cancer of rubber workers was omitted, six more groups of workers were added, and leukaemia was added to the diseases attributable to ionizing radiation. By this date, it had been realized that there were several different lung carcinogens, and that other parts of the respiratory tract could also be affected. But although the lists of both occupations and of cancer sites had lengthened, the number of cases involved still appeared small.

Twenty-one years later, in 1980, the list has doubled in length, and is still being enlarged. Not only have numerous occupations been added, but it has become clear that occupational carcinogens can affect many different sites. Most of the additions on the 1980 list do not in fact represent new risks—rather they are late discoveries of long-established risks or late confirmations of risks long suspected but not fully investigated. For example, it seems likely that an unsuspected nasal sinus cancer risk had existed for many decades in the furniture-making industry, and the lung cancer hazard among makers of zinc chromate pigments was already operative in the 1930s, although unsuspected in this country until forty years later. On the other hand, there were strong indications of a bladder cancer risk among gasworkers from the work of Henry *et al.* in 1931, although confirmation was not received until the 1960s. Also it was clear from the Decennial Supplement on Occupational Mortality for 1951 (Registrar General, 1958) that coal-miners had higher-than-average death rates from stomach cancer, though as their wives were equally affected, it was not clear whether this risk arose from their occupation or from their way of life; in 1977, Rockette provided confirmation of the hazard in the USA.

Eventual discovery or confirmation of old risks has been helped by improved methods of diagnosis (especially in the case of mesothelioma) and by improvements in epidemiological methods, but it has been helped most by the direction of increased effort to the task of deliberately searching for occupational hazards. And the more we search, the more we find. Most recently a suspected but unproven lung cancer hazard for beryllium workers has finally been confirmed. Inevitably, one must suspect that other undiscovered occupational cancer hazards exist. Although a severe risk affecting a large group of workers would be unlikely to go unnoticed, a high risk of a common cancer restricted to a small group can be inconspicuous until investigated, as with the zinc chromate pigment makers; equally, a low risk of a common cancer in a large group may go unnoticed, as with the gastrointestinal cancer of asbestos workers. By now, a great many occupations either have been studied or are currently being investigated, but the task of looking for hidden risks is a long one.

The fact that old risks are still coming to light is sufficient to cause alarm, but it is probably even more alarming to find that whilst these have been slowly discovered and attempts made to eliminate them, new occupational cancer hazards have been created as new chemical substances have been developed and introduced. The lung cancers of workers exposed to BCME or CMME and the liver cancers of VCM workers represent new risks. Fortunately, the numbers of affected workers are small in each instance, but these discoveries have provided clear warnings of what can happen and what will probably continue to happen unless chemicals can be more effectively screened before being brought into industrial use. Of course there have been some successes in avoiding the introduction of carcinogens; notably the English chemical industry recognized that 4-aminodiphenyl (xenylamine) was probably a potent human carcinogen and avoided its use (Walpole *et al.*, 1954); the same prudence was not observed in the USA, and an epidemic of bladder cancer resulted among the workers exposed (Melick *et al.*, 1955).

How much cancer is occupational?

Clearly, there are numerous different substances which are carcinogenic for the workers who make or process them, and there is a very real risk that more such carcinogens may be introduced into use. But just how numerous are occupational cancer cases? As discussed already in this book, there are widely differing estimates, and one sees a paradox here: on the one hand, the idea that such cases are numerous is very alarming, especially to manual workers and their families, but on the other hand, the idea is in a sense attractive, for occupational cancer ought to be relatively easily preventable. Thus it may appear that by passing some laws prohibiting or controlling the use of occupational carcinogens, a significant reduction in cancer death rates could be obtained. Both alarm and wishful thinking may be partly responsible for the belief in exaggerated estimates presently in circulation.

Epidemiologists and government bodies in this country generally accept an estimate of between 1 per cent and 5 per cent of cancer cases being of occupational origin, as suggested by Doll (1977) among others. However, higher estimates may be found in the literature. Sometimes, studies of local areas may suggest high proportions of occupational cancers of one particular site, and such suggestions may easily be taken out of context and treated as general estimates for that site. Currently, the USA report of Bridport *et al.* (1978) has a wide influence. This report suggests that in the near future 20–38 per cent of cancer in the USA will be occupational, and some bodies in this country tend to apply this high figure to cancer in the UK; for example, the trade union ASTMS—the Association of Scientific, Technical and Managerial Staffs (1980)—did so in a recent report which attracted wide publicity.

This high estimate of 20–38 per cent must be borne in mind when considering the differences between the USA and UK approaches to the control of occupational carcinogens: when the UK Government plans legislation, it is trying to prevent at most 5 per cent of all cancer cases, but USA government agencies believe that their impending legislation is crucial in the prevention of a much higher proportion than this.

Mechanisms of cancer prevention

Introduction

This section describes the means by which we seek to prevent occupational cancer in this country; the basic methods, the ascertainment of hazards, the enactment of legislation to control them, the enforcement of this legislation, and the compensation of those affected, including compensation awarded by the courts under common law. Table 6.3 lists these mechanisms.

The part played by compensation in the preventive process may be questioned; its contribution is not a direct one, but in the author's opinion it plays a key role. In the first place, it provides a powerful incentive for the ascertainment of individual cases of occupational cancer by all those concerned with the welfare of affected workers and their families; although our present knowledge of the numbers of people affected is certainly deficient, without the case-finding incentive provided by compensation it would undoubtedly be far more deficient, and

Table 6.3 The mechanisms of occupational cancer prevention

Identification of carcinogens
    Provision of funds for research
    Laboratory testing of new or suspect substances
    Use of epidemiology to search for unrecognized cancer hazards
    Epidemiological studies of defined groups of workers

Enactment of legislation
    Classification of recognized and suspect carcinogens
    Prohibition of certain recognized carcinogens
    Control of recognized and suspect carcinogens
    Legislation for enforcement and compensation

Enforcement, monitoring, screening
    Inspection of working conditions
    Definition of workers exposed to specific carcinogenic hazards
    Monitoring of these workers' exposures
    Epidemiological follow-up of certain exposed workers
    Screening for early diagnosis of disease
    Coroners' inquests on occupational cancer deaths
    Prosecution of employers failing to comply with the law

Compensation of affected workers and common law actions
    'Prescription' of industrial cancers under the Industrial Injuries Acts
    Awards of 'prescribed disease' payments to affected workers
    Awards of legal damages to some affected workers under common law
    Compensation of some affected workers under employers' schemes

knowledge of numbers is essential for effective prevention. Equally or more important is the fact that common law established by court actions finding negligence on the part of the employers of affected workers has had an important and generally salutory influence on the practices of firms whose production may involve the exposure of employees to carcinogens.

Basic methods

In basic practical terms, the prevention of industrial cancer can be effected in four ways once a risk has been identified. First, the carcinogen in question can be removed by ceasing to use it as a raw material, or ceasing to manufacture it as an intermediate or end-product, or modifying production processes so that it no longer occurs as a by-product; prohibition of a substance requires action of this kind. Secondly, plant machinery and/or processes and/or handling procedures can be modified in such ways that the amount of the carcinogen released into the atmosphere is reduced to acceptable (permissible) levels. Thirdly, individual worker's exposures may be reduced to acceptable levels by the use of protective clothing and masks; regulations 'controlling' substances generally require action by these two methods. Lastly, it might be thought that there is scope for employing only 'low-risk' workers on jobs which may be hazardous, but in practice there is at present little promise in this method of preventing industrial cancer, for currently very little is known about individual susceptibility to cancers of relevant sites. Any measures taken by prudent employers at the present time are probably confined to excluding men with pre-existing respiratory disease from any job which might involve exposure to a respiratory carcinogen and, similarly, excluding those with any form of urinary disease or proneness to skin disorders from work which might involve a risk of bladder cancer or skin neoplasm.

As described later, the tendency of the USA Government is to favour prohibition or 'zero levels' of carcinogens (which may scarcely be feasible), whereas in this country, prohibition is officially regarded as a last resort for the most potent carcinogens such as benzidine and β-naphthylamine. Here the emphasis is on the use of the second and third methods to achieve low levels of exposure which are considered safe. As Pittom (1980) of the Health and Safety Executive (HSE) has expressed it, 'The emphasis is and must be on means of control, that substances should be used safely, not that all substances should be safe in themselves ... It is impractical to expect we could ever reach a point when no dangerous substances were in use.' This approach takes into account that prohibition of a substance (unless it presents a potent hazard) might lead to its substitution by a new and possibly equally dangerous material.

'Safe' levels are determined following procedures described later, taking into account all available epidemiological and other evidence. The onus is then on employers to meet the prescribed standards by means of modifying factory plant or acquiring new machinery, extending the use of 'closed' processes, improving dust extraction, enforcing the use of respirators and using appropriate monitoring equipment—all of which may prove very expensive. There is also an onus on employees to make proper use of protective clothing and to observe safety precautions.

Can a recognized industrial cancer hazard be effectively removed or controlled by these means? Both successes and failures are on record. Epidemiological studies where workers have been subdivided by level of exposure or by date of entering employment may be able to show that, below a certain exposure level or after a date when process changes were made, workers have not suffered excess cancer mortality. For example, Doll et al. (1977) studied the mortality of workers at a nickel refinery; for men first employed before 1930, there was a dramatic excess of deaths from nasal sinus cancer (0.195 expected, 56 observed), but no deaths from this cause had occurred among men starting work since 1930—when relevant process changes were being made. When Newhouse (1969) studied the mortality of men employed at an asbestos factory making textiles and insulating material, she found a significant excess of lung cancer among those with 'heavy' exposure, but no excess of this cancer among those with 'low' or 'moderate' levels of exposure. New asbestos regulations are aimed at reducing exposure below the levels which give rise to excess lung cancer mortality. On the other hand, it may not be feasible to reduce exposures below the very low levels which may induce mesotheliomas. A notable failure in cancer control concerned specially designed British plants to manufacture benzidine and α-naphthylamine. These enclosed plants were built to the most advanced design and were thought to provide the workers operating them with complete protection against the risk of contracting bladder cancer. But both plants were closed down in 1965, following the diagnosis of bladder tumours in one worker in each plant—and neither worker had any previous exposure to bladder carcinogens (Lancet, 1965).

The setting of exposure standards for proven or possible carcinogens will always prove difficult, and must take into account not only considerations of workers' safety, but also the feasibility of checking whether the standards are being observed, the economic feasibility of continuing production if the standards require drastic cost rises, and the life-saving properties (if any) of the substances; the latter consideration arises particularly in respect to asbestos.

The identification of occupational carcinogens

We are powerless to prevent occupational cancer unless we can identify carcinogens so as to remove or control them, but how certain of a risk must we be before taking action—how do we define a carcinogen? The whole question of the definition and identification of carcinogens is currently controversial, and the following is a much simplified summary of the issues dealt with in more detail elsewhere in this book.

Relatively simple, quick and cheap tests can identify which of a series of chemicals tested are mutagenic, and it is known that many mutagens are also carcinogens—at least in laboratory animals. Longer and more expensive laboratory experiments on rodents can show whether the substances tested are animal carcinogens, but it is suggested that a full-scale testing procedure for a new substance could cost a quarter of a million pounds (Chemistry in Britain, 1980). By no means all animal carcinogens are in practice carcinogens for man, and ultimately only epidemiological research can finally confirm whether or not a substance causes cancer in man under normal conditions of use. Such research often takes the form of a follow-up mortality (or morbidity) study of a group of workers exposed to the suspect substance, but, because of the long latent intervals that are characteristic of occupational cancer, epidemiology can generally provide a quick result only for 'old' substances which have already been in use for twenty or more years. There is no way in which epidemiology can provide a quick answer to queries about new substances—it can only study past experience. Not only is this a crucial limitation, but it is an emotive one: Epstein (1976) protests that 'In the absence of "pre-testing", the worker himself or herself, is unwittingly used as an involuntary test subject', and the Trade Union ASTMS (1980) asserts that 'Put crudely, proof of cancer causation by epidemiological methods means proof by counting bodies', even though a great deal of medical research has always functioned by learning from past experience and 'counting bodies' in one sense or another. Apart from the delay aspect, the other main limitation of mortality studies of workers exposed to suspect substances is that if the number of exposed workers is small, no clear-cut answer may emerge unless the substance is a potent carcinogen which has created a severe hazard; it may not be possible to distinguish between an absence of risk and the possibility of a weak risk.

Clearly, epidemiology alone cannot provide a solution to this problem of identifying occupational carcinogens, and many people see expanded laboratory testing on animals as the answer. Undoubtedly, animal tests have an important role with new substances, but in general in this country we look to epidemiology to indicate which 'old' substances are carcinogenic to man. Here there is an important difference between official attitudes in the UK and the USA: we do not usually label a substance as carcinogenic in relation to man unless there is evidence that it has caused human cancer, but in the USA positive results from animal experiments are enough to warrant the label 'carcinogen', and may even be given more weight than negative epidemiological results.

At best, epidemiological hypothesis-testing studies may give a clear answer as to whether or not a substance is an occupational carcinogen, and may even give some indication of the threshold dose. At worst, such studies may be unable to provide any clear answer at all. In some instances a study may incriminate individual substances, but in others it may only be shown that an occupation involves a hazard without the exact source of the hazard being identified; for example, the precise causes of the nasal sinus cancer risks for woodworkers and leather workers are not known (Acheson *et al.*, 1968; Acheson *et al.*, 1970). In such cases of doubt, laborious and expensive laboratory testing on animals may provide the answer, but in the meantime the authorities have to attempt to control an ill-defined hazard: legislation for the control of occupational carcinogens is no easy task!

It should also be pointed out that through chance or human error, a hypothesis-testing study may occasionally produce an incorrect answer, though there is no reason to suppose that this happens very often. On the other hand, hypothesis-generating studies may easily produce 'false positive' results and groundless 'cancer scares'. Studies which generate hypotheses of fresh occupational cancer hazards should receive critical appraisal; it may be difficult for the authorities to decide whether to take action on them or to await the results of further confirmatory studies.

Legislation

Relevant types of legislation

The most relevant Act of Parliament is the Health and Safety at Work (etc.) Act of 1974, which sets out general principles and policies. Detailed implementation of the Act by Regulations (etc.) is by 'delegated legislation'. Common law, reached by judges' decisions in court cases, is dealt with under the subsection concerned with compensation. In the future, an increasing part of our law will derive from the EEC, whose law takes precedence over the domestic law of member countries. The legislative situation in the USA is described because of the wide repercussions of developments there.

The Health and Safety Act of 1974

This Act lays on employers the duty of ensuring the health and safety of their employees as far as is reasonably practicable, and of conducting their undertakings so that those outside are not harmed—eg. by neighbourhood risks. Manufacturers must ensure that the substances they supply are safe in use, and must carry out appropriate tests to ensure this. Employees must be given full information on health and safety issues. In turn, along with their right to know to what risks they are exposed, workers have a duty to co-operate with the employer in controlling those risks. Provision is made for regulations on mechanisms of consultation.

The Act establishes the Health and Safety Commission (HSC) and the Health and Safety Executive (the enforcement agency). The HSC comprises a chairman and between six and nine others, all appointed by the Secretary of State for Employment, but nominated by and representative of employers, employees, local authorities and professional bodies. The HSC has a major research, education and advisory role, but its most important function is that of preparing draft regulations and codes of practice under the 1974 Act, and generally preparing proposals for revising and extending statutory provisions on health and safety at work.

Delegated legislation

Sets of regulations concerning carcinogens were already in force prior to 1974, and some of these have been summarized by Montesano and Tomatis (1977) in a paper describing legislation on chemical carcinogens in fourteen industrialized countries. The earliest of these regulations were concerned with risks of cancers of the skin and scrotum. There were Patent Fuel Manufacture (Health and Welfare) Special Regulations in 1946, and Mule Spinning (Health) Special Regulations in 1953; the latter require that all oil used for oiling mule spindles be entirely of animal or vegetable oil or be white oil, with the intention that the oil be free of carcinogenic polycyclic hydrocarbons. The Carcinogenic Substances Regulations of 1967 prohibit (with exceptions) the manufacture or use of the bladder carcinogens β-naphthylamine, benzidine, 4-aminobiphenyl, 4-nitrobiphenyl, and their salts. The same regulations control the manufacture or use of the less potent bladder carcinogens α-naphthylamine, o-tolidine, o-dianisidine, dichlorbenzidine, and their salts, and the manufacture of auramine and magenta. Workers exposed to the 'controlled substances' must undergo six-monthly urine cytology tests. Separate regulations deal with the import of the 'prohibited substances'. The Asbestos Regulations of 1969 control exposure to asbestos dust in factories, and supersede the earlier 1931 Regulations; interpreting the 1969 Regulations, HM Factory Inspectorate set standards for asbestos dust concentrations of 2 fibres/ml for asbestos dust in general, and 0.2 fibres/ml for crocidolite (Department of Employment and Productivity, 1970). There are also regulations limiting exposure at work to ionizing radiation; these follow the recommendations of the International Commission on Radiological Protection (ICRP).

However, the further life of some of these regulations is likely to be short, for various new sets of regulations have either been drafted or are under active consideration. It is one of the functions of the HSC to prepare draft regulations in the form of consultative documents, which after a due process of consultation and revision may be approved by the Secretary of State for Employment, and become law. To this end, the HSC appoints expert advisory committees, and its Advisory Committee on Asbestos reported recently and made proposals which would place tighter curbs on crocidolite, lower exposure levels for other types of asbestos, require medical examinations and registers of exposed workers, and achieve better control of asbestos emissions likely to affect the public. The HSC also has an Advisory Committee on Toxic Substances which has been preparing new and more comprehensive carcinogenic substances regulations, which will be additional to existing statutory provisions. The new regulations will follow the general recommendations of the 1974 Convention of the International Labour Organization (International Labour Organization, 1974), and scheduled carcinogens will be classified as either 'prohibited', 'authorized' or 'controlled'. The regulations will be augmented by detailed supporting documents such as codes of practice and guidance notes (Douglas, 1979); an important code of practice which preceded the setting-up of the HSC is that on vinyl chloride (Health and Safety Executive, 1975). It remains to be seen how wide a range of substances will be regulated, and it is possible that events may be overtaken by EEC legislation.

There is also a proposed scheme for notification of toxic properties of substances, designed to detect at an early stage those toxic substances—especially new ones— which are likely to present serious health hazards. The scheme will give manufacturers guidance on the information to be notified, and on the nature of the testing and research considered necessary under the 1974 Act.

Mention must be made of another important set of regulations which came into force in 1978; these put into effect the intentions of the 1974 Act with regard to Safety Representatives and Safety Committees. The Act imposed a duty on employers to consult safety representatives, and the regulations set out their functions. Representatives are appointed by recognized trade unions, and among their functions are: to investigate potential hazards and employee complaints, to consult the employers as necessary and to represent the employees at meetings of safety committees and in consultations at work with HSE inspectors. Safety representatives have a right to inspect any part of the workplace, and employers have a duty to make information available to them that relates to the employees' health and safety at work, including technical data on hazards, statistical records of the occurrence of industrial diseases etc. Employers are also required to set up safety committees if requested to do so by safety representatives; such committees have a general function of keeping under review the measures taken to ensure the employees' health and safety. All levels of management should be represented in safety committees, but management representatives must not outnumber those for the employees. Thus, for perhaps the first time, legislation is actively encouraging and assisting the process of consultation between both sides of industry on matters of health and safety, and is in fact requiring that trade unions take a more active role than ever before. The 1974 Act provides a great impetus for unions to acquire more knowledge and expertise in the field of industrial diseases, including cancer.

EEC legislation

Membership of the EEC will in future have an increasing effect on health and safety legislation in the UK; EEC law is binding on member states, and where it conflicts with the domestic law of a member state, the European law prevails. Descriptions of EEC legislation on health and safety issues are available in publications by Hunter (1978) and the Confederation of British Industry—CBI—(1980).

The Commission of the European Communities (CEC) has an Advisory Committee on Safety, Hygiene and Health Protection at Work, which was set up to assist in preparing and implementing initiatives on all topics falling under this heading except those concerned with mining and ionizing radiations, which are dealt with by separate bodies. The Advisory Committee comprises six members from each member state—two each from government, employers and employees. It is likely that 'directives' will be produced on many substances including carcinogens, under the framework of a draft general directive on the protection of workers from harmful agents at work. A 'directive' is a statutory instrument binding on member states which sets out principles which have to be observed, but which leaves the means of implementation to the discretion of national governments.

The formulation and implementation of legislation by the EEC are inevitably very slow processes, but the EEC clearly has every intention of gradually introducing comprehensive legislation on toxic substances (including carcinogens), and in the future much of our UK legislation will derive from this source.

Legislation in the USA

In the USA, passions run higher over occupational cancer than they do here, and there is a long-standing controversy over legislation to control carcinogens. Bingham (1980) has outlined the USA approach and pointed out how the country had previously lagged behind in matters of occupational health. In 1970, after much controversy, the Occupational Safety and Health Act was passed, giving workers strong legal rights, placing the responsibility for providing a risk-free work environment firmly on employers, and establishing two important agencies. The National Institute for Occupational Safety and Health (NIOSH) conducts research on work hazards and recommends new health and safety standards to the Occupational Safety and Health Administration (OSHA), which sets and enforces health and safety standards.

Standards may be of three kinds. Initially, OSHA in effect adopted *en bloc* the Threshold Limit Values (TLVs) previously drawn up by ACGIH—the American Conference of Governmental Industrial Hygienists, an industry consensus group. 'Emergency temporary standards' can be adopted for immediate control of serious hazards, and 'permanent standards' are developed after a lengthy rule-making process. But when OSHA attempted to regulate one by one the numerous substances needing consideration, it was found that each standard took over a year to prepare and many months to litigate; similar issues were debated each time, and the process was slow and inefficient. Litigation continues to play an important role in the USA in this field—the courts have helped to define OSHA's legal authority, and many proposed standards have been disputed in court.

So OSHA turned to a generic approach, seeking to establish certain basic principles so that a number of substances could then be classified and regulated at the same time. In 1977, OSHA published draft rules for the 'Identification, Classification and Regulation of toxic Substances posing a potential occupational carcinogenic Risk'. Early in this lengthy document, it was noted that OSHA recognized that some 1500–2000 agents had been identified by NIOSH as being 'suspect carcinogens', but that since 1971 OSHA had completed regulatory activity for only 17 of these. A system of categories was proposed: Category I would comprise 'potential occupational carcinogens', and emergency temporary standards followed by permanent standards would be mandatory and, if suitable substitutes were available, the substances might be prohibited. Category II would include substances where evidence of carcinogenicity was only suggestive, based on an unreplicated experiment on one mammalian test species; standards would be set which would prevent known acute or chronic effects, and further research would be instigated.

Because of the simplistic manner in which OSHA planned to interpret existing research data, it was able quickly to prepare a preliminary list of no less than 261 chemicals which were likely to fall into Category I and 196 chemicals in Category II (Maugh, 1980). The proposals met with a storm of protest from American industry, and a typical industrialist's view was to term the proposals 'scientifically unsupportable, administratively unsound, legally wrong, and economically infeasible'. More than ninety USA companies and thirty trade associations have banded together to form the American Industrial Health Council (AIHC), specifically to try to modify the regulations following public hearings, and AIHC put forward a number of proposals for alterations.

Three years later (in 1980) OSHA's classification policy was published in its final draft form, following the study of evidence running to 250 000 pages (*Safety*, issue of March 1980). Some concessions were made, but ironically the revised proposals immediately drew lawsuits from both sides of industry. As Weaver (1976) remarked, 'The OSHA Standards for carcinogens epitomize the legalistic approach, and may be considered a bureaucratic triumph or nightmare, depending on one's point of view.'

Controversy and modifications continue, but the time is presumably approaching when increasing numbers of possible occupational carcinogens will be regulated in the USA, perhaps at the rate of about ten per year. The UK and European situation on carcinogen regulation cannot be fully appreciated without knowledge of the evolving situation in the USA, for what happens there has a profound influence elsewhere. Some European countries tend to follow where the USA leads on toxic substances rather than have to devise their own sets of regulations. If the USA officially declares that a substance is a 'potential occupational carcinogen', some groups in this and other countries may find it hard to believe that it can be safely used with appropriate precautions. On a strictly practical level, UK firms which export chemicals and related products to the USA, or other countries which adopt USA regulations, may find that some of their products are no longer acceptable because they contain 'classified' substances.

Enforcement, monitoring and screening

Enforcement of the 1974 Health and Safety at Work Act and of the regulations under the Act is the duty of the Health and Safety Executive (HSE), which derives medical expertise from the Employment Medical Advisory Service (EMAS). The HSE issues numerous Guidance Notes and Codes of Practice on health and safety precautions for toxic substances, and is often called on to make *ad hoc* decisions about the safe handling of suspected carcinogens. The HSE administers six inspectorates covering agriculture, alkalis and clean air, factories, mines, quarries, and nuclear installations. Local authorities also have enforcement duties under the Act. It would probably be agreed by all concerned that these inspectorates do not have sufficient staff to inspect premises as often as desired, and currently the HSE has incurred cut-backs in spending in common with other government departments. Where conditions of work are controlled by specific sets of regulations or codes of practice, it is the duty of the HSE to ensure compliance with requirements for controlling levels of toxic substances in the air, use of protective masks or clothing, personal monitoring—e.g. of radiation exposure—and the carrying out of statutory medical examinations. If an inspector believes that conditions at a place of work are such that the Act is being contravened, he may serve an 'Improvement Notice', requiring that the situation be remedied within a specified period. If he believes that activities being carried on involve a serious risk of personal injury or damage to health, he may serve a 'Prohibition Order', which takes immediate effect. As a final resort, an inspector may prosecute an employer before a Magistrates Court.

Some regulations require employers to maintain and preserve records of exposed workers, which must be available to the HSE. Examples are registers of persons exposed to 'Controlled Substances' under the Carcinogenic Substances

Regulations of 1967, and records of certain workers covered by the Vinyl Chloride Code of Practice; one possible use of such records is for epidemiological studies.

Large numbers of workers with past exposure to carcinogenic aromatic amines in the chemical, rubber and cable-making industries undergo regular exfoliative urine cytology tests for early diagnosis of urinary tract tumours. For workers exposed to 'prohibited' or 'controlled substances' under the 1967 Regulations, these tests are mandatory at six-monthly intervals, and if they leave employment, workers must be given an approved 'cautionary card' which recommends contin-ued screening. The chemical industry pioneered urine cytology in this country, and most screening is carried out by the relevant industries; the Health Research Unit of the British Rubber Manufacturers' Association (BRMA) provides a service for rubber factories. Where statutory requirements do not apply, employ-ers such as rubber manufacturers who had used carcinogens would be negligent under common law if they failed to provide screening tests.

There is no effective system in this country (or elsewhere) for collecting statistics on the numbers of occupational cancer cases, many of which go unnoticed and unrecorded. The HSE keeps records of all cases of rare tumours, such as meso-thelioma or liver angiosarcoma, that are likely to be occupational. The DHSS notifies the HSE of claims for Prescribed Industrial Disease, but these probably represent only a small fraction of occupational cases (cf. below). In theory, a coroner's inquest should be held in every case of death from industrial cancer, and may help to draw attention to such cases; in practice, however, inquests are held in only a small minority of cases.

Compensation

The State scheme

The National Insurance (Industrial Injuries) Acts constitute a scheme of insur-ance against 'Prescribed Industrial Diseases' (PDs) as well as injuries sustained at work, and the 'benefit' payable by the DHSS for prescribed disease is higher than ordinary sickness benefit. Moreover, the benefit relates to disablement rather than inability to work, and thus applies to retired persons as well as those of working age. As with so much legislation in the field of occupational health, the scheme is currently under review, but although some changes are likely, the general prin-ciple of higher payments to those disabled at work is unlikely to be altered.

Table 6.4 lists the neoplastic diseases included among some fifty prescribed diseases; some are recent additions to the list, which is kept under review.

Montesano and Tomatis (1977) have listed most of the occupational cancers for which state compensation is given in different countries, and from their list it appears that the UK compares unfavourably with some other countries in that our scheme does not specify lung cancer in relation to arsenic or asbestos exposure or bichromate manufacture, or leukaemia in relation to benzene exposure. But in practice, typical English compromise prevails: the authorities are unwilling spe-cifically to prescribe lung cancer as an industrial disease because it is such a common form of cancer, but it may be treated as a complication of arsenic poisoning or asbestosis (which are both prescribed) and hence be effectively covered for many affected workers; similarly, leukaemia may be regarded as a form of benzene poisoning, which is also prescribed. As for affected workers in bichromate manufacture, they are numerically few and the industry has

Table 6.4 Summary of neoplastic diseases prescribed for benefit under the National Insurance (Industrial Injuries) Act, 1946

Diseases which are specifically included

23b, c   Localized neoplasm of the skin, or squamous-cell cancer of the skin (including scrotum) following exposure to arsenic, tar, pitch, bitumen, mineral oil, etc.

25   Skin cancer or bone cancer following exposure at work to x-rays or ionizing radiation

37   Cancer of the nose, nasal sinuses, or lung following work associated with certain nickel-producing processes

39   Tumour of the urinary bladder, renal pelvis, ureter or urethra following exposure to certain carcinogenic aromatic amines, including beta-naphthylamine and benzidine

44   Mesothelioma of the pleura or peritoneum following exposure at work to asbestos

45   Adenocarcinoma of the nose or nasal sinuses following work associated with the manufacture of wooden furniture

50   Angiosarcoma of the liver following exposure to vinyl chloride monomer in the polymerisation process.

51   Cancer of the nose or nasal sinuses following work in the manufacture or repair of leather footwear

Additional diseases which are covered in practice

4   Lung cancer following arsenic poisoning

—   Lung cancer following asbestosis

7   Leukaemia following benzene poisoning

25   Leukaemia as a form of radiation sickness

---

undertaken to compensate them for their disability. It is to be hoped that when the scheme is revised these anomalies will be removed.

The prescribed disease scheme does not work entirely satisfactorily. The onus is on the patient to submit a claim to the DHSS, and this implies knowledge of a possible link between his illness and his past employment on the part of either the patient, or his clinician, or his trade union. Because of the long latent interval which generally occurs between exposure to a carcinogen and the subsequent development of an occupational tumour, this possible link is often overlooked. Somerville *et al.* (1980a) have described some of the complications of claiming for PD 39 (bladder cancer), and both Somerville *et al.* (1980b) and Leon (1980) have pointed out that there appears to be marked under-claiming for PD 39. There is probably also under-claiming for other prescribed occupational cancers, though one hopes it is less severe. Apart from under-claiming through unawareness of an occupational aetiology, there are not infrequently cases where PD claims are contraindicated for technical reasons too detailed to describe here; all these cases help to render statistics of awards of PD benefit for industrial cancer of very little use as indicators of the numbers of occupational cancer cases that occur.

Employers' schemes
As pointed out by Gardiner (1980), some employers in the dyestuff-manufacturing industry have for many years operated compensation schemes for workers who develop bladder tumours, whether or not those affected are still current employ-

ees. Such compensation does not preclude workers from also claiming state payments in the form of PD benefit, but it may preclude them from seeking legal damages. It has already been noted that workers in the bichromate-producing industry who develop lung cancer may obtain compensation from their employer, but cannot obtain PD benefit.

Common law

The cancer risk in many rubber and cable-making factories arose from the use until 1949 of an anti-oxidant manufactured by Imperial Chemical Industries (ICI) called 'Nonox S', which contained as impurities small amounts of uncombined α- and β-naphthylamine. In 1971, with the help of their trade union, two rubber workers who had contracted the disease brought legal actions for negligence against both ICI and their employer (Dunlop Ltd). These were test cases, and the plaintiffs won their cases; ICI appealed against the verdict, but their appeal was dismissed (British Medical Journal, 1971, 1972). ICI were found negligent on the grounds that the firm was in a position to know by about 1943 that Nonox S was very likely to prove dangerous in use, and that they should have taken appropriate action some six years before they finally withdrew the product in 1949. The court emphasized the important principle that the manufacturer's responsibility extends to the purchaser's employees. Dunlop Ltd was found negligent for not making cytological urine screening available to the plaintiffs until 1965 and 1966, although this could readily have been done several years earlier; had the plaintiffs been screened sooner, the disease might have been diagnosed at an earlier date, and the delay had affected treatment adversely. The plaintiffs were awarded damages of £6000 and £15 000 respectively against ICI and £1000 each against Dunlop. Following these test actions, many similar cases against ICI have been settled out of court; the size of the sums awarded depends on the severity of the disease at the time. Widows have also obtained damages. In 1972 it was suggested that as many as 450–500 chemical and rubber workers or their widows might be expected to claim against ICI. A key part of the judgment in this case was: '... the duty of the manufacturer to the purchaser's workmen ... is the same as the duty of the manufacturer towards his own workmen, subject only to one proviso. That proviso is that the manufacturer knows how the goods are going to be used by the purchaser' (Court of Appeal, reported in the *Times* of 2nd November 1972). This judgment had a wide impact with its definition of the manufacturer's responsibility towards workers using his products, and preceded by two years the statute law which imposed similar obligations: 'It shall be the duty of any person who manufactures, imports or supplies any substance for use at work ... to ensure, so far as is reasonably practicable, that the substance is safe and without risks to health when properly used' (Health and Safety at Work, (etc.) Act 1974, Chapter 37). There can be no doubt that the 1972 judgment caused many UK firms to check whether their practices met this obligation, and to modify their practice where necessary. The Chemical Industries Association, for example, issued a statement to its members following the judgment, clarifying the implications of the case for chemical manufacturers, and indicating that they might need to communicate additional data on their products to those using and distributing them (Chemical Industries Association, 1976). The judgment against Dunlop stimulated rubber manufacturers to check that cytological screening was being made available to all their workers who should be covered.

In the asbestos industry also, large sums have been paid to claimants as compensation for asbestosis with or without lung cancer following work in conditions considered to involve negligence on the part of the employers. The October 1979 issue of *Safety* reported that, in 1973, Cape Asbestos (the largest UK group in this industry) had made a provision of £3.5 million (£1.7 million before tax relief) for compensation, hoping that this sum would cover all future claims.

In 1968, the widow of a man who died from scrotal cancer brought a successful court action against her husband's employers, and was awarded £10 000 damages (Weekly Law Reports, 1968). The deceased man had been employed as a tool setter by an engineering firm, and it was not contested that he had been exposed to carcinogenic mineral oils. His cancer was diagnosed too late for effective treatment, and the employers were found negligent in failing to institute six-monthly medical examinations or to issue appropriate warnings to workers about the risk of skin cancer. This judgment was widely considered to be controversial in respect of six-monthly examinations for skin cancer, the encouragement of self-examination being held to be more practicable. But doubtless the judgment led to a review by many firms of their measures for the prevention and early detection of skin cancer. For example, the British Rubber Manufacturers' Association (1969) issued a pamphlet for member firms, setting out advice on the use of mineral oils in rubber-manufacturing operations.

Another feature of court cases like these is that they attract publicity and draw attention to the problems of industrial cancer; further cases that might otherwise have gone unnoticed may come to light as a result of increased awareness. Publicity also results (usually more locally) from inquests on cases of death from industrial disease. Strictly speaking, all such deaths should be reported to the Coroner and inquests should be held, for they are not 'natural' deaths; in practice, however, many such deaths do not get reported. The purpose of an inquest is to establish the cause of death; an inquest is not directly concerned with compensation or with issues of legal liability, but the verdict may be very relevant to both and, where important issues are involved, both relatives and employer may be legally represented. In December 1979, for example, there was a controversial inquest on a worker at the atomic weapons research establishment at Aldermaston who died aged 49 years from a rare form of cancer, and who had been exposed to more than the maximum permitted dose of plutonium. Expert witnesses disagreed as to whether the man's disease was caused by radiation, and an open verdict was returned (*Safety*, issue of January 1980). In the meantime, the man's trade union was pursuing a High Court action for compensation on behalf of the relatives— one of numerous claims for compensation made in connection with exposure to radiation at work and the development of leukaemia or cancer.

In certain other countries too there have been important court cases concerned with industrial cancer. For example, in 1977 the owners and general manager and doctor at an Italian synthetic dye factory were sued by relatives of men dying from bladder cancer, and were charged with multiple manslaughter; at least 132 workers were said to have died from the disease at the 'cancer factory' near Turin over a twenty-year period (*Observer*, issue of 19th June 1977). Prison sentences resulted from this case, which set an important precedent in Italy.

Attitudes

Employers

Organization
On tripartite committees representing government, unions and employers, the latter are generally represented by employers' associations. Examples of these important bodies are the Chemical Industries Association (CIA)—formerly the Association of British Chemical Manufacturers (ABCM)—the British Rubber Manufacturers' Association (BRMA)—formerly the Rubber Manufacturing Employers' Association (RMEA)—and the Institute of Petroleum (IP). Such associations are formed to look after the interests of member firms and to represent them *vis-a-vis* the Government and the public in matters of health and safety, as in other spheres; they generally have committees or divisions specifically devoted to health and safety. For example, the CIA has a 'Chemical Industry Safety and Health Council' with various specialist committees, and the BRMA has a 'Health Advisory Committee'. Manufacturers' associations issue information and guidance to member firms and act on their behalf; this is a particularly valuable service for small firms with limited expertise in health matters. Associations have frequently issued codes of practice for dealing with hazards, although nowadays such codes are more often produced by the HSE after tripartite consultations. Associations may initiate and fund research into possible hazards.

Examples of many codes of practice or information and guidance notes are those on bladder tumours in the chemical industry issued by the ABCM in 1953 and the CIA in 1976, and those on bladder tumours in the rubber industry (Rubber Manufacturing Employers' Association, 1961) and on the use of mineral oils in the same industry (British Rubber Manufacturers' Association, 1969). In the knowledge that a severe bladder cancer hazard existed in the dyestuffs-manufacturing industry, the ABCM sponsored the research of Case *et al.* (1954) which measured and defined the risk; some twenty years later, the Institute of Petroleum (IP) decided to sponsor a mortality study of oil refinery workers as a precaution to check whether any unsuspected hazards existed (Rushton and Alderson, 1980), an enlightened decision in which the ICI court case was not without influence. The BRMA Health Research Unit carries out some epidemiological research of its own, as well as performing another important function: that of carrying out cytological screening for thousands of rubber workers formerly exposed to bladder carcinogens.

Only the largest firms have the resources and medical expertise to be independent in matters of occupational health and, at best, these firms may set standards for a whole industry. For example, Scott and Williams, who in 1957 wrote a Code of Practice approved by the dyestuffs industry, were medical officers for the two largest firms in that industry.

Attitudes
Since it is employers who own and run factories and manufacture goods, it is they who have to take responsibility for health hazards resulting from any exposure to carcinogens involved in these operations. It is all too easy to view the industrial cancer scene as a drama with two sets of characters: the uncaring and even villainous employers, and the innocent workers kept in ignorance of the risks to

which they are exposed. The employers may be seen as bent only on making a profit at any cost to the workers, as unwilling to spend money on improving conditions or compensating those affected, and as ready to suppress evidence of hazards; Peto (1980) has recently expressed such a view of industry's past record: '... where ... industries have been found to cause cancer ... in their workers or in the consumers of their products, their immediate response has usually been to delay acceptance of the findings, to minimise their relevance to current practice, and in general to delay or obstruct any hygienic measures which will cost money'. But is the situation as simple as this? Is the polarization between 'them and us' so clear-cut? After all, who are the 'employers'? If one had to make a distinction between 'employers' and 'workers', it would probably correspond roughly to a 'staff'/'operatives' division, with 'employers' including directors, managers, works doctors and works chemists. But it is perhaps not generally appreciated that, in various industries, staff such as these have themselves been affected by the same occupational cancers as the operatives. Among the many cases of occupational bladder cancer known to the author are several such cases, including the following: director of a family-owned rubber factory; assistant works manager of another rubber factory; works chemist at a cable factory; technical officer at the same cable factory; works chemists at two dyestuffs factories; director of another dye-stuffs factory. Mesothelioma cases known to the author have included at least three 'staff': a building supervisor, a marine surveyor, and the owner of a small factory.

In general, 'staff' such as those listed (with the possible exception of the chemists) would have been less severely exposed than operatives, but clearly they were exposed and they were affected. Cases such as these should lead us to examine the factors which have led industrial managements to behave in a culpable manner; in the author's experience, these factors include ignorance, wishful thinking, alarm and denial on the part of management, which have caused the very staff who should have perceived and dealt with a hazard to be so blind to it that they have been affected by it themselves. Moreover, both authorities such as the factory inspectorate and even researchers must share the blame for industry's ignorance and slowness to act, for often these authorities have failed to enforce hygiene standards, and information on possible hazards has not been adequately disseminated. It is easy for outsiders to express righteous indignation about industry's past record, but how many of us would have done better had we been factory managers and directors?

It is important to remember two points. Firstly, the long latent interval of occupational cancers may be readily grasped theoretically by researchers, but researchers are not personally involved. When those who are personally involved are told of a possible cancer hazard, disbelief is a common reaction in both workers and management; it is equally difficult for both groups to grasp that a disease may develop twenty or more years after the cause, for this is so far outside normal experience as to appear unreal. Secondly, when a cancer hazard does become real, the employers and the trade unions will ask different questions, for a factory means something different to the two. To the trade union, the purpose of the factory is to provide jobs, whereas to the employer, its purpose is to manufacture certain products, and to do so profitably. So the trade union will ask: 'How many workers have been affected? Will they get compensation? Can they have medical screening? Is the risk still there? Are our jobs safe?' For the employers the priority questions may be: 'Have we removed the risk? Can we still make this product? Can we keep the factory open? Can we afford to make the necessary improvements and remain competitive? Will our insurers cover us for compensation payments?' The employers have to take decisions based on the answers to these questions, and the conflict of interests that can arise is illustrated by a second quotation: 'Whilst the protective measures and the alternative processes which have to be used inevitably increase manufacturing costs, this must in the interests of human welfare be a secondary consideration even in the face of world competition' (Association of British Chemical Manufacturers, 1953). However, this quotation is nearly thirty years old, and one would not expect to read such a statement today, with its reluctant concessions to 'human welfare'. Undoubtedly many employers have been negligent in this matter of occupational cancer, and most still have much to learn about how to deal with a 'possible hazard' situation, but attitudes are changing fairly rapidly, and the greater consultation introduced by the 1974 Act and the wider dissemination of information must surely contribute to a continued improvement.

Trade unions

At times in the past, it seemed that the role of trade unions in industrial cancer situations was limited to assisting affected members and their relatives to obtain compensation—though the importance of this role should not be underestimated. Great credit is due to the Transport and General Workers' Union (TGWU) for bringing the influential test action against ICI, for they stood to lose a very large sum of money indeed had the case been lost; no individual worker could possibly have brought such a case unaided.

But 'The sleeping giant is beginning to stir' (McGinty, 1980)—unions are increasingly adopting a much broader role, aided by the 1974 Act. They participate in decision-making committees, and raise questions in Parliament; they appoint national health and safety officers and try to acquire expertise in industrial health subjects; they may promulgate their own policies on industrial cancer, and occasionally they may effectively ban the use of suspect substances.

Statements by union spokesmen in some recent publications illustrate both unions' bitterness about the past history of industrial cancer and their determination to prevent future hazards. Escanez (1976), speaking for French trade unionists, has suggested that workers have had to incur cancer risks with as little choice as hostages held by terrorists, and Blyghton of the TGWU (1976) has stressed his union's concern that more effective medical screening is not possible for workers already exposed to risk. Gee (1980), national health and safety officer of the General and Municipal Workers' Union (GMWU), has given a bitter account of the consequences of the old 'innocent until proved guilty' attitude to workplace substances, and has urged instead 'the assumption that substances are more likely to be harmful than harmless'; thus he reported that the message from the 1979 Congress of the GMWU was: 'Regard fibre-glass, rocksil, rockwool, calcium silicates, etc. as dangerous materials and treat them like asbestos.' In similar vein, the *Daily Telegraph* of 9th June 1980 reported that the Bakers' Union is calling for a government inquiry into the use of chemical additives in flour and dough, and questioning whether long-term chemical hazards might be a factor causing premature retirement and death among members. McGinty (1980) reported that the National Union of Agricultural and Allied Workers was repeating the TUC's call for a ban on the pesticide 2,4,5-T.

The Association of Scientific, Technical and Managerial Staffs (ASTMS) has gone a step further, and issued its own policy document entitled 'The Prevention of Occupational Cancer' (1980). Coming as it does from a union better equipped than most to make a balanced assessment of the situation, it is a pity that this lengthy document is emotional and over-partisan in its approach, and makes the assumption that 40 per cent of cancer in the UK is occupational (based on the USA estimate).

Clearly, some unions may be adopting extreme attitudes on occupational cancer, exaggerating the size of the problem, and being over-ready to condemn substances as carcinogenic. But could one realistically expect it to be otherwise? Past experience of industrial cancer has been deplorable, and it is union members who have suffered in their thousands. Moreover, the painful legacy of the past is still with us and will be for decades to come; the long latent intervals of the disease mean that there must inevitably be thousands more dormant cases caused by past exposures which will develop up to the end of the century and beyond, with asbestos the main cause. How can one expect the trade unions, still inexperienced in their role of power and decision making, to be any less biased in their approach at present than the employers have been in theirs?

The Health and Safety Executive

It has already been emphasized that the HSE does not support the rigid USA criteria for defining carcinogens, or their predilection for 'nil exposures' or prohibition, or their assessment of the scale of the industrial cancer problem. The British approach emphasizes the need for safe working limits for carcinogens, and for assessing each potential hazard separately with critical evaluation of all available evidence. McGinty (1977) complained that 'Typically, the British approach is more pragmatic and opaque ... The whole UK scheme ... reeks of the nanny-knows-best syndrome.' Certainly this approach is more pragmatic, and it is more 'opaque' in that it is an 'outline' policy, not a detailed one. McGinty expresses above the view of unions which see the HSE as too much aligned with employers, as over-inclined to believe substances safe, and over-ready to expect their own assessment of possible hazards to be automatically accepted.

Trade unions do not automatically accept the HSE's opinion that a substance is not carcinogenic in proper use. Their mistrust of the HSE derives mainly from past failures of the factory inspectorate to prevent the existence or continuation of hazardous factory conditions; a case in point concerns Acre Mill, an asbestos factory at Hebden Bridge in Yorkshire, the subject of an Ombudsman's report which was critical of the inspectorate's approach (*Safety*, issue of October 1979). It is to be hoped that such omissions will not be repeated in the future, though as a result of government economies the HSE inspectorates may be over-stretched. Fears about the effects of spending cut-backs have been expressed in Parliament (*Safety*, issue of April 1980), and the Institution of Professional Civil Servants has complained that Nuclear Installations Inspectorate staffing levels have fallen dangerously, with 22 out of 104 posts vacant (*Nature*, 1980).

A subject of current conflict between the HSE and the National Union of Dyers, Bleachers and Textile Workers (NUDBTW) is the safety or otherwise of benzidine-based dyes. Whilst the HSE believes that the dyes used today are safe, and points to negative evidence (including some from research it has sponsored itself), the NUDBTW is encouraging local agreements for the withdrawal of these dyes, and appears to place more reliance on the research and attitude of NIOSH in the USA (*Health and Safety at Work*, March 1980). The HSE must expect more such conflicts in the future, as USA legislation on carcinogens proceeds.

Research workers

Although the Office of Population Censuses and Surveys, the HSE, and industry itself carry out some research on occupational cancer, most such work in the UK is carried out in universities and research institutes. Major studies are generally funded by the Medical Research Council or the Cancer Research Campaign, or are sponsored by industry. Learned societies, such as the Royal Society of Medicine and many others, play a part by organizing conferences for the exchange of information, and the International Agency for Research on Cancer has an influential role.

In the USA, the situation with regard to research on industrial cancer is disturbing, for many research groups appear to be aligned with either industry or the environmentalists and to be under pressures to produce results acceptable to their lobbies. Correspondence in the *Journal of Occupational Medicine* entitled 'Industry's Credibility' (Johnson, 1974) and 'Are Medical Ethical Practices Sufficient in Industrial Medicine?' (Morton, 1973) show how much distrust there has been of both industry and government departments. Recently there has been bitter controversy over the carcinogenicity of beryllium and over epidemiological studies of this possible hazard, with NIOSH officials suggesting that industry might be tampering with or destroying worker records, and industry suggesting that NIOSH was 'gerrymandering' its research data to produce a positive result (Science, 1977). Apart from such distrust, the USA estimate that 20–38 per cent of cancers would be occupational, coming as it did from official bodies, appears to many UK epidemiologists to indicate a widespread lack of judgment and tendency to exaggeration in the USA which is disquieting.

Fortunately, such distrust is unusual in the UK, and researchers are generally unaligned. McGinty (1980) has suggested that some scientists studying hazards inhabit 'ivory towers', but as Doll (1979) has pointed out, it is important that the research process be separate from the decision-making process in the field of industrial cancer: 'Research workers can only be expert witnesses; it is the layman, the civil servant, the jurist or the politician who must take a decision. . . .' For this reason, the merits of research being carried out by either industry itself or by the HSE may be open to some question, since a conflict of interests may arise. ASTMS (1980) has implied that research workers may align themselves with the employers sponsoring their research, but experienced researchers should be well able to resist any pressures which almost inevitably occur from time to time. One type of pressure may arise because epidemiological studies cannot generally provide direct answers to the sort of practical questions that employers ask about possible hazards, and study results may appear abstract to industry; the epidemiologist must avoid any tendency to over-interpret his results, and may also have to attempt to dissuade others from doing so.

Pressure groups

Table 6.1 lists the pressure groups most relevant to industrial cancer, but these bodies are very numerous. An example of a local group is the Hebden Bridge Asbestosis Action Group, set up in 1975 in connection with the Acre Mill asbestos factory near Hebden Bridge in Yorkshire, which was the subject of publicity following an Ombudsman's report in 1976. The mill was closed in 1970, but some 2199 people had worked there since 1939 according to the owners (Cape Asbestos). Conditions had been exceedingly dusty there, and estimates of the number of men affected range from 70 cases of asbestosis and 3 of mesothelioma known to Cape Asbestos in 1977, to 400 or more affected in the opinion of the solicitor advising the Action Group. The Group was set up to campaign for adequate compensation, and to lobby locally against asbestos exposure, especially in the form of asbestos waste tips. Almost all the members are ex-workers at the Mill, and several have died from asbestos-induced diseases since the group was founded; their concern extends to mesothelioma and other cancers as well as asbestosis (*Safety*, issue of October 1979).

A national pressure group also concerned with asbestos is the Society for the Prevention of Asbestos-Induced Diseases (SPAID), which again has the dual function of assisting patients and their relatives, and campaigning against the dangers of the material. The principal founder member was Nancy Tait, and it was again bitter personal experience when her husband died from mesothelioma which led Mrs Tait to mount her campaign. Personal experience of an occupational bladder tumour and of difficulties in having his illness recognized as occupational led Edward Rushworth, a former factory inspector, to found the Cancer Prevention Society, based in Glasgow. The Society is concerned mainly with industrial cancer, and aims to assist affected workers and their relatives, and to campaign for better recognition of the extent of occupational cancer and identification of individual cases. The 'Friends of the Earth' is one of several groups which campaigns against the use of nuclear power and the attendant radiation hazard to workers and those in the vicinity of nuclear installations.

The effectiveness of pressure groups like these in influencing the authorities and research workers must depend in part on the extent to which they are seen as biased and partisan. It is inevitable that the groups be partisan to a degree, but it is a pity that the Cancer Prevention Society appears to accept the USA estimate of the extent of occupational cancer uncritically and apply it to the UK: 'The extent of occupational cancer must be determined. Probably 20 per cent of all cancers are occupationally related, at least in part' (Cancer Prevention Society, Press Notice 1980). The same press notice suggests that around 30000 deaths a year are due to this cause, and many epidemiologists would feel that such statements can cause unnecessary alarm and that the Society's campaign is based on faulty assumptions. A quotation from Nancy Tait's *Asbestos Kills* (Tait, 1976) reflects an idealistic but unrealistic approach: 'Only when the myth that the causes of cancer are unknown has been discarded and replaced by a determination that future generations shall not be subject to this largely man-made disease, will measures be taken to control industrial carcinogens.' Unfortunately, it is not a myth that the causes of cancer are unknown—for most cancers it is an unpalatable but true fact.

But pressure groups like these have formidable adversaries in industry-controlled and financed bodies such as the Asbestos Information Council and the Nuclear Power Information Group. Perhaps Peto (1980) is right when he says '... it may be that where adversary politics operate one needs views at both extremes in order to get a balanced outcome'.

Conclusions

How successful are our efforts to prevent occupational cancer? The past record is not one to be proud of, for preventive action has nearly always come late rather than early. In the recent past and even to some extent today, dangerous exposures to substances recognized as carcinogens decades ago are still occurring. Hopefully, more stringent procedures will make the introduction of new industrial carcinogens less likely, but constant vigilance will be needed.

At present there are tendencies to over-reaction and exaggeration of the industrial cancer problem, but this represents a swing of the pendulum. Probably in five or ten years time perspectives will be clearer.

Those who hope that measures to prevent occupational cancer can achieve a significant reduction in overall cancer mortality are probably doomed to disappointment; it would be a pity if too much attention were diverted from the need to deal with carcinogens such as cigarettes, with their far greater death toll and current immunity from any control. However, such measures at least have the advantage that they are imposed by authority, and generally require little effort or initiative on the part of the individual at risk. Measures to prevent industrial cancer thus have a greater chance of success than those dependent on changes in individual behaviour, and despite their limited scope, they should be given a high priority.

References

Acheson, E. D., Cowdell, R. H., Hadfield, E. and Macbeth, R. G. (1968). *British Medical Journal* **2**, 587.

Acheson, E. D., Cowdell, R. H. and Jolles, B. (1970). *British Medical Journal* **1**, 385.

Association of British Chemical Manufacturers (1953). *Papilloma of the bladder in the chemical industry*. ABCM, London.

Association of Scientific, Technical and Managerial Staffs (1980). *The Prevention of Occupational Cancer. An ASTMS policy document*. ASTMS, London.

Bingham, E. (1980). *Annals of Occupational Hygiene* **23**, 79.

Blyghton, A. C. (1976). In *Environmental Pollution and Carcinogenic Risks*, p. 425. IARC Scientific Publications, No. 13. IARC, Lyon.

Bridport, K., Decoufle, P., Fraumeni, J. F., Hoel, D. G., Hoover, R. N., Rall, R. N., Saffiotti, U., Schneiderman, M. A. and Upton, A. C. (1978). *Estimates of the Fraction of Cancer in the United States related to Occupational Factors*. Unpublished report prepared by the National Cancer Institute, National Institute of Environmental Health Sciences, and National Institute for Occupational Safety and Health.

British Medical Journal (1971). *British Medical Journal* **1**, 411.

British Medical Journal (1972). *British Medical Journal* **2**, 437.

British Medical Journal (1974). *British Medical Journal* **1**, 590.

British Rubber Manufacturers' Association Health Advisory Committee (1969). *Mineral Oils*. BRMA, Birmingham.

Cancer Prevention Society (1980). Press Notice 12.1.1980. Cancer Prevention Society, Glasgow.

Case, R. A. M. and Hosker, M. E. (1954). *British Journal of Preventive and Social Medicine* **8**, 39.

Chemical Industries Association (1976). *Tumours of the bladder in the chemical industry*. CIA, London.

Chemistry in Britain (1980). *Chemistry in Britain* **16**, 235.
Confederation of British Industry (1980). *Safety and health legislation in the European communities—an employers' guide*. CBI, London.
Davies, J. M. (1965). *Lancet* **ii**, 143.
Davies, J. M. (1979). *Journal of the Oil and Colour Chemists Association* **62**, 157.
Department of Employment and Productivity (1970). Technical Data Note 13. *Standards for Asbestos Dust Concentrations for Use with the Asbestos Regulations, 1969*. HMSO, London.
Doll, R. (1977). *Nature* **265**, 589.
Doll, R. (1979). In *Carcinogenic Risks: Strategies for Intervention*, p. 277. IARC Scientific Publications No. 25. IARC, Lyon.
Doll, R., Fisher, R. E. W., Gammon, E. J., Gunn, W., Hughes, G. O., Tyrer, F. H. and Wilson, W. (1965). *British Journal of Industrial Medicine* **22**, 1.
Doll, R., Mathews, J. D. and Morgan, L. G. (1977). *British Journal of Industrial Medicine* **34**, 102.
Douglas, D. B. (1979). In *Carcinogenic Risks: Strategies for Intervention*, p. 81. IARC Scientific Publications No. 25. IARC, Lyon.
Epstein, S. S. (1976). In *Environmental Pollution and Carcinogenic Risks*, p. 389. IARC Scientific Publications No. 13. IARC, Lyon.
Escanez, J. (1976). In *Environmental Pollution and Carcinogenic Risks*, p. 431. IARC Scientific Publications No. 13. IARC, Lyon.
Figueroa, W. G., Raszkowski, R. and Weiss, W. (1973). *New England Journal of Medicine* **288**, 1096.
Gardiner, J. S. (1980). *British Medical Journal* **1**, 867.
Gee, D. (1980). *Chemistry and Industry*, p. 180, 1st March 1980. The Society of the Chemical Industry, London.
Health and Safety at Work (1980). Maclaren Publishers, Croydon.
Health and Safety Executive (1975). *Vinyl Chloride: Code of Practice for Health Precautions*. HSE, London.
Health and Safety Executive (1980). *Mortality in the British Rubber Industries, 1967–76*. HMSO, London.
Henry, S. A., Kennaway, N. M. and Kennaway, E. L. (1931). *Journal of Hygiene* **31**, 125.
Hunter, D. (1959). *Health in Industry*. Penguin, Harmondsworth.
Hunter, W. J. (1978). *Journal of the Society of Occupational Medicine* **28**, 101.
International Agency for Research on Cancer (1973). *Biological Effects of Asbestos*. IARC Scientific Publications No. 8. IARC, Lyon.
International Labour Organization (1974). *Control and Prevention of Occupational Hazards Caused by Carcinogenic Substances and Agents*. ILO, Geneva.
Johnson, W. M. (1974). *Journal of Occupational Medicine* **16**, 645.
Lancet (1965). *Lancet* **ii**, 1173.
Legge, Sir T. (1934). In *Industrial Maladies*, p. 3. Ed. by S. A. Henry. OUP, Oxford and H. Milford, London.
Leon, D. (1980). *British Medical Journal* **280**, 1053.
McGinty, L. (1977). *New Scientist*, 22/29 December 1977.
McGinty, L. (1980). *New Scientist*, p. 810, 13th March 1980.
Maugh, T. H. (1980). *Science* **201**, 1200.
Melick, W. F., Escue, H. M., Naryka, J. J., Mezera, R. A. and Wheeler, E. P. (1955). *Journal of Urology* **74**, 760
Montesano, R. and Tomatis, L. (1977). *Cancer Research* **37**, 310.
Morton, W. E. (1973). *Journal of Occupational Medicine* **15**, 860.
Munn, A. (1974). *Journal of the Society for Occupational Medicine* **24**, 90.
Nature (1980). *Nature* **285**, 125.
Newhouse, M. L. (1969). *British Journal of Industrial Medicine* **26**, 294.
Olin, G. R. (1978). *American Industrial Hygiene Association Journal* **39**, 557.
Peto, R. (1980). *Nature* **284**, 297.
Pittom, L. A. (1980). *Annals of Occupational Hygiene* **23**, 85.
Redmond, C. K., Ciocco, A., Lloyd, J. W. and Rush, H. W. (1972). *Journal of Occupational Medicine* **14**, 621.
Registrar General (1958). *Decennial Supplement, England and Wales 1951: Occupational Mortality, Part II*. HMSO, London.

Rockette, H. E. (1977). *Journal of Occupational Medicine* **19**, 795.

Rubber Manufacturing Employers' Association (1961). *Papilloma of the bladder in the rubber industry*. RMEA, Birmingham.

Rushton, L. and Alderson, M. R. (1980). *An Epidemiological Survey of Eight Oil Refineries in the UK—Final Report*. Institute of Petroleum, London.

Safety (1979, 1980). A British Safety Council Publication, London.

Science (1977). *Science* **198**, 898.

Scott, T. S. and Williams, M. H. C. (1957). *British Journal of Industrial Medicine* **14**, 150.

Somerville, S. M., Davies, J. M., Hendry, W. F. and Williams, G. (1980a). *British Medical Journal* **1**, 540.

Somerville, S. M., Davies, J. M., Hendry, W. F. and Williams, G. (1980b). *British Medical Journal* **1**, 867.

Stocks, P. (1962). *British Journal of Cancer* **16**, 592.

Tait, N. (1976). *Asbestos Kills*. The Silbury Fund, London.

Wada, S., Nishimoto, Y., Miyanishi, M., Katsuta, S. and Nishiki, M. (1962). *Hiroshima Journal of Medical Science* **11**, 75.

Wagoner, J. K., Infante, P. F. and Bayliss, D. L. (1980). *Environmental Research* **21**, 15.

Walpole, A. L., Williams, M. H. C. and Roberts, D. C. (1954). *British Journal of Industrial Medicine* **11**, 105.

Weaver, N. K. (1976). *Journal of Occupational Medicine* **18**, 607.

Weekly Law Reports (1968). Stokes v. Guest, Keen and Nettlefold (Bolts and Nuts) Ltd. p. 1776 (1966 S. No. 7468).

7

Non-governmental approaches to the control of cancer

Michael Calnan

Introduction

In this section the ways in which various agencies, groups and individuals have gone about attempting to control various cancer-provoking agents will be considered. The main focus of attention will be on tobacco and alcohol control policies because these have received a considerable amount of attention and are probably more appropriate subjects for non-governmental policy than the other agents. As will be seen, the nature of tobacco and alcohol dependence and associated problems are distinctly different and the need to be discussed independently.

Non-governmental policy in smoking control

In this section those strategies for smoking control which have been proposed and used at the individual and group level will be examined. However, before these various approaches have been described and evaluated, it is necessary to describe in more detail the nature of smoking.

Explanations of smoking

A variety of factors have been proposed and identified as being significant in the generation and continuance of smoking (Russell, 1971). These explanations have ranged from genetic, psychological, sociological and sensorimotor to pharmacological. While the relationships between the factors are uncertain, it is evident that psycho-social factors play an important part in taking smoking up and psychological and pharmacological factors play a part in the continuance of the behaviour (Raw, 1978).

Recent controversy over explanations of smoking behaviour focuses on the significance of the dependent nature of smoking. For example, Raw (1978) states that psychologists have been guilty of ignoring alternative theories of smoking behaviour. He states:

> 'It is undoubtedly time to focus more attention on the nature of smoking, with a view to incorporating into a treatment model what we now know about its psychology, pharmacology and economics.'

The more recent models of smoking behaviour have not only attempted to incorporate this process of dependence (be it predominantly physiological or psychological in nature) but also have attempted to move away from the more behaviouristic approach of learning theory to an emphasis on the ability of individuals to make rational choices about whether to smoke or not (Eiser and Sutton, 1977). Thus smoking behaviour is not seen entirely as a response to either external or internal stimuli, but may be seen as a form of rational action by individuals, even though it may have some negative consequences.

It is necessary to divide the 'career' of the smoker into two stages, as different factors play a part in the generation and establishment of smoking behaviour and its maintenance and continuance.

A number of models attempting to explain why people start to smoke have been developed (Horn, 1979) but perhaps the most coherent one is that developed by Bynner (1969), called the recruitment model. The model consists of the identification of factors which are barriers to the taking up of smoking and those that increase the chances. Psycho-social factors predominate. The barriers of sensory discomfort and nicotine effects are only temporary; other more important barriers are parental attitude, school attitude, and perceived health risks. On the other hand, the factors that influence a young person starting smoking are: availability of cigarettes, curiosity, rebelliousness, to appear tough, anticipation of adulthood, social confidence, parental example, older siblings and friends smoking. Evidence from other research supports the notion that the young person's social environment plays a crucial part in influencing whether that person takes up smoking or not. The smoking habits of parents, siblings or friends seem to have a bearing on why young people take up smoking (Bewley *et al.*, 1974; Bewley and Bland, 1977; Pearson and Richardson, 1978). Other findings show that boys smoke more and start smoking earlier than girls and that the amount of smoking increases with age (Bynner, 1969). These differences between boys and girls in terms of prevalence of smoking may have decreased over the past decade. A recent study examining the smoking habits of 16-year-olds in a national sample of children (Pearson and Richardson, 1978) supports this contention. The Government Social Survey of 1964 showed that 38 per cent of males and 20 per cent of females were considered to be regular smokers. The National Child Development Study (NCDS) data of 1974 showed that 20 per cent of 16-year-old boys and 24 per cent of 16-year-old girls smoked more than ten cigarettes a week. There was an overall drop between the two surveys for all smokers from 39 per cent in 1964 to 36 per cent in 1974. The NCDS data showed that the frequency of smoking increased progressively from social class I to social class V. The study also showed that smoking was heavier among children attending comprehensive or secondary modern as opposed to grammar schools. Heavy smoking was also closely related to money available and also associated with social activities such as drinking, going to dances and parties.

In a study carried out in 1975, investigating the smoking habits of 10 498 secondary schoolchildren (Rawbone *et al.*, 1978), overall 14.9 per cent of secondary schoolchildren were smoking. The prevalence, however, varied with age, rising from less than 5 per cent in 11-year-olds to over 20 per cent at age 15. The study also showed that children who smoked regularly had a higher prevalence of upper respiratory tract infections, and a higher incidence of respiratory symptoms, cough, phlegm production and shortness of breath compared to non-smokers.

However, perhaps the most crucial finding of them all is the apparent link between smoking in adolescence and smoking in adulthood. A large proportion of all young people who regularly smoke persist in this habit when they grow up (McKennell and Thomas, 1967).

The models explaining continuing smoking in adulthood put less emphasis on psycho-social factors and more on pharmacological and psychological factors (McKennell and Thomas, 1967; Russell, 1971). Russell (1971), extending the typology of McKennell and Thomas, identified five different types of smoker. This classification is based on the motives of the smoker. The psycho-social smoker and the indulgent smoker—i.e. the person who smokes for pleasure—are those whose motives contain a predominantly social element. The tranquillization, stimulation and addictive smokers are dominated by pharmacological rewards. According to this model, the career of the typical smoker starts off with socially orientated motives and moves on to the stages where smoking is nicotine motivated (see Russell, 1976). How accurate such a model is, is difficult to tell, but it seems to be based on the assumption that dependence on smoking is almost entirely due to psychological or pharmacological rewards. The idea that dependence may be reinforced by the social environment in which a smoker lives, such as through images created by advertising, or within the cultural environment itself is seen to be of minimal importance. Certainly, the recent shift in the climate of opinion in favour of non-smoking in our society may make it easier for smokers to try to stop. As we shall see, the significance of social support in the process of smoking withdrawal may suggest that social elements of dependence may have been undervalued. The reasons given by smokers for wanting to discontinue are varied but in general, for young people, expense is the main reason, and ill-health is the main reason in older people (Royal College of Physicians, 1977).

For those concerned with developing smoking control policies, one problem with these models is that there is no explanation of why individuals have different levels of cigarette consumption. The difference between the heavy and light smoker may be an artificial distinction which has been created purely to suit the needs of epidemiological research. However, it would be useful to find out, if possible, how a light smoker becomes a heavy smoker and vice versa.

The second problem concerns the reasons people give for smoking or not. It has been argued in the above that many smokers are strongly influenced by psychological or pharmacological dependence. However, whilst this might be the case, many smokers state that they smoke more when they are under stress (Schachter, 1978).

It could be argued that the dependent smoker's stress is caused by the pharmacological or psychological sensations caused by the addiction itself. However, it could also be that stress or believed feelings of stress have some origin in some social settings or social circumstances. Thus, certain life events such as bereavement, divorce or unemployment may induce stress. The ability to cope with stress may be influenced by an individual's psychological state and the level of social resources available. As yet, there is no evidence to support these propositions; however, it does raise an important point for policy. If, in fact, smokers smoke heavily because they believe it eases tension, anxiety or stress, which in themselves are produced by certain social events, then smoking is not only meeting an individual's perfectly rational need for coping with stress, but also the stress is generated by 'events' out of his control. So, policies aimed at stopping people smoking should either provide a substitute coping mechanism or attempt to eradicate the sources of stress. If there is a link between stress and smoking, then present-day smoking control policies may create more problems than they solve because they are not aimed at eradicating the root cause of smoking or providing the smoker with a means for coping with stress.

Medical and psychological treatments for smoking withdrawal

It is not surprising that the vast majority of methods for smoking withdrawal are either pharmacologically or psychologically orientated, given that these two disciplines have provided the predominant explanations or theories of smoking behaviour. It is only recently, when social factors have been seen to play a part in smoking behaviour, that the approach to smoking withdrawal has been more collectively orientated.

Raw (1978), in his review of the treatment of cigarette dependence, has identified the following different types of treatment:

(i)   drug therapy;
(ii) hypnosis;
(iii) aversion therapy;
(iv) self-control approaches;
(v)   smoking withdrawal clinics and group approaches;
(vi) miscellaneous.

This is not the place to discuss each of these methods in detail. However, a little detail on each approach and its effectiveness may be useful. Raw (1978) identified two main approaches to drug treatment: (i) treatment of withdrawal symptoms by tranquillization, and (ii) the substitution, or replacement, of nicotine or its pharmocological action. Included under the latter heading is nicotine chewing gum which is now available to the general public through prescription from family doctors (Toynbee, 1980). Results from a recent study (Raw et al., 1980) show that nicotine chewing gum, in comparison with other psychological treatments for dependent smokers, was more successful. At a one-year follow-up, 38 per cent of the 69 people taking chewing gum were still abstinent, compared with 14 per cent of the 49 people who received other psychological treatments. Abstinence was confirmed by the measurement of carboxyhaemoglobin or expired air carbon monoxide. The blood nicotine concentrations when patients used the gum averaged half the smoking values and side-effects were few. Addiction occurred in two of the subjects. The authors conclude that nicotine chewing gum is a useful aid to giving up smoking and is probably acceptable even for people with cardiovascular disease. Once again, however, this leaves untouched the problem of preventing relapse. Raw concludes:

> 'The drug treatments are best thought of as short-term aids and as useful, not because of especially high success rates, but because they require so little therapist time and effort to administer, compared with psychological or large clinic approaches.'

Raw's conclusion about the value of hypnosis is similarly critical and he argued that the apparently high success rates found for hypnosis are derived from studies using no controls and highly selected samples. He argued that there is no evidence to say that hypnosis is better than any other technique.

Aversion therapy is the single most used approach of all the behavioural psychological approaches in smoking, either in the form of electric aversion therapy, convert aversion therapy, rapid smoking or satiated. Once again, Raw concludes that there is little evidence to show whether aversion therapy has a specific effect over and above the effect of support.

Of the self-control approaches (see East and Towers, 1979), Raw (1978) concludes:

'The only self-control approach which merits serious attention is stimulus control. It is important because it deals with real-life smoking situations straightaway because it minimises dependence on the therapist, because it seems to generate treatments which are acceptable, cheaper and more readily available.'

Smoking withdrawal clinics have been set up in some areas to deal directly with smoking modification. Most clinics are run by area health authorities but private clinics are run by the British Temperance Society and the Seventh Day Adventists. There was an increase in the number of clinics during the early part of the 1970s. In the Second Report of the Royal College of Physicians (1971) there were fewer than 10 such clinics, but by 1975 a survey carried out by ASH showed at least 50 were operating. Apparently this number fell to 35 in 1980 (Toynbee, 1980). The clinics carry out a variety of treatments, both pharmacological and psychotherapeutic, but the basic function is to provide psychological aid.

Raw described the group approaches used in these clinics (1978):

'apart from drug therapy, specific treatments take second place to the general processes of dissemination of health information, group discussion and support, and general advice'.

The long-term success rate in some studies has been 15–20 per cent of treated clients still abstinent a year after treatment. Raw concluded:

'If a client's resources are mobilised (the effect of a placebo) and they are given very basic support and advice, a fair proportion of them can stop smoking permanently.'

With regard to the other treatments, (i) systematic desensitization is no more effective than support, (ii) there are no data to evaluate psychoanalysis, and (iii) sensory deprivation is effective but the reasons for its success are unknown (Raw, 1978). Raw's overall conclusion about these treatments was that there is not much to choose between them. The average success rate is 15–20 per cent at six months and the relapse rate is about 70 per cent. He suggests that the reason for the success of some treatments and combination of treatments in the short term may lie with motivation, structure and support. In a previous paper (Raw, 1977b) he has suggested that no treatments are better than support, although both treatment and support groups do better than clients told to stop unaided.

Raw's (1978) major criticisms of the approaches to smoking control that he reviewed were that they were too treatment or curative orientated rather than orientated to the clients' needs. He suggested that treatments should be tailored to individuals' needs and that pharmacological treatments and psychological treatments should be integrated and used either in combination or individually, depending on the type of client involved. He also argued that the psychological approach up to now has been too concerned with externally or overt measurable phenomena to the neglect of motivation and the degree and nature of dependence.

According to Raw, as much concern must be placed on relapse as on the initial stopping of smoking; thus a treatment package could contain treatments aimed specifically at short-term withdrawal and relapse. Finally, he argued that individual counselling is better than group counselling and that, in the context of rapid smoking treatment, individual rather than group treatment is more beneficial.

Information and advice giving in smoking control

Information and advice about smoking have been given in both individual and group forms and have been directed at adult smokers with the intention of reducing or stopping cigarette smoking and at young people with the intention of preventing them starting.

Attempts to prevent children taking up smoking have been mainly carried out in the form of group methods in schools. Thompson (1978) reviewed the educational programmes on youth behaviour and smoking and concluded:

'Attempts to change the smoking behaviour of young people have included anti-smoking campaigns, youth-to-youth programmes, and a variety of message themes and teaching methods. Instruction has been presented both by teachers who were committed or persuasive, and by teachers who were neutral or presented both sides of the issue.' He continues: 'Didactic teaching, group discussion, individual study, peer instruction and mass media have been employed. Health effects of smoking, both short term and long term effects, have been emphasised. Most methods used with youth have shown little success. Studies of other methods have produced contradictory results.'

Such a conclusion seems to be accurate (Biener, 1975; Dale, 1978). Although some programmes have had little impact on behaviour, some have increased knowledge but not always improved attitudes. Watson (1968) compared four different methods of health education for schoolchildren in Scotland and showed that only the didactic method produced a significant decrease in smoking.

Other studies may have highlighted the reason for the failure in many health education campaigns. As Bland et al. (1975) state:

'One reason may be that the words used to describe the health consequences of smoking are not fully understood by children.'

This approach to changing people's behaviour is a clear example of an assumption in much health education that individuals can be influenced by information given by official agencies and totally ignores the findings that the greatest influences on young people in the field of smoking are through informal influences such as their parents, peers and friends. Thus, perhaps health education methods should try to utilize these social networks for social change, or at least recognize that health education can only work if the social context in which people live is taken into account (see Green, 1970). Perhaps the reason for the reduction in the number of smokers in the age group 16–21 years, is due to a reduction in the number of their parents smoking.

Martin and Stanley (1965, 1966) carried out two intensive anti-smoking campaigns in two Scottish towns—one in 1963 and one in 1965. The emphasis was on education through promotion and publicity. The only positive change was found in one town which showed a significant decline in smoking rates.

Group methods of health education have been tried with adult smokers. Results from evaluations of smoking clinics have been reported previously and the evidence suggested that they are no better than any other of the techniques reviewed. Other methods that have been tried are those by Bernstein (1970) who attempted to modify smoking behaviour principally through social pressure. Eight sessions of twenty to twenty-five minutes over two weeks were held for small groups; subjects kept a record of their smoking for one week before the programme and were followed up by telephone for five to sixteen weeks after the programme. Although social pressure, group and individual placebos and individual effort methods are all effective at reducing smoking in the short term, there is no evidence of long-term success. More successful results were found in a study by Janis et al. (1970) who looked at the facilitating effects of daily contact between partners who make a decision to cut down on smoking. The aim was to measure the effects of contact between partners. All groups reduced smoking during the period of the clinic but the high contact group reduced the most. The control group (the group of people who had a different partner at each session) relapsed by one year to the initial level—32 cigarettes a day—the low contact group relapsed to about 22 cigarrete a day, but the high contact group maintained the initial reduction to 8 cigarettes per day.

These results are interesting in the sense that interaction is almost reduced to a one-to-one encounter between people who were beginning to get to know each other. However, a later study showed that increased contact alone did not lead to lasting reduction.

Some of the most effective methods of modifying smoking have been through advice or health education carried out on an individual level between professional and client. When discussing individual treatments, it was concluded that there was no better treatment than support. Giving and continuing to give advice may be another form of this. Some studies have been carried out to evaluate the effect of advice or instruction on those patients with chronic conditions such as heart disease. In these studies (Burt, 1974; Croog, 1977) results showed that previous experience of a heart attack reduces smoking but a close relationship to someone who has had an attack does not. This indicates the importance of advice by professionals to 'motivated' people. In these studies people were motivated for reasons of health. It must be remembered that motivation and dependence have been identified as two of the most important factors in understanding why people stop smoking.

Other studies have examined the general practitioners' role in counselling about cigarette smoking. Porter (1972) gave vigorous advice to an experimental group of smokers in his practice and compared the outcome with a control group of smokers who received no advice. Of the total 191, 9 gave up smoking—5 from E group and 4 from C. Manual workers were more likely to give up than non-manual. Whilst these figures were not very optimistic, Russell, in a more recent study (1979), has shown more favourable results from general practitioners giving advice and health education. He suggests that, compared with smoking withdrawal clinics, this is a more economical and more effective (in terms of access to numbers) method. Handel's study of general practitioners and changing smoking habits (1973), also showed good results. One year after being given advice by their general practitioners, 37 per cent of the men and 11 per cent of the women had stopped smoking.

Self-help groups and lay methods of smoking control

The evidence on how many people stop smoking without any professional help is difficult to find, as is the evidence to explain why or how this can be achieved. Models have been developed which attempt to explain individual compliance with recommended health actions, but much of this research has concentrated on take up or regular compliance with preventive health services (Rosenstock, 1974; Becker and Maiman, 1975). Little evidence is available to explain why people take regular exercise for health reasons, follow strict diets for health reasons or carry out regular breast self-examination. Perhaps the health belief model can be applied to these patterns of behaviour or maybe other factors, which have been identified as important in the previous literature—such as social support— should be included (Becker, 1979). The dependent nature of cigarette smoking complicates the picture even further.

Raw (1977a) suggests that in smoking withdrawal clinics, abstinence rates are quite a lot higher than the spontaneous stopping rate, although whether this is due only to the degree of attention given to the individual smoker is difficult to decide. An alternative method, not so much for getting people to give up smoking but to prevent relapse, is self-help groups (Baric, 1978). These involve continual meetings of a group of ex-smokers who have recently given up smoking. The value of these groups is still uncertain, but their evaluation might identify whether social support is as crucial a factor in the maintenance of health behaviour as has been suggested. Thus, there is a need for a controlled evaluation study of self-help groups for smokers. In addition, detailed evidence is needed on the beliefs and feelings of those smokers who are successful at giving up smoking without any kind of formal intervention, as well as the circumstances that surround their giving up. Also, further evidence is needed on the most appropriate settings for group work, particularly comparing clinical settings to occupational settings (see East and Towers, 1979).

The work of non-governmental institutions in smoking control

The Government has provided funds to ASH and the Health Education Council to implement some of its policies directed at smoking control and has funded some research to examine factors influential in the process of cigarette dependence. However, other bodies who have no direct link with the Government have been involved in the smoking control debate. The one body which seems to have made a significant contribution to smoking control is the Royal College of Physicians, with the publication of their three reports (1962, 1971, 1977). Not only do they seem to have provided the stimulus for government action but the publicity given to them may have played a part in influencing the consumption of cigarettes (Peto, 1974). This influence, particularly in the eyes of the public, may have been due to the degree of publicity given to the reports through the mass media, or it may reflect the authority given by the public to the College pronouncements on matters of health.

Summary

A number of alternative smoking control strategies have been tried on small groups and individuals. Of the medical and psychological treatments, no one stands out above the rest in terms of long-term success rates. The real problem with these treatments is in maintaining abstinence or preventing relapse. The reasons for even short-term success are difficult to find and it may be nothing more than the effect of the therapists' support. This might be the reason why general practitioners do as well as some other treatments in getting people to give up.

Educational methods aimed at preventing young people from starting have showed little success, as have group methods of influencing adult smokers. The most successful results occurred when individuals were interacting on a one-to-one basis. It could be that the reason why individual methods on smoking control appear to be more successful than group methods is the intensity of support given in one-to-one encounters. It may be possible to obtain that degree of support in groups, particularly amongst smokers in self-help groups which might prevent relapse. It is difficult to know whether the reasons for the lack of success in smoking control methods are mainly due to the dependent nature of smoking or are mainly due to the social context which may not enhance the pursuance of any health practice.

Non-governmental approaches to the control of heavy drinking and its associated problems

In this section, non-governmental policies for the control of heavy drinking will be considered. It is evident that the efficacy of any control policy will be based, at least in part, on the validity of the assumptions that are made about drinking behaviour. So it is necessary to give a brief outline of the various theories of drinking behaviour which are available.

Theories of the causation of drinking problems

Three different types of 'causal' theory of heavy drinking and associated problems have been identified (Robinson, 1976). They are:
   (i)   biochemical theories;
   (ii) psychological theories;
   (iii) sociological theories.

Biochemical theories of drinking problems

These theories emphasize the significance of physiological and biochemical mechanisms in the determination of heavy drinking problems. Shields (1977) explains the basis of the interest in the area:

'In pharmacogenetics one searches for individual genetic differences in response to the drug and endeavours to elucidate the mechanisms by means of animal models where appropriate. In this respect, genetic studies of alcoholism might be thought to hold particular promise.'

In his review, Shields (1977) identifies the significance of genetics in sex differences in the incidence of alcoholism, although he recognizes that social factors may have a lot to do with these variations. In discussing family studies, he suggests:

'The presence of an alcoholic parent in the home, whatever problems this creates, does not seem to be a specific cause of alcoholism—or if it is, one would have to argue that it also has the effect of driving some of the children to teetotalism.'

Genetic (Shields, 1977) as well as biological factors (Littleton, 1977) have been suggested to have an influence on ethanol metabolic rates and to be influential in the development of personality disorders which are supposed to predispose people to alcoholism. Certainly, the evidence for the latter type of explanation is weak. Whilst some writers (Shields, 1977) emphasize the importance of genetics as a causative factor in alcoholism, there appears to be little consistent evidence available, at least at present, to support these contentions.

Psychological theories of drinking problems

Other types of explanations which also place emphasis on intrinsic defects or disorders within the individual as causative factors in the development of drinking problems are those that can be broadly termed 'psychological' theories. Some of these theories, like the genetic theories, appear to accept the disease concept of alcoholism. These psychological theories have been divided into three different types (Robinson, 1976). They are personality trait analyses, learning theory and psychoanalytic theory. Evidence to support the idea of an alcoholic personality is weak (Robinson, 1976; Orford, 1977) and there appears to have been a shift away from this approach to one that attempts to integrate individual differences such as vulnerability or susceptibility with pharmacological and social factors which might generate or reinforce heavy drinking. Orford (1977) states:

'On the basis of psychological factors, it is going to be extremely difficult to predict who is going to be most susceptible to some forms of pharmacological or social reinforcement from drinking.'

Learning theories of different types have been used to explain drinking behaviour. Robinson explains their general approach (1976):

'Some theorists see alcohol consumption as a reflex to certain kinds of stimulus or as a way of reducing anxiety or fear. Operating on the pleasure–pain principle, such theories hold that people are drawn to pleasant situations and repelled by unpleasant or anxiety arousing ones.'

These theorists, according to Robinson (1976), account for the persistent attraction of alcohol to heavy drinkers, given the acute pain and distress that it can produce, in terms of the immediate relief it can provide from those feelings of guilt or anxiety that drinking has produced. So, in effect, the heavy drinker appears to be involved in a process which contains an inherent reinforcement mechanism. However, this reinforcement is predominantly partial, in that reinforcement does not occur every time a response occurs (Orford, 1977). The probabilistic nature of the process has also been emphasized (Orford, 1977), in that some responses become more probable and other responses become less probable. Finally, as Orford states (1977):

'There is the gradient of reinforcement, a fact which may go quite a long way to explaining paradoxical behaviour; reward which follows immediately upon behaviour is more effective in shaping behaviour and making it more probable or less probable in future, than is reinforcement that occurs later on.'

The third type of psychological theory that has been identified is psychoanalytic. Tendencies such as self-destruction, oral fixation, latent homosexuality and power struggles have been emphasized as being important determinants of drinking problems (Robinson, 1976) although, as always with this approach, empirical evidence to support such propositions is difficult to obtain.

Sociological theories of drinking problems

Sociological theories of drinking problems have been divided into three different approaches (Robinson, 1976). They are the societal–cultural, the aetiological–pathological and the ethnographic or processual approach.

The societal–cultural approach, according to Robinson (1976), attempts to identify what alcohol means to a society at a general level and what functions it fulfils. For example, societies have been classified in terms of their cultural orientation to drinking or they have been classified in terms of the potential integrative or disintegrative functions of alcohol for that society. Robinson (1976) suggests that there is a need to understand the meaning of alcohol or drinking for members of society as it is an essential part of explaining why people drink in the way that they do. However, Robinson (1976) does confess that this approach is directed at such a general level that it could never be appropriately evaluated.

The aetiological–pathological approach involved the identification of social or socio-demographic factors such as age, sex, social class, marital status, education and religion as predictors of drinking problems. Other more detailed variables, such as individual orientations towards drinking, have also been used in analysis (Robinson, 1976).

This approach has been criticized on a number of grounds. First, that definitions of drinking problems are constructed by the researchers without any recourse to the feelings of the respondents about drinking (Robinson, 1976). This means that the definitions of drinking problems may be derived from the prior assumptions of the researcher, which may bear no relation to what the respondents define as a problem. Another difficulty with this approach has been identified (Robinson, 1976). He states:

> 'The range of any possible causal links which epidemiologists can forge is determined by the range of social areas which are built into the investigation before it starts. As a result it is a characteristic of such studies that they usually cover a great deal of ground rather "superficially".'

The ethnographic or processual approach represents a shift away from the approaches which explain alcoholism or drinking problems in terms of some attribute of an individual or of a culture, towards a perspective which sees the label 'alcoholic' as a product of certain social processes or is related to social settings. Using this perspective, it is as important to examine who labels an individual as being an alcoholic as it is to examine why certain people are labelled as such. This perspective, therefore, appears to represent a movement away from the treatment of alcoholism as a disease to one that sees it as a product of societal classification. Studies adopting this approach have been carried out in other areas of deviance, but little of this kind of work has been carried out in the area of alcoholism (Robinson, 1976).

One study which would be classified as adopting a processual approach was carried out by Plant (1979), although in his study the emphasis was placed on examining the impact of different social settings on drinking behaviour. He looked at alcohol-related problems amongst different occupational groups. He found that those involved in occupations related to alcohol production drank more and experienced more problems with their drinking than those engaged in other types of occupation. He found that eight of the ten heavy drinkers had previous records of 'high-risk' employment—i.e. employment in alcohol production. Plant also found that most men did their heaviest drinking at the weekend, so their drinking problems were not normally visible to their employers.

Plant (1979), in examining the determinants of drinking behaviour, found that people changed their drinking habits sometimes to fit the context in which they worked. He found that drinking habits increased markedly when men moved from low-risk to high-risk employment and from low-risk jobs to unemployment. He concludes:

> 'On the strength of the evidence of this study it would appear that, of the items examined, current occupation was the most influential in determining an individual's current drinking habits and consequent alcohol-related problems.'

This study clearly points to the importance of the influence of the social setting in which people live and work on their drinking patterns. Other settings, apart from occupation, may be important, such as family and marital life (Orford and Edwards, 1977).

In summary, there is little evidence available which could be used to evaluate these different theories. However, it is evident that researchers from all three different perspectives emphasized the social nature of drinking and drinking problems. Therefore, further research is necessary to identify the nature of the social processes and conditions that are associated with drinking problems.

Alcohol control strategies

This section consists of three different parts. The first two parts will contain an examination of the various treatments used for controlling excessive alcohol use and the third part will be concerned with the impact of health education on prevention.

The treatment approaches have been divided into two, according to whether they focus on the individual or the group (Robinson, 1976).

Individual approaches

These approaches usually begin with the use of drugs and medications aimed at controlling withdrawal symptoms. This is followed by medical treatments aimed at treating the physical effects of excessive alcohol consumption. These treatments sometimes occur in detoxification centres, which have been a more recent development in the UK, although the value of such centres in terms of reducing drunkenness arrests is still open to doubt (Hore, 1977). In fact, the value of medical treatments as a whole has been brought into question (Orford and Edwards, 1977).

Following these initial treatments for withdrawal and physical effects of alcohol, various forms of treatment are used. Some concentrate on controlling the drinking itself, others are aimed directly at the cause of the problem, as heavy drinking is seen to be only a symptom.

One treatment which could be classified in the former group of treatments is behaviour therapy. A number of methods of modifying excessive drinking through behaviour therapy have been developed (Hodgson, 1977), although each is based on the assumption that excessive drinking is a compulsive habit. Each method of investigation is derived from learning theory.

The methods are classified by Hodgson (1977) as follows.

1. The development of skills which give the alcoholic the ability to cope with the pressures and stress which induce heavy drinking.

2. Contingency management which attempts to modify behaviour by altering some of the circumstances that reinforce drinking. The circumstances that are referred to are mainly environmental, and the methods of treatment advocated are: vocational counselling, marital and family counselling and social counselling. Each of these different types of counselling aims at reducing those environmental contingencies that reinforce drinking. For example, social counselling methods involve changing the drinker's social environment so that more interactions occur with people who are non-drinking acquaintances and less with those friends who have drinking problems. However, this moves into the more group-orientated approach to the control of excessive drinking. Hodgson (1977) also includes aversion therapy under this heading, even though it is a purely physical method of making drinking unattractive. Aversion therapy can either come in the form of electric shocks or by the use of a drug which is an emetic. Hodgson (1977) suggests that there is no evidence to tell whether either type of aversion therapy is effective or not.

3. Exposure involves the alcoholic being exposed to the cues that induce heavy drinking and the therapist helping him to resist these cues.

Hodgson (1977) is very tentative in advocating the effectiveness of any of these three different modes of treatment without further evidence from more rigorous research. However, he does cite an example where these various methods of behaviour therapy were more successful than the more medical and physical approaches. This occurred in a study where the treatment goal was not total abstinence but controlled drinking. After a two-year follow-up, where the goal was total abstinence, behaviour therapy was found to be no better than other conventional techniques but, in a controlled drinking programme, after two years behaviour therapies were more effective.

Group approaches

These approaches involved emphasis being placed on the therapeutic value of the interactions between groups of individuals with drinking problems. Three different group approaches have been identified (Robinson, 1976):

(i)   the therapeutic community of milieutherapy (see Cook and Pollak, 1976);

(ii)   group psychotherapy;

(iii)   treatment regimes of groups and organizations such as Alcoholics Anonymous (AA).

Once again, the evidence of the long-term success or failure of each of these approaches is difficult to find, although more recently the approach of Alcoholics Anonymous appears to have received some support (Leach, 1973). Edwards *et al.* (1976) suggest that AA is as much a supportive organization as it is a treatment orientated organization. They also suggest that AA, despite its overt open door policy, covertly 'selects' by offering a strongly characterized 'ideal' member with whom not all potential members will be able to identify.

Robinson (1979) argues that although AA has received considerable support, it is not clear for whom it works and how it works. He carried out an observational study of various AA groups and came to the conclusion that, through the use of 'talk' in the groups, members managed to change their identity from alcoholic to non-drinker. Robinson (1979) argues that drinking problems were not specifically treated or solved but that the members managed to talk their way out of their alcoholism and into a new status position. Their previous history of drinking with its associated problems is taken over by a new identity.

The relative value of these treatments, whether they are individual or group orientated, is difficult to assess. Certainly, there has been a shift in policy away from more specialized treatment units to more community approaches. Although, as Orford and Edwards (1977) point out:

'There is therefore in the previous literature no very substantial evidence that any intensive conventional treatment is of proven superiority to a less intensive approach.'

They conclude that, irrespective of the pattern of care being offered to the alcoholic, there is still a question mark against whether any of it has much effect.

Other agencies also play a part in the treatment and rehabilitation of people with drinking problems.

Professional workers, such as general practitioners (Rathod, 1967; Parr, 1977), social workers, priests/clergymen and probation officers, amongst others, are all involved in providing help for people with drinking problems (Robinson, 1976). There is no available evidence to show whether any of these different professionals have a significant effect on the control of drinking problems. Certainly, their supportive roles cannot be underestimated particularly in the area of rehabilitation and the maintenance of abstinence. However, it is also becoming increasingly evident that alcoholics are viewed as 'trouble', particularly by medically trained personnel (Strong, 1979) who are not equipped to deal with deviant behaviour which is essentially social in nature.

Approaches to education

Apart from the mass education campaigns carried out by central government-sponsored agencies, a number of more small-scale and intensive programmes have been carried out.

Engs (1977) carried out small group education on student volunteers on topics of concern such as drinking and sexuality. Students were divided into experimental and control groups. The experimental groups received two- to three-hour sessions beginning with a film and continuing with a discussion on alcohol only. The control group had a similar type of training but concentrated on sexuality only.

Each student filled in a questionnaire pre- and post- the course and also at three months after. The results showed no significant change in drinking behaviour between the two groups after three months, but the experimental group's knowledge was better at post-test and at the three months follow-up.

Another study (Biener, 1975), which has been reported previously, examined the influence of health education on the use of tobacco and alcohol in adolescence. Results showed that of the group who received education, 27 of the 34 who were abstinent before the education remained abstinent afterwards, compared with only 5 of the 31 in the control group. The education consisted of exhibits, discussions, literature, provision of leisure activities etc. This evidence indicates the value of health education, although more long-term evaluation is necessary.

Other groups have been proposed as having a valuable role to play in alcohol education (such as general practitioners), although no evidence is available to support these contentions (Acres, 1977; Davies, 1977).

Drew (1978) suggests that educational programmes should consist of a combination of approaches. First, he suggests the need for a community education programme which aims to develop a positive balanced orientation to alcohol; secondly, a programme emphasizing the value of early intervention; and thirdly, central government controls such as price control should be introduced.

The work of non-governmental institutions in alcohol control

A number of other bodies have played a part in the formulation of alcohol control policies. For example, the Royal College of Psychiatrists (1979) produced a report on *Alcohol and Alcoholism*. They emphasized the sociological nature of alcoholism and followed the Ledermann approach, arguing that there is a strong association between national per capita consumption and the prevalence of alcohol-related disability. They recommended:

(i) that 4 pints of beer, 4 large spirit drinks or 1 bottle of wine per day should be regarded as the upper limit of alcohol intake, and that it would be unwise to habitually drink those amounts regularly;

(ii) that the availability of inexpensive spirits is a potential hazard;

(iii) that public revenues should be used in the interests of health, and that special preventive programmes should be set up for those in high-risk occupations in collaboration with trade unions and professional organizations.

It is difficult to judge how far these reports influence government thinking and public opinion on alcohol control. Judging from the impact of the equivalent reports on smoking, the influence of such groups should not be underestimated.

Summary

Non-governmental approaches to alcohol control have been as varied as are the theories of causation of drinking problems. No evidence is available which could provide the basis of an assessment of the relative merits of one treatment over another. While alcoholism is a multi-faceted problem, it has become clear that the disease concept of 'alcoholism' is outmoded. Alcoholism is essentially a 'social problem' which requires solutions which are predominantly socially orientated.

Conclusions

This chapter has clearly illustrated the vast array of approaches that have been used to try to explain and control both smoking behaviour and heavy drinking. The problem of smoking is compounded by the pharmacological nature of dependence. Psychological and medical treatments appear to have a degree of success in stopping people smoking, though 'relapse' presents different problems which have yet to be solved. More evidence is needed on why such treatments are effective and whether factors such as support and motivation are important.

One policy which was recommended was the tailoring of treatments, both psychological and medical, to meet individual needs. More evidence is needed on the value of professionals in smoking control and also of lay remedies and non-professional bodies such as self-help groups.

In contrast to smoking, medical and psychological approaches to alcohol control appear to be giving way to approaches with an essentially social orientation. The social nature of alcohol dependence appears to suggest that alcoholism could be reversible, although it is unclear as to the social conditions necessary to facilitate such an outcome. The relative merits of the different approaches to control are difficult to estimate, given the lack of hard evidence. Obviously, further evidence on this issue is needed and also on the relative value of professional, self-help and lay methods of coping with alcohol problems.

References

Acres, D. I. (1977). In *Alcoholism*, pp. 321–8. Ed. by M. Grant. Croom Helm, London.

Baric, L. (1978). *Journal of the Institute of Health Education* **16**(4), 103.

Becker, M. H. (1979). In *New Directions in Patient Compliance*, pp. 1–31. Ed. by S. J. Cohen. Lexington Books, New York.

Becker, M. H. and Maiman, L. A. (1975). *Medical Care* **13**, 10.

Bernstein, D. A. (1970). *Behavioural Research and Therapy* **8**, 133.

Bewley, B. R. and Bland, J. M. (1977). *British Journal of Preventive and Social Medicine* **31**(1), 18.

Bewley, B. R., Bland, J. M. and Harris, R. (1974). *British Journal of Preventive and Social Medicine* **28**(1), 37.

Biener, K. J. (1975). *Preventive Medicine* **4**, 252.

Bland, J. M., Bewley, B. R., Banks, M. H. and Pollard, V. (1975). *Health Education Journal* **34**(3), 71.

Burt, A. (1974). *Lancet* **i**, 304.

Bynner, J. M. (1969). *The Young Smoker—The Government Social Survey*, HMSO, London.

Cook, T. and Pollak, B. (1976). In *Alcohol Dependence and Smoking Behaviour*, pp. 124–35. Ed. by G. Edwards, M. A. H. Russell, D. Hawks and M. Maccafferty. Saxon House, London.

Croog, S. H. (1977). *American Journal of Public Health* **67**, 921.

Dale, J. J. (1978). *Health Education Journal* **37**, 142.

Davies, D. L. ((1977). In *Alcoholism*, pp. 345–51. Ed. by G. Edwards and M. Grant. Croom Helm, London.

Drew, L. R. (1978). *Health* **28**(3–4), 23.

East, R. and Towers, B. (1979). *No Smoke: a psychologically based manual of information and self-applied exercises for use in giving up smoking.* East and Towers, London.

Edwards, G., Russell, M. A. H., Hawks, D. and Maccafferty, M. (Eds.) (1976). In *Alcohol Dependence and Smoking Behaviour*, pp. 115–23. Saxon House, London.

Eiser, J. R. and Sutton, S. R. (1977). *Addictive Behaviors* **2**, 129.

Engs, R. C. (1977). *Journal of Alcohol and Drug Education* **22**, 39.

Green, L. W. (1970). *Health Education Monograph* **30**, 25.

Handel, S. (1973). *Journal of the Royal College of General Practitioners* **23**, 149.

Hodgson, R. (1977). In *Alcoholism*, pp. 290–307. Ed. by G. Edwards and M. Grant. Croom Helm, London.

Hore, B. D. (1977). In *Alcoholism*, pp. 313–20. Ed. by G. Edwards and M. Grant. Croom Helm, London.

Horn, D. (1979). *N.I.D.A. Research Monograph* **23**, 24.

Janis, I. L. and Hoffman, D. (1970). *Journal of Personality and Social Psychology* **17**, 25.

Leach, B. (1973). In *Alcoholism: progress in research and treatment*, pp. 245–84. Ed. by G. Bourne and R. Fox. Academic Press, New York.

Littleton, J. M. (1977). In *Alcoholism*, pp. 107–116. Ed. by G. Edwards and M. Grant. Croom Helm, London.

McKennell, A. C. and Thomas, R. K. (1967). *Adults' and Adolescents' Smoking Habits and Attitudes.* Government Social Survey. HMSO, London.

Martin, F. M. and Stanley, G. R. (1965) *Health Bulletin* **23**, 84.

Martin, F. M. and Stanley, G. R. (1966). *Health Bulletin* **24**, 13.

Orford, J. (1977). In *Alcoholism*, pp. 88–99. Ed. by G. Edwards and M. Grant. Croom Helm, London.

Orford, J. and Edwards, G. (1977). *Alcoholism: A comparison of treatment and advice with a study of the influence of marriage.* Maudsley Monographs 26, Oxford University Press, Oxford.

Parr, D. (1977). *British Journal of Addiction* **54**(1), 25.

Pearson, R. and Richardson, K. (1978). *Public Health* **92**(3), 136.

Peto, J. (1974). *British Journal of Preventive and Social Medicine* **28**, 241.

Plant, M. A. (1979). *Drinking Careers.* Tavistock, London.

Porter, A. M. W. (1972). *Practitioner* **209**, 686.

Rathod, N. H. (1967). *British Journal of Addiction* **62**, 103.

Raw, M. (1977a). In *World Smoking and Health* **1**, 4. American Cancer Society.

Raw, M. (1977b). In *Contributions to Medical Psychology*, pp. 189–209. Ed. by S. Rachman, Pergamon, London.

Raw, M. (1978). In *Research Advances in Alcohol and Drug Problems*, Volume 14, pp. 441–85. Ed. by Y. Israel, R. J. Gibbins, H. Kalunt, R. E. Popham, W. Schmidt and R. G. Smart. Plenum, New York.

Raw, M., Jarvis, M. J., Feyerabend, C. and Russell, M. A. H. (1980). *British Medical Journal* **281**, 481.

Rawbone, R. G., Kelling, C. A., Jenkins, A. and Cruz, A. (1978). *Journal of Epidemiology and Community Health* **35**, 53.

Robinson, D. (1976). *From Drinking to Alcoholism: A Sociological Commentary.* John Wiley, London.

Robinson, D. (1979). *Talking out of Alcoholism—the Self-help process of Alcoholics Anonymous.* Croom Helm, London.

Rosenstock, I. M. (1974). *Health Education Monograph* **2**(4), 328.

Royal College of Physicians (1962). *Smoking and Health.* Pitman, London.

Royal College of Physicians (1971). *Smoking and Health Now.* Pitman, London.

Royal College of Physicians (1977). *Smoking or Health, Third Report.* Pitman, London.

Royal College of Psychiayrists (1979). *Alcohol and Alcoholism.* Tavistock, London.

Russell, M. A. H. (1971). *British Medical Journal* **2**, 330.

Russell, M. A. H. (1976). In *Research Advances in Drug and Alcohol Abuse*, pp. 3–21. Ed. by R. Gibbins, Y. Israel, H. Kalunt, R. E. Popham, W. Schmidt and R. G. Smart. John Wiley, London.

Russell, M. A. H. (1979). *British Medical Journal* **2**, 331.

Schachter, S. (1978). In *Smoking Behaviours*, pp. 208–28. Ed. by R. E. Thornton. Churchill Livingstone, Edinburgh, London and New York.

Shields, J. (1977). In *Alcoholism*, pp. 117–35. Ed. by G. Edwards and M. Grant. Croom Helm, London.

Strong, P. (1979). *Sociology of Health and Illness* **2**, 1.

Thompson, E. L. (1978). *American Journal of Public Health* **68**(3), 250.

Toynbee, P. (1980). *The Guardian*, 12th June, p. 12.

Watson, L. M. (1968). *Health Bulletin (Scotland)* **24**, 5.

8

Screening for early detection of cancer: general principles

Jocelyn Chamberlain

Introduction

Screening for early signs of disease is sometimes referred to as 'secondary prevention' since its aim is not to prevent the occurrence of disease but to prevent its
gross later manifestations which, in the case of cancer, means prevention of death.
In other words, its aim is to reduce mortality rather than to reduce incidence, and
this is how it must be judged. For some cancer sites, however, screening is able to
indentify biological changes thought to precede the development of invasive
disease. In such cases, surgical removal of the affected epithelium should reduce
the *incidence* of invasive cancer as well as reducing *mortality*. This will be the
expected outcome if the entire organ is removed, as, for example, in performing
total hysterectomy for carcinoma-in-situ of the cervix. It is often possible, though,
to excise an area of affected pre-cancerous epithelium without removal of the
entire organ, for example by removal of bladder papillomata or adenomatous
polyps of the colon. This less radical treatment has clear advantages for the patient
but it should be noted that the individual concerned, far from being cured of his
cancer, must be regarded as being at especially high risk, since the same carcinogenic influences which caused the first lesion are very likely to have acted, or to
continue to act, on other epithelial foci within the organ concerned. Thus screening can seldom prevent the development of cancer, but it can in theory prevent
much of the morbidity and mortality associated with it.

For the many cancers whose aetiologies are not fully understood and which are
therefore not susceptible to primary prevention (e.g. breast cancer), and for others
such as lung cancer, in which application of primary prevention is difficult,
screening to control morbidity and mortality is an attractive proposition. Experience has shown, however, that evaluation of its effectiveness is not simply a
straightforward matter of counting the presymptomatic cases detected by a
screening test, but involves examination of the underlying theory of development
of cancer. Moreover, various practical considerations are likely to influence both
the amount of good which can be achieved and the amount of harm which might
be caused (Wilson, 1970). It has been pointed out by McKeown (1968) that, as
with other public health measures, doctors offering screening are in a different
ethical position from that of doctors being consulted by individual patients with
problems. In the latter case, the doctor is under no obligation to be able to cure
the patient's complaint, but where the doctor takes the initiative and offers a
service such as screening to the public at large, he does have a clear responsibility

to be sure that the service he is offering will benefit its recipients. This means that he must have scientific proof that early detection and treatment do influence prognosis for the better and that they do not have serious harmful side-effects on the people screened. Moreover, the doctor—or more accurately the health authority providing the service—should have some evidence that this is a more appropriate way of using scarce resources than other competing areas of need. Therefore, before going on to look at screening for specific cancer sites, this chapter considers in general terms some of the theoretical problems in evaluating cancer screening, some of the practical considerations which must be taken into account, and ways of evaluating the advantages and disadvantages of screening programmes.

Theoretical considerations

The natural history of cancer

The idea of screening for early detection of cancer springs from the common clinical experience that cancers diagnosed and treated at an 'early' stage stand a much better chance of being cured than those which are diagnosed 'late', when local or metastatic spread is already evident. 'Early' and 'late' in this context refer to stages in the natural history of the cancer and are not necessarily synonymous with early and late in a temporal sense. For example, in the case of a cancer with a very variable length of natural history such as breast cancer, it is possible for one tumour, known by the patient to have been present for five years or more, to be still at Stage I when medically diagnosed, while another may already be far advanced in Stage III or IV even though it has been present only a few weeks.

It is therefore not the time for which a tumour has been present which determines its natural history, but its rate of growth. Growth rates of tumours are commonly expressed in terms of volume doubling times. This concept was first put forward by Collins et al. (1956), who suggested an exponential model of tumour growth starting with one malignant cell which divides to become two, four, eight, sixteen and so on. According to this hypothesis, they estimated that a single cell, taken to have an average diameter of $10\,\mu$ would grow to a nodule 1 mm in diameter in twenty doublings, 1 cm in thirty doublings and that a further ten doublings would result in approximately 1 kg of cancer tissue. If the change in volume in a given time interval were known, the average growth could be determined in terms of its doubling time. If this was assumed to be constant, the duration of a given tumour and the time of its inception (i.e. the one cell stage) could be estimated by extrapolating backwards. To test this model of cancer growth, Collins and his co-workers examined serial x-rays of untreated pulmonary metastases from a variety of primary sites, and calculated doubling times ranging from 11 days (for a testicular teratoma) to 164 days (for an oesophageal carcinoma). If these doubling times were assumed to be constant, the depressing conclusion was reached that the metastasis was established often many years before the primary lesion could possibly have been detected, with the implication that early diagnosis of the primary was extremely unlikely to have any capability of altering prognosis.

There are several reasons for doubting the relevance of this simple exponential model to the complexity of growth and spread of human tumours. Geddes (1979) drew attention to the fact that some tumours have doubling times which are so long that backwards extrapolation leads to the absurd conclusion that the tumour began long before the individual was conceived! Animal studies (Dethlefson *et al.*, 1968) show a tendency for growth rates to slow as the tumour gets larger, probably because of decreased vascular supply to the central part of the tumour causing necrosis of some cells. This suggests that growth rates are not exponential but more likely to be Gompertzian, with slower rates of growth in the early and late stages than in the middle period of their existence (Fig. 8.1, from Forrest and

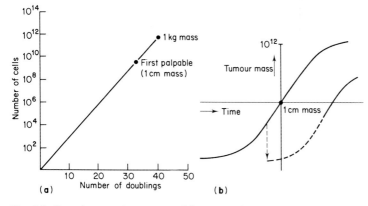

Fig. 8.1 Growth curves for tumours: (a) exponential; (b) Gompertzian.

Roberts, 1980). A further criticism of the exponential doubling time model is that the hypothesis is based on the behaviour of pulmonary metastases which may not be typical either of the primary tumour or of metastases in other sites, such as bone, where there may be different physical and vascular constraints on the size reached by the lesion (Steel, 1977). Smithers (1968) also pointed out that some cancers are liable both to fast maturation and to spontaneous regression, indicating that their behaviour may be influenced by immunological or other factors acting at different periods in their lifetime.

Alternative methods of estimating the natural history of the early stages of cancer depend on follow-up of patients in whom a microscopic 'preneoplastic' lesion has been identified. The theory of this approach is illustrated in Fig. 8.2. A

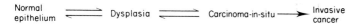

Fig. 8.2 Hypothetical stages in the natural history of cancer.

group of epithelial cells becomes proliferative—*the dysplasia stage*; some of these cells develop malignant characteristics but are still contained by an intact basement membrane—*the carcinoma-in-situ stage*; and eventually the lesion breaks through the basement membrane to infiltrate the surrounding tissue—*the invasive stage*. It is assumed that metastatic spread cannot occur before the tumour has become invasive locally. Animal experiments indicate that earlier lesions in this postulated natural history are reversible (Butler and Jones, 1976), and carcinoma is not an inevitable outcome. It is still not known, however, whether earlier changes are obligatory in the development of every invasive cancer.

Most of the human work on this topic is based on preneoplasia of the uterine cervix. In the original series of Peterson (1952), a group of symptomatic women with carcinoma-in-situ diagnosed by cytology, followed by limited biopsy of the affected area, was followed and 35 per cent of the women developed invasive cancer within the ensuing fifteen years. A more recent series of asymptomatic women, diagnosed on cytology and punch biopsy, is reported by Green (1974), who found that only 8.5 per cent developed invasive cancers in an eight-year period of follow-up. However, the findings of all such follow-up surveys must be interpreted with caution because, on the one hand, it is possible that the diagnostic biopsy removed the entire area of affected epithelium in some women and hence reduced the subsequent incidence of invasive cancer and thus caused the proportion which progressed to be underestimated, or that the biopsy missed an area in which invasive cancer was already present, thus causing an overestimation of the proportion which progressed.

Studies have also been done on women with dysplasia of the cervix, to estimate the proportion which progress to carcinoma-in-situ or invasive cancer, and the proportion which regress. Many cytological studies (e.g. Richart, 1967; Spriggs et al., 1971; Burghardt, 1973) support the hypothesis of a temporal progression from mild to moderate to severe dysplasia and eventually to carcinoma-in-situ, but also suggest that not all invasive cancers go through a recognizable pre-invasive phase. Ratios of detection rates of dysplasia to those of carcinoma-in-situ have been used to estimate the proportion of dysplasias which regress (e.g. Koss, 1970), but this provides no evidence that the carcinomas-in-situ have in fact progressed through a dysplasia phase. It has also been shown that the subsequent incidence of carcinoma is very much higher in women previously diagnosed as having dysplasia (Stern and Neely, 1964) than in the general population.

Attempts to follow-up women with dysplasia directly, by repeated smears but no biopsy, have been bedevilled by the very substantial losses to follow-up, occurring principally in the first year after an abnormal (dysplastic) smear. Using a life-table technique, Armstrong (1980) studied 666 women with dyskaryosis and estimated that the probability of development of carcinoma-in-situ or invasive cancer was 13.6 per cent over a four-and-a-half-year period. Twenty-four per cent of women in this study were judged to have lesions which regressed, as defined by three normal smears with at least six months interval between each. From these various sources, it may be concluded that there is circumstantial evidence of a natural history which progresses from one phase of abnormality to another and, as far as 'earlier' lesions are concerned, that regression or lack of progression are both possible. But direct evidence of the natural history of early neoplasia in humans remains impossible to obtain because histological confirmation of the diagnosis requires that the lesion be at least partly removed, and ethical constraints require that the more advanced lesions be treated.

Intervention by screening

At what point in the natural history of cancer should a screening test be aimed in order to be most effective in changing the prognosis? Cole and Morrison (1980) propose that the components of natural history be subdivided into various intervals. That between the inception of the cancer and the time of symptomatic presentation and diagnosis they term the *total preclinical phase*. With present knowledge, the beginning of this phase is impossible to define and the end of it—when the patient seeks care for signs or symptoms—differs from person to person according to factors such as their perception of the severity of their symptoms and the availability of medical care. Within this total preclinical phase is the *detectable preclinical phase*, which has the same end-point but which starts at the time when the disease could first be detected by the relevant screening test. For example, in the case of cancer of the cervix, the detectable preclinical phase starts when affected cells first start to exfoliate; in the case of breast cancer, it may be the time when malignant calcification can first be identified on a mammogram. The aim of screening is not to intervene at the earliest point in the detectable preclinical phase, but to intervene at the latest point at which cure, by a procedure causing least morbidity, can be achieved. If the natural history were clearly understood, and the effectiveness of treatment were known, then screening could be applied at the appropriate point.

Length bias

Within a given population of people with preclinical cancer, there is likely to be a case-mix of differing durations of the preclinical phase. Some cancers will be about to present symptomatically, while others will have only just developed. Moreover, there may be a wide distribution in the length of the total preclinical phase, some cancers progressing very quickly through it, while others may be very slow-growing or non-progressive. Screening at a single point in time is likely to pick up a disproportionate number of slow-growing lesions because prevalence is a function of duration, and the slowly progressing cancers have a longer duration. On the assumption that their rate of growth after clinical presentation is directly related to that in the preclinical phase, these slow-growing cancers are those which, even in the absence of screening, have the best prognosis. This results in the so-called *length bias* (Feinleib and Zelen, 1969) which influences comparison of prognosis of screening-detected cases with symptomatic cases, in favour of the former.

Lead time

Another bias influencing comparisons of prognosis is *lead time*, which is simply the time between detection by screening and the end of the preclinical phase—i.e. the time when diagnosis would otherwise have been made. Even if the date of a patient's death is unaltered by the fact that his cancer was detected by screening, his survival (the interval between diagnosis and death) will appear to be longer, giving the erroneous impression that screening-detected cases have a better prognosis. In reality, all such a patient has gained is knowledge of his illness, with consequent anxiety and morbidity from its treatment for a longer period than would otherwise be the case. The lead time gained by screening is only beneficial if it allows a greater proportion of cancers to be cured by early treatment. An adjustment for average lead time of cases detected by screening should always be made in evaluating screening programmes by survival comparisons, as in the case of Shapiro's trial of breast cancer screening (1977), in which an average lead time of one year for cases detected at screening (Shapiro *et al.*, 1974) was used. This meant that six-year survival of screening-detected cases was compared with five-year survival of symptom-detected cases.

The average lead time in a group of screening-detected cancers depends on the variability of duration of the detectable preclinical phase, the sensitivity of the screening test and the frequency with which it is repeated.

Sensitivity of the screening test

The ideal screening test is one which, for every subject tested, tells the truth, the whole truth (no false negatives), and nothing but the truth (no false positives). Sensitivity measures the ability of the test of tell the whole truth and is expressed as the proportion of people with detectable preclinical cancer in whom the test is positive (Thorner and Remein, 1961; Table 8.1). The theoretical method for

Table 8.1 Classification of results of a screening test

Test result	True diagnosis Cancer	No cancer	
Positive	True positives	False positives	All positives
Negative	False negatives	True negatives	All negatives
	All cancers	All non-cancers	All tested

$$\text{Sensitivity} = \frac{\text{true positives}}{\text{all cancers}}$$

$$\text{specificity} = \frac{\text{true negatives}}{\text{all non-cancers}}$$

$$\text{Predictive value of a positive test} = \frac{\text{true positives}}{\text{all positives}}$$

measuring sensitivity is to compare the result of the test with that of a definitive diagnostic work-up of each person tested. In the case of cancer, the definitive diagnosis can only be made on histological grounds and implies a biopsy. It would obviously be completely impractical, as well as unethical, to biopsy a sample of subjects with negative test results. A compromise solution is therefore used in estimating sensitivity of screening tests for cancer, whereby a sample of subjects with negative results is followed carefully and those with cancers diagnosed within a defined interval, either by repeat screening or by symptomatic presentation, are regarded as false negatives to the original screen (Yule, 1973; Chamberlain *et al.*, 1979). The interval cases may be a mixture of some which were present but undetected by the original screen—genuine false negatives—and some fast-growing tumours which arose *de novo* in the interval. Although the decision to classify them all as false negatives is purely arbitrary, it does have some practical importance in defining the proportion of cancers which will escape detection by screening unless the latter is repeated within that interval. Moreover, some cancers detected at second screening may have been detectable but missed at first screening; de Waard *et al.* (1978) devised a theoretical method for distinguishing between 'missed' cases (previous false negatives) and new cases among those detected at second screening. However, this model depends on certain assumptions unlikely to be true in practice. These include a constant exponential growth rate for all cancers, an infallible detection system at second screening, and a sensitivity which does not vary between first and subsequent screens.

On first screening a population, the mixture of cases in the detectable preclinical phase will contain a relatively high proportion which are about to present symptomatically and which may therefore be more easily detectable. At repeat screening, there will be relatively fewer of these obvious lesions and more of those at an earlier stage in the preclinical phase, thus resulting in a poorer sensitivity at repeat screening. It should be remembered, however, that this poorer sensitivity is not necessarily a disadvantage if the lesions missed at first screening are still eligible for cure when detected at subsequent screening. In theory, both numerator and denominator for estimating sensitivity should consist of lesions within a defined band of the detectable preclinical phase in which minimal treatment results in cure. Lesions earlier than this should count as false positives since they do not yet need treatment; lesions later than this are not the objective of the screening programme since treatment is not sufficiently early to influence their prognosis.

Frequency of screening
Even if infallible sensitivity could be assured, a negative screening test does not guarantee that an individual is free of cancer forever. It follows that any cancer screening service must offer repeated screening at intervals. The choice of an optimum interval depends on the distribution of the detectable preclinical phase and the proportion of cases in it which are curable by early treatment. Immediately after initial screening, the only cases left in the detectable preclinical phase will be those which gave false negative results. As time passes, new cases will enter this phase at a rate identical to the incidence of the symptomatic clinical phase in the absence of screening. If this is known (for example from recent cancer registration data), an estimate of the number of new cases entering in a given time interval can be made. Depending on the average lead time in which curative treatment can be applied, a decision on the optimum interval for rescreening could be made, such as to give the maximum yield of curable cases for the least disadvantage in terms of false positives and use of resources. The optimum rescreening interval need not be constant but might perhaps vary from a short interval between first and second screens to compensate to some extent for poor test sensitivity, to a longer interval between second and third and subsequent screens (Spriggs and Husain, 1977). Different rescreening intervals could also be used for subdivisions of the population at different risk (Knox, 1975).

Screening policies

These various considerations of the interrelationships between the natural history of early cancer and the lead time, test sensitivity and frequency of screening, illustrate some of the difficulties encountered in formulating a screening policy and evaluating its effects. None of these factors can be measured directly in humans, but estimates have to be derived from theoretical assumptions which seem to be plausible explanations of observations in screened populations. As well as these theoretical considerations, however, there is also a number of practical measurable parameters which influence both the benefits and costs of screening programmes.

Practical aspects

In this section, further factors which may influence both benefits and risks of screening are considered. These practical aspects are inevitably intertwined with the theoretical issues already discussed and the distinction between the two is to some extent artificial, but these are more directly measurable and can often be deliberately manipulated in order to achieve a more favourable balance of benefits versus risks. Briefly, the factors which influence the amount of benefit which a screening service can achieve are:

(i)   acceptance of screening by the population at whom it is aimed;
(ii) validity of the screening test;
(iii) effectiveness of medical management;
(iv) patients' compliance with recommended management;
(v)   financial savings from 'early' versus 'late' treatment.

The principal risks and costs arise from:

(i)   hazards of the screening test;
(ii) lack of specifity of the test;
(iii) financial costs of screening and follow-up of positive results.

The balance between benefits on the one hand, and risks and costs on the other will be influenced by the *cut-off point* chosen to separate positive test results from negatives, and by the *yield* of curable cancers in the screened population.

The acceptance of screening

Whenever cancer screening clinics have been set up, open to anyone who chooses to attend, it has been common experience that a waiting list of would-be subjects for screening rapidly builds up. This has led to claims that there is a wide public demand for screening, and acceptability is no problem. However, when such clinics are considered in relation to the catchment population they serve, it is often salutary to learn of the very small proportion of eligible people who have actually attended. For example, a breast cancer screening clinic set up in West London for a research study of the value of mammography (Chamberlain *et al.*, 1975) was open to any woman over the age of 40 years living in the borough, who wished to attend. Although in the early stages a waiting list of several months built up, eventually difficulty was experienced in reaching even the study target of 2500 women—a mere 5 per cent of borough residents in the relevant age group. A similar clinic in Bath was estimated to have screened only 4 per cent of eligible women over a fifteen-month period (Simpson, unpublished thesis). In north-west England, Sansom *et al.* (1972) reported that the proportion of the eligible female population who had had a cervical smear from any source within a period of six years from the introduction of a cervical cancer screening service was 17 per cent. The relationship between supply and demand is of course a two-way process and these low acceptance rates must, to some extent, reflect the availability of the service. Nevertheless, it indicates that mere provision of the screening facility without any inducement or education to attend is only going to reach a small proportion of the would-be target.

Probably the single most important step which can be taken to improve acceptance is to invite subjects individually either by letter, telephone call, or personal visit. Computerized invitations to attend for cervical cancer screening in West Sussex resulted in acceptance rates of around 50 per cent among women over the age of 35 years (Carruthers *et al.*, 1975); acceptance rates of invitations to attend for breast cancer screening issued by the women's own general practitioners range from 57 per cent (Hobbs *et al.*, 1980) to 82 per cent (Edinburgh

Breast Screening Clinic, 1978). Most experience in Western countries suggests that among middle-aged women, response to invitations for initial cancer screening will be of the order of 65 per cent, although there seem to be some international differences, with women in Scandinavian countries standing out as being particularly willing to comply. In Sweden for example, acceptance rates for breast cancer screening of well over 90 per cent of women aged 35 to 74 years have been reported (Lundgren, 1979; Tabar et al., 1980) and in Finland, Hakama et al. (1979) report participation rates of 75 per cent to 97 per cent for cervical screening.

Characteristics of responders and non-responders

These international differences probably reflect socio-cultural differences in attitudes towards preventive health care. Numerous comparisons of users and non-users of preventive services in general, such as immunization of children (Bloor and Gill, 1972) or dental check-ups (Haefner et al., 1967), have consistently shown that the people who make use of the service tend to come from more educated, higher social class groups, and (among adults) from younger age groups rather than older. The Cardiff Cervical Cytology Study (1980) reported that among 71 000 married women between the ages of 25 and 69 years, acceptance rates of an invitation personally given by a visiting field worker to attend a clinic for a cervical smear ranged from 95 per cent for women aged 25–29 years in social class I to only 20 per cent for women aged 65–69 years in social class V. Similarly, Wakefield and Sansom (1966) contrasted the age and social class distribution of women in the Manchester area who had had cervical smears, with those in the general population and showed a marked deficit in numbers who had been tested from the older and lower social class groups. These differences have also been found in the acceptance rates of breast cancer screening (Fink et al., 1968; Hobbs et al., 1980). Little is known of possible differences between men and women in their acceptance of cancer screening because the great majority of studies have concentrated on breast and cervix screening. However, higher screening rates have been reported in men than in women for stomach cancer screening in Japan (Hirayama, 1978), although it is not clear whether comparable methods of enrolling the two sexes were used.

Reasons for non-response

The reasons underlying people's decisions to participate or not in preventive health programmes have been extensively investigated by behavioural scientists. In the United States, the Carnegie Grant Subcommittee on Modification of Patient Behavior for Health Maintenance and Disease Control (Becker et al., 1977) conveniently summarized the findings of these investigations in a Health Belief Model. This postulates that a person's decision to take health action (e.g. to be screened) is influenced by the following factors:

   (i)   readiness to be concerned about health matters;
   (ii)   perception of vulnerability to the illness concerned;
   (iii)   belief about the severity of the illness;
   (iv)   belief about the effectiveness of treatment;
   (v)   belief about possible harm or cost;
   (vi)   reactions to cues (e.g. invitations) which might trigger a response.

   Becker and his colleagues suggest that the approach to people to participate in a preventive health programme should incorporate an educational element most appropriate to the perceptions of the target population. For example, in cancer screening the approach should attempt to reduce fear of the severity of the illness and persuade people that effective treatment is possible at an early stage but not if the cancer is allowed to progress untreated. It has been shown (e.g. Fink *et al.*, 1968; Carruthers *et al.*, 1975; Hobbs *et al.*, 1980) that belief in early detection and the curability of cancer is considerably less in non-responders than responders to screening programmes.

Methods of improving response

Attempts to increase participation in screening which have deliberately emphasized these points are still hard to find, perhaps because educational techniques for reaching the older and lower social class sections of the community, who are most likely both to hold these adverse beliefs and to be at high risk of most cancers, have not been developed. One promising approach was described by Fulghum and Klein (1967) who, by means of social workers working in an indigent population, identified 'opinion leaders' and personally educated them about the value of cervical screening. The leaders, by example, then persuaded their peers that attendance for screening was normal behaviour. A similar approach is possible if screening facilities with appropriate back-up services are provided in workplaces where, again, screening can become 'the norm' and non-attendance unusual behaviour.

Another successful method of getting a good response from women at high risk of cervical cancer was employed by Osborn and Leyshon (1966) who used a pre-existing register of problem families, and sent home nurses to visit the mothers and take cervical smears then and there. This overcame the women's reluctance to think ahead and make clinic appointments, as well as their dislike of the clinical atmosphere (Bloor and Gill, 1972); moreover, the yield of positive tests was ten times that in women attending clinics.

'Do-it-yourself' screening methods which can be performed by the subject without personal contact with a doctor or other health professional might also increase response. Carruthers *et al.* (1975) carried out a trial in which women living in different districts were randomized to receive either an invitation to a clinic for a cervical smear or a cytopipette to use at home and send the resulting specimen direct to the laboratory. Use of the pipette (53 per cent) was more common than attendance at the clinic (41 per cent), but it was not used more by the high-risk women. A similar 'do-it-yourself' test is the *Haemoccult* test, recently developed for screening for colorectal cancer; an acceptance rate of 48 per cent in a completely unselected population over the age of 45 years has been reported (Hardcastle *et al.*, 1980), but much higher acceptance (81 per cent) among a population of 31 937 people who were willing to enter into a controlled trial of the value of such screening (Gilbertson *et al.*, 1980). It is not clear exactly how the latter group was recruited and it is possible that they represent an unduly health-conscious group.

A widely advocated 'do-it-yourself' method of cancer screening is self-examination of the breast. Gastrin (1976) found that personal teaching of the technique, together with instruction on where to go if an abnormality was found, increased the practice of regular self-examination from 5 per cent to 70 per cent. However, this was in a selected population of women aged 20–80 years who were active members of women's organizations in Finland. Stillman (1977) administered a questionnaire to a sample of 122 women who belonged to similar organizations in a selected suburban community in the United States, prior to the start of a self-examination education campaign. By chance, this survey was done shortly after extensive publicity about breast cancer, resulting from its diagnosis in the wives of both the President and Vice-President of the United States. The population studied was younger and of higher socio-economic status than the general population and hence more likely to believe in and use preventive services. It was found that although almost all these women (97 per cent) believed that self-examination could reduce the threat of breast cancer, and the great majority (87 per cent) thought they were vulnerable, only 40 per cent actually practised regular self-examination. About a quarter of the sample had high beliefs but still did not practice, indicating that behaviour is not necessarily prompted by belief. Particular deterrents to participation were embarassment in performing the examination technique and uncertainty about the distinction between normal and abnormal. In contrast to the 'do-it-yourself' techniques for cervix and colon cancer, in which the subject merely has to return the specimen to the relative anonymity of a laboratory which will firstly make the distinction between positive and negative and secondly initiate appropriate action, in self-examination the responsibility for both these decisions falls entirely on the subject herself. The burden of this responsibility may prove extremely worrying for some women and this subject perhaps deserves more attention in education about self-examination than it has so far been given in the various teaching 'packages' produced on this subject.

Acceptance of self-examination is being compared with that of screening clinic attendance in the UK Trial of Early Detection of Breast Cancer (1981). It is still too early to say whether the proportion of 45- to 64-year-old women practising self-examination will be greater or less than those accepting screening, but preliminary results suggest that attendance for initial screening (65–70 per cent) is considerably greater than attendance at a teaching session to learn about self-examination (30–50 per cent).

Acceptance of repeated screening

Most of the work on acceptability of screening is based on response to an invitation to attend on the initial occasion. But it has already been seen that screening at intervals is necessary for cancer control, so that compliance with repeated invitations is also important. It has been consistently found that a high proportion of first attenders are willing to return repeatedly for rescreening, implying that the decision to attend on the first occasion is a good indicator of subsequent behaviour. Nevertheless, the small 'drop-out' rate at each rescreening is likely to be cumulative and can have quite an important effect on the level of control of cancer mortality which is achieved.

In the study of breast cancer screening by Shapiro et al. (1971), 65 per cent of the original population attended for the initial screen; response rates of these initial attenders to the subsequent second, third and fourth annual rescreens were 80 per cent, 74 per cent and 69 per cent respectively. This is illustrated in Fig. 8.3 in terms of the proportion of the original target population screened on each occasion. It is now apparent that less than half of the target group was maintained in the screening programme beyond the second year. Similarly, in the Cardiff study of cervical cytology, in which rescreening at two-year intervals was

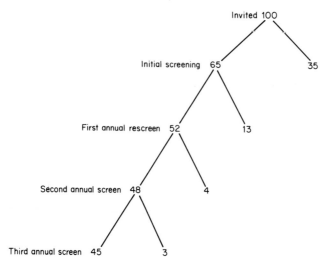

Fig. 8.3 Acceptance of breast cancer screening.

scheduled, the proportions of the original population screened were 65 per cent at the first screen, 51 per cent at the second screen and 37 per cent at the third (Landsman *et al.*, 1977).

In any service provided for a large population, re-attendance rates will of course be influenced by movements in and out of the population. In some countries, such as Sweden, identification numbers for each individual enable such movements to be continuously monitored and each person's whereabouts known so that the person can be re-invited at the appropriate time. A similar but less efficient system based on National Health Service numbers is used in Britain as the basis for recall schemes for screening for cervical cancer and (in selected high-risk men only) for bladder cancer. In a pilot study of the national five-yearly recall scheme for cervical cancer, Allman *et al.* (1974) found that, when valid reasons for non-response were excluded (the principal one being that an intermediate repeat smear had already been taken), 64 per cent of the eligible population re-attended in response to a postal invitation. A personal visit by a health visitor could increase this to 85 per cent. When response was examined according to the source of the initial test, it was found that women whose previous test was taken in a screening clinic, family planning clinic or by a general practitioner were more likely to re-attend than those whose previous test has been in a hospital setting. They suggested that poor response in the latter group might be related to poor communication about the test, its purpose and the need for it to be repeated. Most hospital smears are taken routinely when the woman is having a vaginal examination for some other reason, and unless staff make a special point of telling the patient what they are doing and why, she may even be unaware that she has been screened.

Influence of acceptance on cancer control
The usual steps in developing a screening programme for cancer are firstly, to identify a reasonably sensitive test and secondly, to prove that treatment at an

early stage does alter prognosis. Having reached that stage of development, the major factor influencing the degree of cancer control that can be achieved by early detection becomes the acceptance of screening by the target population. This is illustrated in simplified form in Fig. 8.4, which presents imaginary but

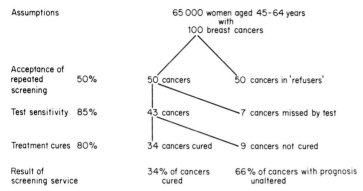

Fig. 8.4 Hypothetical model of the annual benefit achieved by a screening service for breast cancer.

plausible figures for the proportion of deaths which could be prevented by a screening programme for breast cancer with a test of 85 per cent sensitivity and a treatment which is curative in 80 per cent of cases detected at screening. Because poor compliance reduces the number of cancers susceptible to early detection, it accounts for a much greater number of cancers in the 'no benefit' group than the insensitivity of the test or the treatment failures together. This very obvious point is stressed because, although it has no bearing on the benefits or costs which can be expected by the individual person who turns up for screening, it is likely to have a major influence on a health authority considering whether or not to implement a screening service for a whole population.

The simple situation illustrated in the figure assumes that the cancers are evenly distributed in the acceptors and refusers. If, as in the case of cervical cancer, the refusers have a higher probability of cancer, the benefit will be less; if, as perhaps is true of breast cancer, the acceptors have a higher probability of cancer, then the benefit will be greater.

The validity of the screening test

The property of the screening test which influences the amount of benefit which can be achieved is its *sensitivity* which, as has already been discussed, can only be derived from theoretical estimates based on the rate of interval cancers and the yield at repeated screening. However, for some cancers, alternative tests are available and it is important that these should be compared with one another to give relative sensitivities, so that the most efficient test or combination of tests can be employed.

Relative sensitivity
To determine relative sensitivity necessitates the simultaneous application of the tests being studied to a sample of subjects, the results of each being interpreted

independently of one another so that cancers detected by one method but not the other(s) can be distinguished. Table 8.2 shows the relative sensitivities of physical examination and mammography in detection of 683 cancers at initial screening of 148 000 women in the Breast Cancer Detection Demonstration Projects in the United States (Beahrs et al., 1979). The absolute sensitivities of each test will, of course, be lower than those shown here, because cancers missed by both tests are not included in the denominator. Similar tables could be produced for any cancer screening in which there is a choice of alternative tests—e.g. protosigmoidoscopy and haemoccult tests for colorectal cancer—but it is necessary that the alternative tests should be applied to a random sample of screenees on the same occasion and their results independently interpreted.

Table 8.2 Relative sensitivity of alternative screening tests in screening for breast cancer (Beahrs et al., 1979)

Detected by	No. of cancers	Percentage	Relative sensitivity
Mammography only	354	52	91% mammography
Mammography and physical examination	269	39	
Physical examination only	60	9	48% physical examination
Total	683	100	

Test reproducibility

Another aspect of the validity of a screening test is its reproducibility, which measures the extent of agreement in the results of one test applied to the same subject on the same occasion. Variation in the result may be because of biological variation in the subject; for example, in screening for lung cancer by sputum cytology malignant cells may be present in one sample but absent in another (Delarue et al., 1971). Alternatively, the tester may vary in his interpretation of the result—within-observer variation—or different testers may vary from one another—between-observer variation. Variation, whether it originates in the subject or the observer, leads to misclassification of individuals who are screened, and hence implies that the sensitivity of the screening programme will be less than perfect.

Before implementing a screening service, the reproducibility of the screening test should be assessed, and if it is poor some measure of quality control should ideally be incorporated. Reproducibility can be measured by double interpretation of tests, performed independently of one another, on a sample of subjects. In one study of screening tests for breast cancer, women were given two independent physical examinations of the breast—one by a nurse and one by a doctor—and also had mammograms taken which were read independently by two radiologists (Chamberlain et al., 1975). Tables 8.3 and 8.4 show the extent of agreement in the interpretation of physical examination and of mammography, respectively, and also illustrate that the sensitivity of each observer separately is less than that of the two combined. In this case, physical examination detected 9 out of the 12 cancers found in the sample of women tested (sensitivity 75 per cent) but the doctor detected only 8 (sensitivity 67 per cent) and the nurse only 6 (sensitivity 50

Table 8.3 Agreement between nurses and clinic doctors on the need to refer women to a surgeon (Chamberlain *et al.*, 1975)

Action recommended by nurse	Action recommended by clinic doctor		Total
	Referral	No referral	
Referral	43 (5 cancers)	46 (1 cancer)	89
No referral	46 (3 cancers)	864 (3 cancers)	910
Total	89	910	999

Number of referrals: $43+46+46=135$.
Agreement on referrals: $43/135=32\%$.
Agreement on cancers: $5/9=56\%$ (excluding cancers undetected by either observer).

Table 8.4 Agreement between two radiologists interpreting mammograms on the need to refer women for surgical assessment (Chamberlain *et al.*, 1975)

Action recommended by radiologist A	Action recommended by radiologist B		Total
	Referral	No referral	
Referral	39 (10 cancers)	13 (1 cancer)	52
No referral	24 (3 cancers)	1138 (5 cancers)	1162
Total	63	1151	1214

Number of referrals: $39+13+24=76$.
Agreement on referrals: $39/76=51\%$.
Agreement on referral of women with cancer: $10/14=71\%$ (excluding cancers undetected by observer).

per cent). Similarly, mammography detected 14 out of 19 cancers (74 per cent), with radiologist B having a sensitivity of 68 per cent but radiologist A achieving only 58 per cent. It was also noted in this study that the relatively poor reproducibility of physical examination between a doctor and a nurse was even worse when two doctors were used in a small sample of women involved in a pilot study!

In instances where the subject collects his own specimen for testing, as in screening for lung cancer by sputum cytology or colorectal cancer by the Haemoccult test, within-subject variation can be overcome to some extent by testing several specimens on each occasion. Where screening requires a visit to a clinic however, and/or a contact with a health professional, multiple collections or interpretations to reduce subject and observer variation will probably not be feasible in a service situation. Efforts to ensure good reproducibility of the screening test depend on performing it under standard conditions for each subject, training and regular retraining of the staff involved and, if appropriate, incorporating known standards among the specimens screened.

Effectiveness of treatment

Obviously any benefit to be derived from screening depends on a treatment for the cancers or pre-invasive lesions found which is more effective and/or associated with less morbidity than treatment of cancers presenting symptomatically. Usually the treatment will be identical with that of symptomatic cancers, on which evidence of effectiveness already exists in the form of survival rates of treated cases.

Distribution of stage at diagnosis
Survival information is frequently available according to the stage at diagnosis, showing that response to treatment is better for symptomatic cancers diagnosed at an 'early' stage. There is a tendency to assume that screening-detected cancers behave in an identical way, leading some people to assume that the effectiveness of screening can be proved merely by showing an 'earlier' distribution of cases detected at screening. One example of the fallacy of this approach is given by Brett's study of screening for lung cancer (1969) in which 65 per cent of cases in a group of men who were screened were resectable, compared to 29 per cent in an unscreened group; but three years later the mortality rate was identical in both groups. The higher proportion of resectable cancers was merely a reflection of the 'lead time'. It could be said that the men who underwent surgery without any improvement in prognosis suffered *more* morbidity rather than less as a result of screening.

Correcting for bias in comparisons of effectiveness of treatment
It has already been shown that comparisons of results of treatment of screening-detected cases with symptomatic cases are biased by lead time, and also by length bias. Proof of the superior effectiveness of treatment of screening-detected cancers therefore depends on estimates in which a correction for these theoretical biases has been made. One of the few reported instances where this has been done is Shapiro's trial of breast cancer screening (1978) in which a comparison of case fatality rates of breast cancer diagnosed in study and control groups showed that 49.8 per cent of those in the control group had died after eight years, compared with 37.8 per cent of those in the study group. However, it has been estimated that the average lead time gained by screening was one year and when this adjustment was made for those cancers which were diagnosed by screening (i.e. including their nine-year case fatality rate rather than their eight-year rate), the overall rate in the study group increased to 38.5 per cent. In this case, length bias is also overcome by making the comparison between the *whole* study group (including cancers diagnosed in women who refused to be screened and interval cancers) and the control group. Since virtually the same number of cancers were diagnosed in both groups during the study period, it can be concluded that the case-mix of rates of growth of cancers in the two groups was the same.

Evidence, not subject to bias, of the effectiveness of treatment of screening-detected cancers can be inferred if mortality from the cancer is lower in a population which has been offered screening compared with a control population. This is discussed further below on p. 254.

Comparisons of different treatments for cancer detected at screening
If screening is aimed at detection of pre-invasive lesions, a less radical treatment than that used for the invasive lesion may be feasible. The two treatments can be compared with one another in cases detected by screening. Boyes *et al.* (1970) compared cone-biopsy of the cervix with hysterectomy in 3657 women with carcinoma-in-situ of the cervix. The less radical treatment resulted in a greater recurrence rate (12.7 per 1000 per annum compared with 1.8 per 1000 per annum). No information is given on survival, but by implication none of these women died during the follow-up period. The subjects in this particular report were not randomly allocated to one treatment or the other, nor was there any

matching for age or other variables; those who had cone-biopsy tended to be younger and to have been treated in a more recent time period than those who had hysterectomy. Despite the greater recurrence rate following the less radical operation, the authors of this paper conclude that the difference in rates of risk is not sufficiently great to warrant hysterectomy as initial therapy for all cases of carcinoma-in-situ of the cervix.

Need for continued follow-up

The recurrence of neoplastic change following treatment emphasizes again the fact that the success of any screening programme for cancer depends ultimately on reducing mortality. Early treatment may completely eliminate one particular focus of malignant disease, but the same factors which caused the screening-detected lesion apply to any remaining epithelium. This point is aptly made by Weiss (1978) who, in a discussion of problems in screening for lung cancer, terms it 'the final blow' that some of the small proportion of patients successfully treated for lung cancer will develop a second primary 'since cigarette smoke bathes the mucosa of the entire bronchial tree'. These people, of course, also remain at high risk of other smoking-related diseases. Thus, at best, screening for cancer results in some cures, but at the same time labels these patients as being at high risk of subsequent disease and careful, prolonged follow-up is as necessary for them as for symptomatic cancers.

Compliance with recommended treatment

One further practical aspect influencing the amount of benefit which can be expected concerns compliance of both doctors and patients with recommendations made as a result of screening. Although, faced with a diagnosis of possible cancer, the great majority of patients will agree to whatever procedures are recommended, a small minority may not. Moreover, when the action to be taken as a result of a positive screening finding depends on a doctor who was not involved in the screening procedure, he may disagree with the screening finding, or think it insufficiently important to act upon. This is naturally more likely to occur in the case of borderline lesions. Armstrong (1980) followed up 666 women who had been recommended for a repeat cervical smear because of dyskaryosis; only 35 per cent had had the repeat smear taken within six months of the recommended date. A further 33 per cent had not returned for the recommended repeat (patient default) but the largest group (42 per cent) had not been followed because of a failure on the part of the health service to recall them. It was found that this was most liable to happen when the smear showing dyskaryosis had been taken in a hospital department from which the patient had since been discharged, particularly if the woman had been attending hospital for termination of pregnancy or for sexually transmitted disease.

Economic benefits of screening

Both benefits and costs of screening can be assessed by economic analyses at different levels. The first of these is restricted to measurement of the financial impact of the service on health services for management of the particular cancer. This can be extended to consider the consequences in factors such as work productivity for the patients whose cancers are detected early, for their families and for society at large. A yet wider view looks at the value which people attach to screening which, it is assumed, reflects their expectations both in terms of reduction in the risk of death and other intangibles such as reassurance. Only the direct consequences to the health service are considered here and on p. 248.

Financial benefit to the health service

Savings to the health service may accrue if the costs of management of cancers or pre-invasive lesions detected at screening are less than those which would have been incurred had the disease been allowed to progress to a more advanced stage. Thus, this too depends on assumptions about natural history, length bias and lead time. As in any assessment of expenditure occurring at different times, a discount rate has to be applied to future costs to allow for the fact that they are worth less than present costs. One attempt to estimate financial savings in this way has been made by Simpson (unpublished thesis) who made separate estimates for costs of breast cancers diagnosed at different stages of the disease, and then applied these estimates to the stage distribution of a group of cancers detected at screening. He considered the primary treatment costs in considerable detail including, as separate items, costs of out-patient visits, costs of in-patient nursing care and 'hotel' care, costs of investigation and of each specific form of treatment (surgery, radiotherapy etc.). He also looked retrospectively at all the care received by a cohort of breast cancer patients followed up for twenty years (or till death if earlier), using an annual discount rate of 7 per cent. The estimates, according to stage at time of diagnosis, are shown in Table 8.5. These estimates were then applied to

Table 8.5 Hospital costs of treatment of breast cancer at different stages (December 1977)

Stage at diagnosis	Cost of primary treatment (£)	Total cost up to twenty years discounted (£)
I	762	1980
II	988 ⎫	2860
III	969 ⎭	
IV	451	3190

the stage distribution of a group of cancers detected at screening, to give an average cost for treatment of a screening-detected cancer, and the cost of the screening procedure was added to this. The treatment estimates were also applied to a group of symptomatic cancers presenting through the conventional system, and were discounted to allow for an assumed one-year lead time. (No correction was made for length bias.) The estimate resulted in an average cost for a screening-detected cancer of £2401 and for a conventional, symptomatically referred cancer of £2447. These estimates (for the United Kingdom in 1977) should be regarded with caution because the series of cancers—particularly those detected at screening—on which this work was based were not typical of a real screening service. However, the method used is of interest and might be applied in other more realistic circumstances and to other cancers.

Hazards of the screening test

The first practical disadvantage of screening to be considered relates to the safety of the screening test. Safety is one of the criteria of ideal screening tests mentioned by Cochrane and Holland (1971), although it is often omitted in other such lists of criteria to be met for a valid screening programme—perhaps this is because it seems too obvious to warrant mention. However, again the point must be stressed that different safety limits are applicable to a patient seeking help for explicit symptoms, as opposed to mass screening of apparently symptom-free people. For the first, a certain level of hazard is tolerable if the investigation is likely to prove useful in defining the cause of the symptoms and enabling appropriate treatment to be given. For the second, risk is only tolerable if its probability for the individual screened is considerably less than the probability of early treatable disease being found, with consequent improved prognosis. Since screening tests almost invariably develop from diagnostic tests used in symptomatic patients, there is a danger that the degree of risk they entail for an asymptomatic population may be overlooked. In cancer screening the safety of at least three tests has been questioned.

Proctosigmoidoscopy

This has been fairly extensively used in screening for colorectal cancer, although admittedly in volunteers rather than invitees. A recent UICC Workshop (1978) concluded that the morbidity of this procedure appears to be of the order of 1 perforation for every 2500 tests and maybe 1 death for every 10 000 tests. In view of its lack of acceptability, poor sensitivity and absence of evidence that prognosis can be improved in lesions detected by it, the Workshop concluded that it could not be recommended as a routine mass screening test.

Double contrast barium meal

This test is used for screening for stomach cancer in Japan and necessitates an average of six x-ray film exposures and fluoroscopy each time an individual is screened. A nationwide team in Japan has studied radiation dosages received in thirty-eight centres participating in the screening programme, estimating both mean bone marrow dose, to give an estimated risk of leukaemia, and mean gonadal dose, to give an estimated risk of genetic injury. The estimated risks were then compared with estimated values of screening based on certain assumptions rather than on evidence from a trial. It was concluded that, provided screening was restricted to persons aged over 40 years, the likely benefits outweighed the risks (Ichikawa, 1978).

Mammography

Considerable controversy and even public alarm have arisen in North America about potential radiation hazard from the use of mammography in screening for breast cancer (Culliton, 1977). The particular danger here is induction of breast cancer itself rather than leukaemia or genetic damage. Follow-up studies of Japanese atom bomb survivors (McGregor et al., 1977) and various series of women whose breasts have been exposed to ionizing radiation for medical reasons (e.g. Boice and Monson, 1977) have shown an excess incidence of breast cancer becoming apparent five to twenty years after irradiation, and probably continuing throughout life thereafter. Assuming a linear dose response curve, the risk of inducing breast cancer has been estimated as 3.5–7.5 per million women per year, for every rad surface exposure to the breast, starting ten years after irradiation. (It is actually the mean absorbed dose to breast tissue which is important rather than skin dose, but the latter can be reasonably accurately measured and its use errs on the safe side, since the absorbed dose will be smaller.) Standardized monitoring of dose was considered to be important in the United States Breast Cancer Detection Projects which arranged that dosage was measured bi-weekly using thermoluminescent sachets issued to each screening clinic by one of six national centres for radiological physics and, after exposure, returned for testing. The results were regularly reported back to the screening centre and each year the mammography system was checked by an independent physicist. During the first three years of operation the average skin dose for xerography fell from 3.1 to 1.2 rad (3.1 to 1.2 cGy) and that of film-screen mammography from 1.5 to 0.6 rad (1.5 to 0.6 cGy) (Beahrs et al., 1979).

Unlike the situation with regard to screening for stomach cancer, there is experimental evidence of benefit from screening for breast cancer in women over the age of 50 years (Shapiro, 1977). It is not possible to say exactly how much of the reduction in mortality observed in that study was attributable to mammography, but Beahrs et al. (1979) estimate that it was about one-third. Calculations of benefit versus risk (Shapiro, 1978) suggest that, for screening starting at age 50 years, the person-years gained by mammography screening outweigh the person-years lost by at least 4 to 1, but the benefit of mammography below that age is still unproven.

Balance between risks and benefits

Estimates of risk—particularly radiation risk in two of the examples quoted above—are necessarily very imprecise, being based on extrapolations. With our present imperfect knowledge of the effectiveness of screening for most cancers, the estimates of benefit are equally, if not more, imprecise. Nevertheless, it is very important from an ethical point of view that the possibility of damage resulting from the test should be estimated as carefully as possible and contrasted with the likely benefits. This will usually serve to focus attention on particular points requiring further research, and perhaps delay the introduction of unwarranted unsafe screening programmes.

Lack of specificity of the screening test

Whereas *sensitivity* measures the ability of a test to tell the whole truth, *specificity* measures its ability to tell nothing but the truth. A test with poor specificity misclassifies many non-diseased people, necessitating that they go through the worry of thinking that they may have cancer, and the inconvenience and possible morbidity associated with further investigations. Moreover, lack of specificity may place a heavy additional burden on health service resources, thus adding to the costs of a screening programme.

In Table 8.1, specificity is given by the proportion of non-cancers with a negative test result. As already seen, classification of false negatives (i.e., people with cancer but negative results) is difficult, but their number is usually so small in relation to the number of true negatives that for all practical purposes they can be ignored, and specificity can be approximated by the number of people with a negative test out of all who do not have cancer. For example, if the true prevalence of cancer is 5 per 1000 and the test is 80 per cent sensitive, there will only be 1 false negative in every 1000 people screened.

As in the case of hazards associated with the test, lack of specificity is frequently overlooked when a test is being developed from use as a diagnostic tool for individual patients to use as a population screening tool. This occurs principally because greater emphasis is usually given to achieving maximum sensitivity. But sensitivity and specificity are negatively related so that as one increases the other decreases. Thus a change from Haemoccult I test to Haemoccult II in screening for colorectal cancer was introduced to improve sensitivity, but decreased specificity from 99.5 per cent to 97.9 per cent, meaning that an additional 1.6 per cent of subjects without cancer had to undergo proctosigmoidoscopy (Schottenfeld *et al.*, 1978).

Implications of false positive results

This illustrates well the implications for people with false positive results to cancer screening. In many instances, the additional diagnostic investigations needed to establish whether or not a cancer is present, are invasive, unpleasant, and have their own hazards, frequently including anaesthesia and surgery. This applies not only in the case of sigmoidoscopy, barium enema and biopsy for false positives to colorectal cancer screening, but also to excision biopsies for non-malignant breast lumps, cystoscopy for false positives to bladder cytology, gastroscopy for false positives to stomach cancer screening, and bronchoscopy for false positives to sputum cytology. Some medical authorities disagree with the term 'false positives' to describe benign lesions found by screening since they are true pathological entities which, if they presented symptomatically, would require removal. Nevertheless, their discovery by screening has certainly done the patient no good and may have done him harm.

Effect of repeated screening on specificity

It is often assumed that specificity is a fixed property of a test with a given cut-off level between positive and negative, no matter what population is screened. But this is only so if the prevalence and case-mix of lesions causing false positive results are constant in the differing populations. It has already been seen that sensitivity may alter from a population screened on only one occasion and a population repeatedly screened, because the newly incident cases arising since the previous screen are at a different stage of the detectable preclinical phase. The same applies also to specificity. In the case of breast cancer, it has been shown that, after the pool of possibly long-standing benign lesions has been identified and removed at first screening, specificity markedly improves. Presumably this is due to a lower incidence of false positive benign disease as women get older, causing there to be fewer such lesions in the rescreened population, and to the fact that the new benign lesions which do arise are at an earlier, less detectable phase (Clifford and Chamberlain, in preparation). Whether the same applies in screening for other cancers where lack of specificity is a problem, is not yet known. In the case of colorectal cancer screening by Haemoccult for example, specificity on rescreening will depend on the age-specific incidence of the various non-malignant causes of gastrointestinal bleeding. In considering the total effects of an established screening service repeated screening makes a much larger contribution than initial screening, which only applies to new entrants to the programme. In decisions about implementation of screening services, therefore, the properties of the screening test on rescreening are the most important.

Balance between sensitivity and specificity

It has already been seen that as sensitivity increases specificity decreases and vice versa. Thus the benefits of increased sensitivity have to be balanced against the disadvantages of decreased specificity. This balance can be deliberately manipulated by altering the cut-off point used to separate positives from negatives. One approach to deciding the appropriate cut-off point is to plot sensitivity against specificity, thereby constructing a ROC (receiver operating characteristic) curve as used in detection theory (Lusted, 1969). Rombach (1980) plotted such a curve for different cut-off points in interpretation of mammograms (probably benign, possibly malignant, probably malignant, malignant), thus enabling the consequences of each of these cut-off points to be forecast. A similar approach was used by Simpson et al. (1978), who reported the sensitivities, specificities and costs of fifteen alternative combinations of physical examination and mammography, ranging from physical examination on its own performed by a nurse to double physical examination and double-reading of mammograms. These authors pointed out that, even given information on sensitivity, specificity and cost, the choice of the best test (or best cut-off point) is not obvious but depends on the values placed on true or false positive and true or false negative results. They sent the relevant data to a number of community physicians experienced in health policy decisions, and showed considerable disagreement amongst them, some opting for high sensitivity, others for high specificity, and others for low cost.

The examples of decisions between sensitivity and specificity have referred only to breast cancer, probably because the alternative tests for this neoplasm have been studied more intensively than any others, but the principles are equally applicable to other tests no matter whether their basis is biochemical, cytological or in any other diagnostic modality.

Financial costs

Any form of screening in which unsolicited tests are applied to large numbers of people who have not consulted the health service is bound to have considerable financial implications, which ideally should be assessed in a cost–benefit analysis (Pole, 1968). Financial costs occur not merely because the test itself has a certain expense, but also because the further investigations arising from it (particularly those from its lack of specificity) add an extra cost which would not otherwise have occurred. As already seen, there may also be financial savings from less expensive treatment of cases found. If humanitarian aspects are for the moment ignored, even the benefits of cancer screening programmes are likely to add to total health service costs by increasing life expectancy and thereby increasing future use of health and social security services (principally pensions). Some screening programmes for congenital handicap have been shown to be economic, but these involve only a single screen to prevent a lifetime of handicap. It is unlikely that any cancer screening programme would result in actual savings to the public sector, unless it involved a very limited series of repeated tests for a cancer with a young age-specific mortality, since the persons benefiting from such a programme would contribute many years of productive life. Screening high-risk women for choriocarcinoma may perhaps come into this category.

Fortunately, humanitarian considerations are likely to take precedence over financial ones, but it is obviously still relevant for policy makers to be able to estimate the financial costs of screening and to understand which particular aspects of the service have the greatest influence on cost.

Cost effectiveness

Most reports on financial costs of cancer screening have been limited to costs of the screening test per person screened or per case detected (Carruthers et al., 1975; Last and Bailey, 1978). Dickinson (1972), in evaluating cervical cancer screening, took into account the cost of treatment as well, and Kodlin (1972), in breast cancer screening, also included the costs of false positives. Both these papers then balanced the measured costs against the likely effect of screening on mortality to give an estimate of the cost of screening per life saved. Simpson (unpublished thesis) calculated the costs to the health service incurred by a woman screened for breast cancer who fell into each of the four categories, true or false positive and true or false negative, and multiplied this by the probability of each of these outcomes. He then subtracted from this the probable costs of her being treated for benign or malignant breast disease if she had not been screened. For the items which were discounted (i.e. those where costs were borne at different time periods), a 7 per cent discount rate was used and it was assumed that cancers and benign disease, occurring if she had not been screened, were diagnosed on average one year later than those detected at screening, and similarly that false negatives were diagnosed one year later than screening. The resulting estimate (i.e. all health service costs of managing breast disease in a screened women minus those she would have incurred had she not been screened) was termed the 'cost-effect' on the health service of screening one woman on one occasion. This amounted to an average of £18.50 for screening by physical examination and mammography in England in 1977. The variables having most influence on this estimate were the specificity of the test, the cost of the test and the cost of treating benign disease. This emphasizes again that the costs of screening, like its other disadvantages, are incurred by the many people *without* cancer who are screened, while the benefits accrue to the very few people in whom screening detects a malignancy with sufficient lead time to alter its prognosis.

The cost-effect per true positive detected was calculated, and (from a theoretical comparison of survival of true positives with that of conventionally referred symptomatic cancers) the cost per year of life saved was estimated, the latter also being discounted to take the pattern of survival into account and weight the closer years with a greater value than those twenty years hence.

These estimates were considered separately for screening by different methods, with the results shown in Table 8.6. This is of interest because it illustrates how the ranking order of the different alternatives changes according to whether one looks simply at:

(i) *cost per test*;
(ii) *cost-effect per woman screened* (which is principally influenced by specificity);
(iii) *cost per true positive* (which also depends on sensitivity);
(iv) *cost per year of life saved* (which also depends on lead time gained).

Table 8.6 Financial estimates of alternative screening tests for breast cancer

	Cost of test (£)	Cost effect on health service per screen (£)	Cost per true positive (£)	Cost per discounted year of life saved (£)
Physical examination by a nurse	3.50	9.00	1976	1590
Physical examination by a doctor	4.00	9.50	1846	1488
Mammography with no physical examination	9.00	10.50	1703	
Physical by doctor plus mammography	10.00	18.50	2350	1871
Double physical plus double mammography	13.50	25.50	2750	2221

It is also very relevant to decisions about which tests to use to note how the cheaper paramedical test loses its initial advantage because it is both less specific and less sensitive than the alternatives.

The yield of curable cancers

One further factor which can contribute to the efficiency of a screening programme is the prevalence of cancers in the screened population. If prevalence is high, there will be proportionately more individuals in the left-hand column of Table 8.1 (potential beneficiaries) and fewer in the right-hand column (non-diseased). Changes in prevalence of cancers do not affect the sensitivity or specificity of the test but *do* alter the ratio of true positives to false positives. This is sometimes termed the *predictive value of a positive test* and in Table 8.1 is calculated by the true positives as a proportion of all positives. The higher this proportion the greater are the chances of a person with a positive result having cancer. (It should be noted that this predictive value can also be increased by raising the cut-off point of the test to improve specificity.) Increasing prevalence by focusing on a high-risk group not only improves the predictive value of a positive test, but also reduces the number of non-diseased people screened, thus reducing the costs and exposing fewer people to the hazards of the test. It thus automatically increases benefits relative to disadvantages and costs.

Definition of a high-risk group

Virtually all cancer screening programmes intuitively use the risk criterion of age in formulating policy (one notable exception being the instruction of schoolgirls in breast self-examination, which seems to be based more on the 'captivity' of this population than on consideration of their risk of breast cancer). Apart from age, however, the use of other risk indicators depends on prior knowledge of important factors in the aetiology or pathogenesis of the cancer in question. One obvious risk factor, relatively easy to determine, is occupation; others depend on sociodemographic aspects of the previous life of individuals, which can usually only be determined by a 'prescreening' questionnaire; on previous medical history; or on a 'prescreening' test of some biochemical or biophysical property.

Occupation

Where a clear association exists between a cancer and an occupational hazard (as discussed on p. 59), a selective screening programme may be instituted for people in the particular industry. Since there is always a latent interval between exposure and development of neoplasia, past as well as present workers should be included—indeed, since identification of a cancer hazard will presumably be followed by steps to reduce exposure, the risk in past workers is greater than in present workers. This poses difficulties in identifying them retrospectively, tracing their present whereabouts, and then persuading them that they are at risk and should be screened. Examples of screening of occupational risk groups include schemes for detecting bladder cancer in rubber and dye workers, lung cancer in asbestos and nickel workers, and leukaemia in those exposed to ionizing radiation.

If evidence has been obtained that prior exposure to a specific work environment may have increased the risk for a particular malignancy, the suitability of screening obviously requires review. In such a situation, it is important to have firm evidence that screening would not add to morbidity (e.g. by irradiation hazards from regular x-ray outweighing the saving from any element of early detection). Providing this is so, one would not necessarily require a cost–benefit analysis to demonstrate financial saving from the screening programme. The industry may accept that the threat to health in those that have been exposed at work to a carcinogen is sufficient justification to introduce screening, even if the proportion of subjects who benefit from early detection of cancer is low or very low. The point here is that there may be a 'moral' obligation to take every feasible step that might reduce the hazard from past exposure to carcinogens at work.

Sociodemographic history

This broad heading is taken to include a wide range of background variables in a person's past life which have been shown to be involved in the aetiology of cancer. The most clear-cut example is cigarette smoking in the aetiology of lung cancer, and this has been used to identify risk groups for screening, as in the Mayo Lung Project which restricts screening to men aged over 45 years who have smoked twenty cigarettes or more a day at some period during the previous year (Fontana et al., 1975). In this case, the relative risk of cancer between smokers and non-smokers is so large that there is no question that the majority of cancers would be included in the population sub-group to be screened.

This approach is not so profitable, however, when the relative risk of the aetiological factor or factors concerned is not so great. Attempts have been made to define a risk group for breast cancer screening from women's reproductive histories but it has not proved possible to discriminate a group containing more than one-third of the cancers (Shapiro et al., 1973).

Previous medical history

The distinction between selective population screening and good medical practice in following up patients is not always clear-cut in the case of regular routine testing of people with pathological conditions indicating high risk of cancer. This applies to many 'pre-malignant' lesions which may themselves have been identified by unselected population screening—bladder papillomata, colon adenomas, cervical dysplasia and so on. Hakama et al. (1979) looked at risk factors for cervical cancer found at first screening (age, parity, coital and post-menopausal bleeding, and cytological category) in an attempt to define a suitable risk group for subsequent intensive screening. They arbitrarily decided to aim for inclusion of 90 per cent of the cancers, but to achieve this the size of the high-risk group was 70 per cent of the total population. Perhaps the most successful definition of a high-risk group on medical grounds is women who have had a hydatidiform mole pregnancy. Their risk of subsequent choriocarcinoma is about 3 per cent, compared with a risk of about 3 per 100 000 following normal pregnancy. This means that by screening the urinary chorionic gonadotrophin levels of women who have had a hydatidiform mole, half of the cancers can be detected in one-thousandth of the population.

Biological prescreening tests

In studying the aetiology of some cancers, various tests of biological substances, such as hormones or antigens, have been used. These are not themselves indicative of a pathological state but of risk status. Low levels of urinary aetiocholanolone and androstenedione, for example, were shown to be correlated with high risk of subsequent breast cancer (Bulbrook *et al.*, 1971). On their own, they do not discriminate powerfully between high and low risk, but when used in conjunction with sociodemographic factors such as age at first birth, Farewell (1977) has calculated that a sub-group of 43 per cent of the population could be identified, containing 71 per cent of the cancers. Similarly, it has been suggested that women with certain thermographic patterns (Stark and Way, 1974) and certain mammographic patterns (Wolfe, 1976) in their breasts are at particularly high risk of breast cancer, but these findings need to be corroborated by longer follow-up studies.

Evaluation of screening for cancer

There is an understandable optimistic tendency among doctors or paramedical staff engaged in screening to regard each case found as a success, possibly as a life saved, and therefore to evaluate the screening service purely in terms of the number of cancers found, without regard for its other consequences. But the foregoing discussion has shown how many different factors affect the balance between benefits and costs and how some of the most important issues, such as the natural history of the cancer, are imperfectly understood and can only be estimated indirectly. Evaluation of cancer screening programmes is therefore a more complex undertaking than it may first appear. Cole and Morrison (1980) and Shapiro (1978) discuss some of the methods of investigation together with their advantages and drawbacks.

Comparisons of prognosis of cancers detected at screening with those diagnosed by conventional symptomatic presentation

This is only marginally better than a simple count of cases detected. It may look merely at prognostic indicators, such as stage at detection or resectability, or it may go one step further and look at survival. Either way it is invalid because the groups being compared are not comparable and because it takes no account of lead time or length bias. The cancers detected at screening represent only a sub-group of those in the general population because the individuals who take up the offer of screening are self-selected. The comparison group in cases such as this may be taken from cases seen by the same centre in an earlier time period, cases seen concurrently in this or other centres, but which have not had an opportunity to be screened, or—worst of all—cases occurring in people who have refused the offer of screening. There is no way of retrospectively matching or correcting all possible confounding variables which might bias the comparison between any of these groups of patients and the selected group of patients whose cancers were found by screening.

Case-control study

This approach is aimed at determining whether lack of screening can be regarded as a risk factor for cancer. A group of patients with cancer and a group of matched controls are questioned about their screening histories and other risk variables. One such study has been reported which showed that 32 per cent of cases of cervical cancer had been screened compared with 56 per cent of controls (Clarke and Anderson, 1979). This difference was statistically highly significant and indicated a relative risk of invasive cancer of 2.7 in unscreened compared with screened women. In this particular cancer, however, it is already well recognized that the women at greatest risk are least likely to be screened; an attempt was made to overcome this bias by standardizing for risk factors such as marital status, age at first intercourse and age at first marriage, and within each of these risk groups the difference in risk analysis between screened and unscreened women was still maintained. These authors also took into account the control subjects who had had a hysterectomy. They concluded that the Pap smear is an effective screening procedure for prevention of invasive cancer, but extraordinarily did not mention the one fact which would have lent weight to this—the incidence of pre-invasive lesions detected by the smears which were done in both cases and controls. Unless the controls had a higher proportion of treated pre-invasive lesions, it is difficult to see how the Pap smears *per se* could have contributed to their lower risk of invasive cancer. A completely different conclusion could be drawn from this study if one considers the finding that 35 per cent of the cases had been screened in the previous five years but, in spite of this, developed invasive cancer, indicating that they either had false negative results, ineffective follow-up, or that the frequency of rescreening was insufficient to detect their cancers with sufficient lead time to prevent their reaching the invasive stage.

Correlation of intensity of screening with mortality

This approach depends upon comparisons between places or in different time periods, in the number, or preferably the proportion, of individuals screened and changes in mortality. Examples of this method are in papers by Hirayama (1978), concerning screening for stomach cancer in Japan, and by Ahluwahlia and Doll (1968), Kinlen and Doll (1973) and Miller *et al.* (1976) concerning screening for cervical cancer in Canada. In all these cases, screening was introduced at a period when mortality from these cancers was in any case declining, for reasons connected with aetiological factors, and possibly also improvements in treatment; against such a background it is very difficult to assess the impact of screening. Moreover, retrospective data on intensity of screening are usually only available in terms of number of tests per head of population, rather than number of individuals who have had none, one, or more tests; and similarly the denominator for estimating rates is confounded by migrations in and out of the populations being compared. Correction for these factors may be possible in populations with linked record systems and stable populations. Indeed, the most convincing evidence so far available of the benefit of screening for cervical cancer comes from such a population (that of Iceland) in which increasing intensity of screening was associated with reversal of a previous upward trend in mortality (Johannesson *et al.*, 1978).

Quasi-experimental trials

These represent a halfway house between correlation studies, in which existing data from different populations are compared, and randomized controlled trials. In quasi-experimental trials, populations into which screening is to be introduced and comparison populations in which it is not, are identified in advance and all information on cancer incidence and mortality in them prospectively collected for the duration of the trial. Such trials need to be conducted with at least the same rigorous standards of method and analysis as randomized trials, so that all known biases can be taken into account. They avoid the biases inherent in survival comparisons mentioned above because they are able to compare both incidence and mortality in whole populations which are similar in all respects except for the availability of screening. Hence the incidence and distribution of fast- and slow-growing tumours should be the same. This can be verified during the course of the study and earlier mortality trends can provide evidence of the comparability of the groups. Quasi-experimental trials overcome some of the ethical and other problems associated with randomization, but at the price of a lower level of statistical credibility. One example is the UK Trial of Early Detection of Breast Cancer (1981).

Randomized controlled trials

From the statistical point of view, trials in which a whole population is identified and individuals or groups within it are then randomly allocated to be offered screening or not, provided the most convincing evidence of the effectiveness of screening. The classic example, which started in 1963 but still serves as a model study design, is the trial of breast cancer screening conducted in the Health Insurance Plan of Greater New York (Shapiro, 1977). In this trial, 62 000 women aged 40–64 years enrolled with the Plan for comprehensive health insurance, were randomly allocated either to a study group, which was invited to be screened, or to a control group which was not. The study started in 1963, and follow-up is still continuing. Results up to thirteen years from entry to the trial indicate that mortality from breast cancer is reduced by about one-third in the population offered screening compared with the control group.

Randomized controlled trials are ideal in theory because their design ensures that both systematic bias and random bias are avoided in the comparison between the group offered screening and the control group. However, in practice they may have certain difficulties which limit their applicability to a real-life service situation and hence extrapolation of their results may be misleading. For example, randomization of individuals within a single population for invitations to be screened or not cannot be backed up by a general education campaign exhorting people to take up the offer, because this would lead to a demand for screening from the control group. Moreover, even if there is no public awareness of the invitation, 'contamination' of the control group cannot be avoided completely, nor can it be accurately measured in most situations. Consequently, randomization of individuals may minimize true differences because acceptance of screening may be less than if a population-based campaign were possible, and some of the control group may also have sought screening, or at least been made aware of the importance of early detection.

A similar difficulty arises if the individuals enrolled in the trial are volunteers who agree to be randomized to screening or control group. The nature of such a population implies that it is already very aware of health matters in general and early detection in particular, and hence acceptance rates of screening may be atypically high in the study group and symptomatic presentation atypically early in the control group. This may well be the case in a current trial of colorectal cancer screening in Minnesota (Gilbertson et al., 1980).

For public health measures, the ideal unit to be studied is not the individual but the community to which the measure will be applied in practice (Cornstock, 1978). Ideally the unit of random allocation should therefore be a community not an individual. One example of this in cancer screening is the current trial of breast cancer screening in Sweden (Tabar et al., 1980) in which parishes are randomly allocated to screening or control groups. In this case, the study design envisages that the control group will be offered screening whenever an effect of screening on mortality in the study group is shown. This raises an additional difficulty commonly encountered in randomized trials—how much to offer the control group. Since screening studies are almost always initiated by enthusiasts who believe that screening is effective, they frequently feel obliged to offer a limited service to the control group, either in the form of a less efficient screening device, such as a symptom questionnaire (Gilbertson et al., 1980), or less frequent screening (Brett, 1969) or both (Fontana et al., 1975). In these cases the conflict between the wish to offer a new service and methods of proving the effectiveness of the service remains unresolved, since the results will be relevant only to comparisons of different levels of screening not to screening as opposed to nothing.

Mathematical models

Several computer simulations of the effects of screening on mortality have been devised (eg. Knox, 1973; Albert et al., 1978; Shwartz, 1978; Eddy, 1980). These construct mathematical models of the numerous interacting variables that determine firstly the natural history of the cancer in the absence of screening, and secondly the effects of screening both on that natural history and on the people without cancer who are screened. Their eventual use could be a very valuable tool for determining screening policy by forecasting the effects of altering one or more of the variables. At present, though, they are still of only theretical interest and none has been verified in practice. Of necessity, they are based on theoretical assumptions about natural history, all except Knox (1973), assuming that transitions from one state to another in Fig. 8.2 go only in one direction towards development of cancer. They are dependent on more detailed knowledge than is yet available about the social and biological factors influencing the effectiveness of screening.

References

Ahluwahlia, H. S. and Doll, R. (1968). *British Journal of Preventive and Social Medicine* **22**, 161.

Albert, A. P. M., Gertman, T. A. C. and Lui, S. I. (1978). *Mathematical Biosciences* **40**, 1.

Allman, S. T., Chamberlain, J. and Harman, P. (1974). *Health Trends* **6**, 39.

Armstrong, A. E. (1980). *Follow-up of Women with Dysplasia of the Uterine Cervix.* PhD Thesis, University of London.

Beahrs, O. H., Shapiro, S. and Smart, C. (1979). *Journal of the National Cancer Institute* **62**, 640.

Becker, M. H., Haefner, D. P., Kasl, S. V., Kirscht, J. P., Malman, L. A. and Rosenstock, I. M. (1977). *Medical Care* **15**, (Suppl.) 27.

Bloor, M. J. and Gill, D. G. (1972). *Community Medicine* **129**, 135.

Boice, J. D. and Monson, R. R. (1977). *Journal of the National Cancer Institute* **59**, 823.

Boyes, D. A., Worth, A. J. and Fidler, H. K. (1970). *Journal of Obstetrics and Gynaecology of the British Commonwealth* **77**, 769.

Brett, G. Z. (1969). *British Medical Journal* **4**, 260.

Bulbrook, R. B., Hayward, J. and Spicer, C. C. (1971). *Lancet* **ii**, 395.

Burghardt, E. (1973). In *Early Historical Diagnosis of Cervical Cancer*, pp. 15–30. Ed. by E. A. Friedman. Thiewe, Stuttgart.

Butler, W. H. and Jones, G. (1976). In *Scientific Foundations of Oncology*, pp. 1–7. Ed. by T. Symington and R. L. Carter. Heinemann, London.

Cardiff Cervical Cytology Study (1980). *Journal of Epidemiology and Community Health* **34**, 9.

Carruthers, J., Wilson, J. M. G., Chamberlain, J., Husain, O. A. N., Patey, D. G. H., Richards, N. D., Pennicott, A., Rogers, P., Catling, R., Meado, T. W., Saunders, J. and McEwan, P. J. M. (1975). *British Journal of Preventive and Social Medicine* **29**, 239.

Chamberlain, J., Clifford, R. E., Nathan, B. E., Price, J. L. and Burn, I. (1979). *Clinical Oncology* **5**, 135.

Chamberlain, J., Rogers, P., Price, J. L., Ginks, S., Nathan, B. E. and Burn, I. (1975). *Lancet* **ii**, 1026.

Clarke, A. E. and Anderson, T. W. (1979). *Lancet* **ii**, 1.

Clifford, R. E. and Chamberlain, J. (In preparation.)

Cochrane, A. L. and Holland, W. W. (1971). *British Medical Bulletin* **27**, 3.

Cole, P. and Morrison, A. S. (1980). *Journal of the National Cancer Institute* **64**, 1263.

Collins, V. P., Loeffler, R. K. and Tivey, H. (1956). *American Journal of Roentgenology and Radiation Therapy* **76**, 988.

Cornstock, G. W. (1978). *American Journal of Epidemiology* **108**, 81.

Culliton, B. J. (1977). *Science* **196**, 853.

Delarue, N. C., Pearson, F. G., Thompson, D. W. and Van Boxel, P. (1971). *Geriatrics* **26**, 130.

Dethlefson, I. A., Prewitt, J. M. S. and Mendelsohn, M. L. (1968). *Journal of the National Cancer Institute* **40**, 389.

Dickinson, L. (1972). *Mayo Clinic Proceedings* **47**, 550.

Edinburgh Breast Screening Clinic (1978). *British Medical Journal* **2**, 175.

Eddy, D. M. (1980). *Screening for Cancer, Theory, Analysis and Design.* Prentice Hall, New Jersey.

Farewell, V. T. (1977). *Cancer* **40**, 931.

Feinleib, M. and Zelen, M. (1969). *Archives of Environmental Health* **19**, 412.

Fink, R., Shapiro, S. and Lewison, J. (1968). *Public Health Reports* **83**, 479.

Fontana, R. S., Sanderson, D. R., Woolner, L. B., Miller, W. E., Bernatz, P. E., Payne, W. S. and Taylor, W. F. (1975). *Chest* **67**, 511.

Forrest, A. P. M. and Roberts, M. M. (1980). *British Journal of Hospital Medicine* **23**, 8.

Fulghum, J. E. and Klein, R. J. (1967). *Monograph 11.* Florida Department of Health and Rehabilitative Services.

Gastrin, G. (1976). *British Medical Journal* **3**, 745.

Geddes, D. M. (1979). *British Journal of Diseases of the Chest* **18**, 1.
Gilbertson, V. A., Church, T. R., Grewe, F. J., Mandel, J. S., McHugh, R. B., Schuman, L. M. and Williams, S. E. (1980). *Journal of Chronic Diseases* **33**, 107.
Green, G. H. (1974). *New Zealand Medical Journal* **80**, 279.
Haefner, D. P., Kegeles, S., Kirscht, J. and Rosenstock, I. (1967). *Public Health Reports* **82**, 451.
Hakama, M., Pukkala, E. and Saatamoinen, P. (1979). *Journal of Epidemiology and Community Health* **33**, 257.
Hardcastle, J. D., Balfour, T. and Amar, S. S. (1980). *Lancet* **i**, 791.
Hirayama, T. (1978). In *Screening in Cancer*, pp. 264–78. Ed. by A. B. Miller, UICC Technical Report No. 40, Geneva.
Hobbs, P., Smith, A., George, W. D. and Sellwood, R. A. (1980). *Journal of Epidemiology and Community Health* **34**, 19.
Ichikawa, H. (1978). In *Screening in Cancer*, pp. 279–99. Ed. by A. B. Miller. UICC Technical Report No. 40, Geneva.
Johannesson, G., Geirsson, G. and Day, N. (1978). *International Journal of Cancer* **21**, 418.
Kinlen, L. J. and Doll, R. (1973). *British Journal of Preventive and Social Medicine* **27**, 146.
Knox, E. G. (1973). In *The Future and Present Indicatives*, pp. 17–55. Ed. by G. McLachlan. Nuffield Provincial Hospitals Trust, London.
Knox, E. G. (1975). In *Probes for Health*, pp. 13–44. Ed. by G. McLachlan. Nuffield Provincial Hospitals Trust, London.
Kodlin, D. (1972). *Methods of Information in Medicine* **11**, 242.
Koss, L. G. (1970). *Clinical Obstetrics and Gynaecology* **13**, 873.
Landsman, J. B., Jones, J. M., Evans, D. M. D. and Sweetnam, P. (1977). The Cardiff Cervical Cytology Study Part 1, *The Organisation*. Welsh Office, Cardiff.
Last, P. A. and Bailey, A. R. (1978). *British Medical Journal* **2**, 1784.
Lundgren, B. (1979). *Journal of the National Cancer Institute* **62**, 1373.
Lusted, L. B. (1969). *Radiologic Clinics of North America* **7**, 435.
McGregor, D. H., Land, C. E., Choi, K., Tokuoka, S., Liu, P. I., Wakabayashi, T. and Beebe, G. W. (1977). *Journal of the National Cancer Institute* **59**, 799.
McKeown, T. (1968). In *Screening in Medical Care*, pp. 1–13. Ed. by H. Cohen, E. T. Williams and G. McLachlan. Nuffield Provincial Hospitals Trust, London.
Miller, A. B., Lindsay, J. and Hill, G. B. (1976). *International Journal of Cancer* **17**, 602.
Osborn, G. R. and Leyshon, V. N. (1966). *Lancet* **i**, 256.
Peterson, O. (1952). *Acta Radiologica* **38**, 490.
Pole, J. D. (1968). In *Screening in Medical Care*, pp. 141–58. Ed. by H. Cohen, E. T. Williams and G. McLachlan. Nuffield Provincial Hospitals Trust, London.
Richart, R. M. (1967). *Clinical Obstetrics and Gynaecology* **10**, 748.
Rombach, J. J. (1980). *Cancer Detection and Prevention* **3**, 455.
Sansom, C. D., Wakefield, J. and Yule, R. (1972). In *Seek Wisely to Prevent*, pp. 160–72. Ed. by J. Wakefield. HMSO, London.
Schottenfeld, D., Winawer, S. J. and Miller, D. G. (1978). In *Screening in Cancer*, pp. 308–27. Ed. by A. B. Miller. UICC Technical Report No. 40, Geneva.
Shapiro, S. (1977). *Cancer* **39**, 2772.
Shapiro, S. (1978). In *Screening in Cancer*, pp. 133–57. Ed. by A. B. Miller. UICC Technical Report No. 40, Geneva.
Shapiro, S., Goldberg, J. and Hutchinson, G. (1974). *American Journal of Epidemiology* **100**, 357.
Shapiro, S., Goldberg, J., Venet, L. and Strax, P. (1973). In *Host Environment Interactions in the Etiology of Cancer in Man*, pp. 169–82. Ed. by R. Doll and I. Vodopija. IARC publication 7, Lyon.
Shapiro, S., Strax, P. and Venet, L. (1971). *Journal of American Medical Association* **215**, 1777.
Shwartz, M. (1978). *Cancer* **41**, 1550.
Simpson, P. R., Chamberlain, J. and Gravelle, H. S. E. (1978). *Journal of Epidemiology and Community Health* **32**, 166.
Simpson, P. R. Unpublished thesis.
Smithers, D. W. (1968). *Clinical Radiology* **19**, 113.
Spriggs, A. I., Bowey, E. and Cowdell, R. H. (1971). *Cancer* **27**, 1239.
Spriggs, A. I. and Husain, O. A. N. (1977). *British Medical Journal* **2**, 1516.

Stark, A. M. and Way, S. (1974). *Cancer* **33**, 1671.

Steel, G. G. (1977). *Growth Kinetics of Tumours*. Clarendon Press, Oxford.

Stern, E. and Neely, P. M. (1964) *Cancer* **17**, 508.

Stillman, M. J. (1977). *Nursing Research* **26**, 121.

Tabar, L., Gad, A. and Akerlund, E. (1980). *Cancer Detection and Prevention* **3**, 406.

Thorner, W. and Remein, Q. (1961). *Public Health Monographs*, No. 67.

UICC Workshop. (1978). In *Screening in Cancer*, pp. 328–33. Ed. by A. B. Miller. UICC Technical Report No. 40, Geneva.

UK Trial of Early Detection of Breast Cancer (1981). *British Journal of Cancer* **44**, 618.

Waard, F. de, Rombach, J. J. and Colette, H. J. A. (1978). In *Screening in Cancer*, pp. 183–200. Ed. by A. B. Miller. UICC Technical Report No. 40, Geneva.

Wakefield, J. and Sansom, C. D. (1966). *The Medical Officer* **116**, 145.

Wakefield, J. and Sansom, C. D. (1972). In *Seek Wisely to Prevent*, pp. 62–7. Ed. by J. Wakefield. HMSO, London.

Weiss, W. (1978). In *Screening in Cancer*, pp. 216–32. Ed. by A. B. Miller. UICC Technical Report No. 40, Geneva.

Wilson, J. M. G. (1970). *Annales de la Société Belge de Médecine Tropicale* **50**, 489.

Wolfe, J. N. (1976). *American Journal of Roentgenology* **126**, 1130.

Yule, R. (1973). In *Cancer of the Uterine Cervix*, pp. 11–25. Ed. by E. C. Easson. Saunders, London.

9

Screening for cancer of various sites
Jocelyn Chamberlain

Introduction

The foregoing discussion in Chapter 8 has given a number of examples of screening for different cancers in order to illustrate specific points about the theory, practice and evaluation of cancer screening. Inevitably, many of these examples referred to screening for cervix and breast cancer because these two sites have been the target of so much attention. This is probably because of their accessibility, their frequency and the relatively young age group of women affected by them, which gives any potentially life-saving measure a particular appeal.

This chapter systematically considers screening for cancers site by site, looking at the evidence on natural history, the screening tests which are available, the drawbacks and costs, and a summary of the present position, as seen in the United Kingdom. The sites are covered in order of their listing in the International Classification of Disease (ICD).

Stomach cancer (ICD number 151)

As has been seen in Chapter 2, stomach cancer is still a common neoplasm in the UK. However, mortality has been declining steadily, and principally affects a relatively elderly group of the population. Perhaps for these reasons, screening has not been advocated as a means of reducing the number of deaths in Britain or other Western countries, although, with the development of newer diagnostic methods, there has been a plea for more prompt investigation of dyspeptic symptoms in the hope that this might increase the cure rate (Fielding *et al.*, 1980). In the Far East, by contrast, stomach cancer is still very widespread, being the commonest malignant neoplasm in Japan, even though there has been a substantial fall in both incidence and mortality over the past two decades, concomitant with the change to a more Western diet (see Chapter 3). There has also been an extensive screening programme in Japan which has been in existence for twenty years; it is estimated that approximately four million people are now being screened for stomach cancer each year (Ichikawa, 1978) and no discussion of screening for cancer would be complete without reference to the Japanese experience.

Natural history

There is histological evidence suggesting that the early stages in the natural history of stomach cancer consist of multifocal epithelial changes in the gastric mucosa, one or more of which may progress to become invasive (Collins and Gall, 1952). Epithelial dysplasia and carcinoma-in-situ are recognized, but little is known of the extent to which they are pre-malignant (British Medical Journal, 1976). The definition of 'early' gastric cancer is accepted as being those invasive cancers in which the depth of invasion is limited to the mucosa or submucosa (Fielding et al., 1980). In the absence of screening, probably less than 1 per cent of stomach cancers fall into this 'early' category, although the development of fibre-optic endoscopy may result in a higher proportion being diagnosed in this stage. A recent review of 90 'early' cases, out of a total of 13 228 gastric cancers notified to a British Cancer Registry over a ten-year period, found that the age-adjusted five-year survival was 70.4 per cent, compared with a rate of only 4.7 per cent for the whole series and 17.4 per cent for all operable cases (comprising about a quarter of the total) (Fielding et al., 1980). These 90 patients with early cancer were all symptomatic and it was noted that there was a tendency for those with a longer duration of symptoms to have a better prognosis, suggesting that these may have been particularly slow-growing tumours. This series of early cases excluded those with lymph node involvement, but it has been noted elsewhere that some 10 per cent of cases confined to the mucosa and submucosa may already have spread to the lymph nodes (Sogo et al., 1979); however, even if nodes are involved, early cases still have a relatively good prognosis, again suggesting that they tend to be less aggressive than the majority of gastric cancers or they tend to provoke a more efficient immune response in some patients (British Medical Journal, 1976). A very different distribution of histology is found in stomach cancers diagnosed by screening. In the Myagi prefecture in northern Japan, 135 (61 per cent) out of 221 cancers detected by screening were in the early stage (Ichikawa, 1978). Ichikawa also notes that the average age of patients with early cancer detected by screening is some ten to fifteen years younger than the age at diagnosis of a large series of patients who died of gastric cancer. Information such as this, however, cannot answer the essential question concerning the proportion of early cancers detected at screening which, if left untreated, would progress to infiltrate the serosa, nor the average time period over which this would occur. Ten-year survival of early cancers detected by screening in Japan is over 90 per cent but, as discussed in Chapter 8, lead time, length bias, and selection of subjects for screening may all contribute to biasing the apparently favourable comparison between cancers detected at screening and those presenting symptomatically.

Further light on the natural history could be obtained by comparing the incidence and stage distribution of cancers diagnosed at repeated screening of a cohort of people with those diagnosed at first screening. However, the major results, as presented, do not distinguish first screens from repeat screens, although there is anecdotal evidence that late cancers are becoming increasingly rare in populations which are repeatedly screened (Ichikawa, 1978). The proportion of early cases among all screening-detected cancers seems to be increasing over time but some, at least, of this change is attributed to an improvement in sensitivity of the screening test.

Screening tests

The technique used for screening in Japan is x-ray gastrography using barium as a contrast medium. When it was first introduced in the 1960s, the usual technique was one upright view and possibly one prone view with compression. This has now been replaced by the double contrast technique, with an average of six views in different positions. The double contrast technique enables much clearer visualization of the gastric mucosa. Several mobile units have been equipped for screening and can cope with a workload of up to 200 individuals screened per day. The more modern units have indirect equipment with an image intensifier to reduce radiation dose.

In a series of over 33 000 people screened in the Osaka prefecture between 1967 and 1970, Oshima *et al.* (1977) found that the sensitivity of screening was 84 per cent. False negatives were defined as cancer cases presenting symptomatically within one year of a negative screen plus cancers detected at subsequent screening for which examination of previous films showed that a lesion had been missed.

More alarming than false negatives is the remarkably high number of false positives, indicating the lack of specificity of screening. Almost a quarter of screened individuals are referred for further investigation, which involves additional x-rays with fluoroscopy, cytology, endoscopy and possibly biopsy. Large numbers of benign peptic ulcers and gastric polyps are discovered in this way. In the whole of Japan in 1975, the yield of disease detected at screening was 3022 gastric cancers and 79 707 benign conditions (Hirayama, 1978). Hirayama terms this enormous yield of non-malignant disease a 'side-benefit' of screening. This view must surely be open to question since no study of the symptomatology of these 80 000 people is reported, much less any trial of their response to the treatment which was presumably initiated. Moreover, the further investigations required for their diagnosis are themselves uncomfortable and carry a small morbidity. The additional load placed on the health services by the diagnosis and treatment of these incidental benign conditions (many of which might not otherwise have presented for medical care) must be very considerable.

Acceptability

From the various reports in English, it is not clear how the screening programme has been offered to the population in Japan, and there is very little information on its acceptability. Hirayama (1978) shows how the proportion of the total Japanese population who were screened in 1975 varies by age and sex. In that year, 3.4 per cent of adult males and 2.3 per cent of adult females were screened. Screening rates were very low below the age of 30 years, but rose to a peak of 7.5 per cent in men between 45 and 55 years, and 5.4 per cent in women of the same age, before falling off gradually thereafter.

The acceptance of repeated screening in small communities appears to be high, with over 80 per cent of those screened once returning for repeated annual screens over a five-year period (Ichikawa, 1978). Acceptance of further investigations in those with positive screening results was also very high (96 per cent) in the same study.

Hazards and costs

Estimates of the radiation hazard of screening have been made both in terms of induction of leukaemia and cancer, and in terms of genetic damage (Ichikawa, 1978). To this has been added an estimate of death and injury resulting from endoscopy and biopsy in those who screen positive. (It is interesting to note that the estimate of risk of injuries from endoscopy and biopsy is greater than that from radiation.) The results of these calculations indicate that by annual screening of people over the age of 40 years, for an assumed benefit of 100 man-years, 2.5 man-years would be lost; for women the ratio is somewhat less beneficial, at 7.5 woman-years lost per 100 gained. Under the age of 40 years, the ratio is much less favourable, partly because of the risk of genetic damage. (In 1975, nearly 20 per cent of people screened were under the age of 40.)

There is no information on the cost of the screening programme, nor on its manpower requirements, beyond the fact that the films are taken by technicians and read by doctors. The costs of investigating the very large number of false positives must add very substantially to the cost of the whole programme.

Effectiveness

No controlled trial of screening for stomach cancer has been done and there is therefore no direct evidence of the benefit which could be achieved. Indirect measurements of benefit are severely hampered by the fact that both incidence and mortality have in any case been declining quite rapidly, probably because of dietary changes. Between 1963 and 1973 in Osaka, for example, the incidence of gastric cancer fell by 21 per cent in both sexes, and mortality fell by 18 per cent in men and 12 per cent in women (Hanai and Fujimoto, 1977). Hirayama (1978) cites, as evidence of the effectiveness of screening, the fact that the decline in mortality is greatest in the age group with the highest screening rate. He analysed forty-six prefectures, classifying them by their consumption of milk and eggs, the proportion of their 40- to 74-year-old population screened, and the decline in their stomach cancer mortality rates in the same age groups. The decline in mortality was greatest in those with the highest milk and egg consumption and the highest screening rate, but no mention was made of possible biases resulting, for example, from different social class distributions in the different prefectures. Ichikawa (1978) compares mortality in screened subjects with that in the general population, and concludes that screening reduces mortality by about 20 per cent, but again these results make no allowance for selective differences between the screened population (less than 5 per cent of the whole) and the remainder. This estimate of benefit is then used in the benefit : risk estimates quoted above in the subsection on hazards and costs.

A more critical assessment of the effects of screening has been reported by Oshima et al., who set up a computerized record linkage system to collate the file of a cohort of people screened in Osaka between 1967 and 1970 with the population-based cancer registry. The original screened population consisted of 33 221 individuals in whom 123 cancers were found at initial screening (prevalence 3.7 per 1000), and 51 cancers at subsequent screens in the ensuing five years. (The number attending for repeat screening on each occasion was not given.) A further 89 cancers were diagnosed symptomatically. During the ensuing seven years, all cancer deaths were noted and the observed number (131) was compared with that expected from the general population of Osaka (149.5). The ratio of observed to expected (0.88) was not statistically significant, and after making a correction to allow for the fact that perhaps 5 per cent of the screened group had left the population during the follow-up period, the O : E ratio was close to 1.

Conclusions

In many respects, the Japanese experience of screening for stomach cancer can be likened to the Western experience of screening for cervical cancer. Both were started with enthusiasm and conviction but without any plans for evaluation, and both were set in the context of a falling incidence and mortality. An extensive and sophisticated service has been built up over a twenty-year period, but it still reaches only a small proportion of those at risk. It is only in recent years that attention has turned towards evaluating its effectiveness and towards formulating a screening policy that will maximize the benefit and minimize the risk. Questions about establishing an appropriate rescreening interval, and defining high-risk groups, are only now beginning to be asked. The disadvantages of this screening programme in terms of both risk and cost are substantial. It seems highly unlikely that the value of screening for stomach cancer can ever be established from the work in Japan, and unless other high-incidence areas undertake controlled trials, perhaps the essential answers will never be known.

Colorectal cancer (ICD numbers 153 and 154)

Natural history

There is still some controversy surrounding the pre-invasive stages of the natural history of colon cancer, perhaps because there are different histological types of benign colonic lesions, only some of which are associated with invasive cancer (Sherlock et al., 1975). There is increasing evidence, however, that multifocal polypoid adenomas are precursors of malignancy (Day and Morson, 1978), showing the same gradation of cellular changes as that illustrated in Fig. 8.2. This model of natural history of development of colorectal cancer is backed up by animal experiments in which the sequence has been directly observed in chemically induced colon carcinoma in rats (Cole, 1978), and by epidemiological comparisons of the distribution of adenomatous polyps and colorectal cancer (Correa, 1978). Within the broad group of adenomas, both size and histology are related to risk of malignancy, the larger lesions and those with a villous component having the greater potential for malignant change (Morson, 1979). A large majority of adenomas, however, do not progress to invasion within the affected individual's lifetime. Thus the picture of natural history that emerges is similar to that of other cancers, in which multifocal areas of dysplasia develop throughout the epithelial surface, one or more of which go through an in situ phase and eventually become invasive. Little is known about the time sequence of these early changes but, having become invasive, the majority of colorectal cancers progress rapidly through the intestinal wall to invade lymphatics and metastasize to the liver; over 70 per cent of registered cases in England and Wales die within five years of diagnosis (OPCS, 1980).

Screening tests

Two tests have been used in screening for colorectal cancer—proctosigmoidoscopy and faecal occult blood.

Many screening centres in the United States have screened asymptomatic volunteers by rigid proctosigmoidoscopy. Maximum benefit of this procedure is often not obtained; properly inserted, the instrument should be able to visualize 25 cm, but often the examiner is unable to insert it beyond 15–18 cm (Schottenfeld et al., 1978). Since only about half the cancers of the large bowel are in the last 25 cm, the sensitivity of this test is at best 50 per cent and in practice probably considerably less. Its specificity is unknown. It also carries a substantial hazard due to accidental perforation. For all these reasons it is no longer considered suitable as a screening test. The flexible fibre-optic sigmoidoscope overcomes many of these objections but is unsuitable for screening because of the expertise needed in its use, and its initial and maintenance costs.

Faecal occult blood has, in the past, been considered unsuitable for screening because of its poor specificity (Ostrow et al., 1973). False positives occur because the test may detect the small quantity of blood lost through the intestinal mucosa in normal individuals, because of meat in the diet, or because of other dietary peroxidases which may increase with storage of faeces.

Recently a guaiac-impregnated filter paper test has been developed which is much less sensitive to small amounts of blood (and hence more specific as a cancer screening test) and can be stored for several days between the contact with faeces and being tested. This enables it to be used by subjects at home and sent by post to a laboratory for testing. Because colorectal cancers bleed intermittently and the blood is not uniformly dispersed in the stool, testing of two different parts of the stool on three consecutive days is recommended. The sensitivity of this method for cancer detection has been studied by Gnauck (1977), who concluded that it was no more than 90 per cent sensitive and possibly less; its sensitivity for adenoma detection was much less, at only 50–75 per cent. Its specificity in a recent British study was 96.8 per cent (Hardcastle et al., 1980).

Acceptability

Much of the research so far done in colorectal cancer screening has come from American or German cancer screening clinics attended by highly motivated volunteer subjects, among whom 85–90 per cent have been willing to use the test, compared with only 15 per cent when test kits were randomly distributed in New York. Hardcastle et al. (1980) found an overall acceptance rate of 48 per cent in a population aged over 40 years, registered with an English general practice. The test itself is relatively easy and harmless, but distaste for the subject of defaecation and adverse beliefs about cancer detection and cure may contribute to poor response rates. It is likely that the feasibility of a screening service for colorectal cancer will depend very largely on its acceptability.

Hazards and costs

The hazard and expense of proctosigmoidoscopy as the initial screening test has already been mentioned. Assuming that screening is done by the guaiac filter paper method, the principal disadvantage arises from the further investigations required to diagnose the cause of positive results. People with positive test results have to undergo sigmoidoscopy and, if this is negative, a repeat occult blood test after dietary restriction. Full colonoscopy and barium enema are often required. These further investigations are unpleasant for the patient and expensive for the health service.

Effectiveness

There is ample evidence that stage at diagnosis is earlier and five-year survival rates of cancers detected by screening are very much better than those of symptomatic cases. For example, Sherlock and Winawer (1977) report survival rates of 88 per cent, and Gilbertson and Nelms (1978) survival rates of 65 per cent. However, these figures make no allowance for lead time or length bias and they come from a highly selected group of patients, so they cannot be taken as proof of the effectiveness of screening. In a randomized trial of different frequencies of a multiphasic screening package which included sigmoidoscopy, one of the few beneficial effects noted in the frequently screened group compared with the control group was a reduction in mortality from colorectal cancer (Dales *et al.*, 1973). This paper, however, gave insufficient detail to interpret whether this small reduction was attributable to sigmoidoscopy screening or not.

The removal of polypoid adenomas, detected at screening, may in the long term prove an effective measure for reducing the incidence of carcinoma and hence its mortality. Gilbertson and Nelms (1978) attribute an abnormally low incidence of adenocarcinoma of colon and rectum in a group of 21 000 subjects who had been screened annually, to the fact that all polypoid lesions found at successive screens had been removed.

In summary, there is considerable circumstantial evidence that screening could be effective in reducing both incidence and mortality from colorectal cancer but, because of the selected nature of the participants in most screening programmes for which follow-up is reported, and because of the inherent biases in comparisons of survival, its effectiveness is still open to question.

Conclusion

Screening for colorectal cancer appears to have considerable potential but is still at a relatively early stage of development, requiring further research on its acceptability, the validity of the occult blood test, the implications of further investigations of those with positive tests, the economic costs and benefits, the optimal frequency of screening and, especially, on its effectiveness in reducing incidence and mortality. A randomized trial in an unselected population is needed to provide direct evidence of its effectiveness and to assess the long-term benefits and disadvantages of identification of a particularly high-risk group of patients with multiple polypoid adenomas.

Lung cancer (ICD number 162)

Natural history

The classical study by Auerbach *et al.* (1961), of bronchial epithelium from 1522 autopsies, demonstrated the presence of multiple pre-malignant lesions, suggesting the pattern of natural history shown in Fig. 8.2. In 405 men, 63 of whom had died of lung cancer, there was a clear association between the number of (a) lesions with atypia, (b) carcinomas-in-situ, and (c) micro-invasive carcinomas, and the number of cigarettes they had smoked. Multiple lesions were found in the lungs of heavy smokers who had died of other causes as well as those who had died of lung cancer. This is probably the only primary carcinoma in humans for which growth rates have been reported, because it has been possible to observe doubling times from serial chest x-rays, although Spratt (1963) has estimated that twenty-five doublings, or 60 per cent of the tumour's life span, has occurred before it reaches a size of 1.0 cm, when it is reasonably certain of being visible on x-ray. Weiss (1971) reported on 52 cancers for which serial x-rays were available: 29 per cent had doubled in less than three months and the remaining 71 per cent within six months. From what is known of its natural history, therefore, lung cancer (at least in smokers) appears to be a bilateral disease of the whole bronchial tree, with a fast growth rate, neither of which characteristics make it an ideal candidate for screening.

Screening tests

Two tests have been used in screening—chest x-ray and sputum cytology. In a detailed study of their validity when applied at six-monthly intervals to a population of 14 600 Veterans Administration Domiciliaries in the United States, Lilienfeld *et al.* (1966) concluded that the sensitivity of x-ray alone was 42 per cent, that of cytology alone 33 per cent, and that of both tests combined 63 per cent. The denominator for calculating sensitivity consisted of 138 cases detected at screening plus one-third of 118 deaths (39) from lung cancer in the ensuing three years among people who had had negative screening results to both tests. These authors also studied the reproducibility of both tests and noted that the proportion of agreed positives for chest x-ray was 50–60 per cent (Lilienfeld and Kordan, 1966) and agreement on cytology (positives, suspicious and negatives combined) about 75 per cent (Archer *et al.*, 1966). Although this particular study was conducted over twenty years ago (between 1958 and 1961), there have not been any major developments in either test which would be likely to make a substantial alteration to these estimates. In an attempt to improve sensitivity, however, the Mayo Lung Project has increased the frequency of screening to four-monthly. This results in a sensitivity of x-ray of 69 per cent, cytology 25 per cent and both tests 88 per cent (Table 9.1). Also, in order to reduce within-subject variability in sputum cytology, the test is now applied to a three-day pooled specimen (Fontana and Taylor, 1978).

The hazards and disadvantages of screening relate more to lack of specificity of the tests than to the radiation hazard of repeated chest x-rays. The x-ray doses given in these circumstances are very low, and the subjects to be screened are almost always at particularly high risk by virtue of their smoking histories

Table 9.1 Validity of screening tests for lung cancer

	Sensitivity (%) Six-monthly[1]	Four-monthly[2]	Specificity (%)
X-ray alone	42	69	98
Cytology alone	33	25	98
X-ray and cytology combined	63	88	96

[1] Lilienfeld *et al.* (1966).   [2] Fontana and Taylor (1978).

as well as their ages. Presumably it is felt that radiation risks are so tiny in comparison to the subject's risks of death from other causes that they can be ignored.

Lack of specificity, however, is more of a problem because of the difficulty of distinguishing false positives from true and—where cytology is positive but x-ray negative—the difficulty of localizing the lesion. Follow-up procedures for positive results include additional x-rays, tomography, bronchoscopy, separate cytological washings from each side and—as a last resort—exploratory thoracotomy. However, the development of the flexible fibre-optic bronchoscope has helped greatly with the problem of localization (Fontana and Taylor, 1978), although the multiple sites of early lesions from which cells may be exfoliated must still cause problems. An additional disadvantage arises in management of multifocal true positives which are found to be bilateral.

Acceptability and compliance with treatment

Screening for lung cancer has not been reported in a completely unselected population, so that general acceptance of initial screening is unknown. It is worth noting, however, that by virtue of age and socio-economic group, the high-risk group for this disease is also that least likely to attend. The frequency with which screening is advocated may also cause problems with compliance. In the Philadelphia Pulmonary Neoplasm Research Project, Weiss (1978) noted that the average probability of having two consecutive semi-annual chest films was 57 per cent and the proportion of men who made uninterrupted semi-annual visits for ten years was only 18.5 per cent of those still eligible. Moreover, non-compliance with recommended follow-up procedures was also a problem in 14 per cent of the 121 men who developed lung cancer in this project. In the Mayo Lung Project, by contrast, where screening is offered to men who are heavy smokers aged over 45 years and who are enrolled with the Mayo Clinic (possibly an atypically health-conscious group), compliance with four-monthly screening is reported as 83 per cent over a one- to six-year period (Fontana and Taylor, 1978).

Effectiveness of screening

The only controlled trial of screening so far completed is that of Brett (1969), who compared 29 723 men aged over 40 receiving six-monthly chest x-rays at their place of work for three years, with 25 311 men from different workplaces who were screened by x-ray only at the start and the finish of the project. Excluding the first (prevalence) screen, the subsequent annual incidence was similar in study and control groups (1.1 and 1.0 per 1000 respectively). Of 101 lung cancers diagnosed in the study group, 65 were detected by screening. Two-thirds of these were resectable, compared with less than one-third in the control group. Five-year survival was only 6 per cent in the control group, compared with 15 per cent in the whole study group and 23 per cent in those detected by screening. However, neither the survival nor resectability proportions have made any allowance for lead time in cases detected by screening, and it is assumed that length bias has been overcome by excluding the prevalent cancers detected at first screening. The best measure of effectiveness—that of lung cancer mortality—unfortunately showed no significant difference, with 0.7 deaths per 1000 in the study group and 0.8 per 1000 in the controls.

Nash and his co-workers (1968) compared survival rates of lung cancers diagnosed in men attending mass x-ray units with survival rates of all lung cancer patients in the same region. The results were very similar to those of Brett and again no allowance was made for lead time. Comparison of mortality rates was impossible because the men did not come from a clearly defined population.

A further controlled trial is now under way in the United States (Fontana *et al.*, 1975) in which a high-risk group of men was screened by sputum cytology and chest x-ray and then randomly allocated to four-monthly repeat testing or to annual questionnaires. Subsequent incidence of lung cancer was higher in the rescreened group (4.4 per 1000 per year) than in the controls (2.9 per 1000 per year) in the initial three years of the project, and especially in men over 70 years of age. Multicentric tumours were diagnosed in 14 per cent of the four-monthly surveillance cases and 3 per cent of the controls.

As in Brett's study, resectability rates and survival rates (with no lead time allowance) have been greater in the four-monthly surveillance group than the controls, but so far no benefit has been shown in mortality rates (1.7 per 1000 man-years in each group). This study is continuing and longer-term results are awaited with interest.

Conclusions

In favour of lung cancer screening is the relatively easy identification of a high-risk group (which, if future studies are undertaken, should surely also include women since lung cancer is now the second commonest cause of cancer death in women). There are, however, a number of factors militating against it. These include the rapid growth of lung cancer; its multifocal distribution in an organ essential to life; poor levels of acceptance of screening and follow-up from the high-risk group; rather low levels of test sensitivity; difficulties in follow-up of positive cytology; and problems in management of multicentric disease found by screening. In the controlled trials which have so far been reported, there has been no reduction in mortality in the group offered screening compared with the controls, but one of these studies is still in progress and later follow-up may alter this gloomy picture. Unless that happens, there is no case for provision of lung cancer screening as a service, and resources for control of this disease should be directed towards primary rather than secondary prevention.

A special case may, however, exist for selective screening within particular industries, where occupational exposure is added to the risks of smoking. Relevant industries include those using asbestos, coke ovens, nickel, uranium, mustard gas, halo ethers and probably many other chemicals. However, no studies demonstrating benefit from screening occupational groups for lung cancer are known, and the possible disadvantages—particularly those associated with unpleasant or dangerous investigations or forms of treatment which make no difference to the eventual outcome—would, on present evidence, seem to out-weigh the advantages. There may be a case though for experimental studies of screening within certain occupations.

Malignant melanoma of the skin (ICD number 172)

Rapidly rising incidence and mortality from malignant melanoma among white-skinned people have been apparent for several years and there is evidence to suggest that this increasing frequency of melanoma is associated with exposure to sunlight (Knut, 1977; Swerdlow, 1979). Knut (1977) concludes that measures to control mortality from this cause by primary prevention (i.e. limiting exposure to sunlight) and by early diagnosis (i.e. self-screening) should be possible, although difficult to implement in practice. Similarly, the *Lancet* (1978) speaks of 'the continued lethality of the melanomas, against which earlier diagnosis seems to offer the only solid hope of progress'.

Screening by regular self-inspection, and by educating people to be aware of the early signs of malignant change, is advocated, particularly in sunny climates with a large White population, such as the southern United States, and Northern Australia. There has, however, been very little study of the effects of health education on this topic. Smith (1979) cites the experience in Queensland in which an intensive educational campaign, in schools, clinics, doctors' premises, libraries and radio programmes, has been in progress for about fifteen years. During this time, the crude annual incidence of malignant melanoma of the skin has doubled from 16 per 100 000 population to 34 per 100 000, but the five-year survival of cases notified to the Cancer Registry has improved from about 40 per cent before the campaign started to 88 per cent in women and 74 per cent in men. Mortality data are not given, and no allowances are made for lead time or length bias. Hedley (1979) noted that the distribution of histological categories in the Queens-land series of cancers shows them to have been *more* advanced biologically than other published series (Clark *et al.*, 1969; Wanebo *et al.*, 1975), and yet their prognosis was better. He suggests that the natural history of the Queensland tumours is different from that in America, and that within each histological grade they have a lower metastatic potential. This could be a reflection of length bias in the tumours detected by self-examination, although an equally plausible explan-ation could be variability in reporting histology. Until more definitive study is made of the effectiveness of education in reducing mortality in a defined popula-tion, the case for self-screening for malignant melanoma remains unproven.

Breast cancer (ICD number 174)

Natural history

Breast cancer is remarkable because of the very variable natural history it may follow after diagnosis. If the doubling time hypothesis is accepted, there would seem to be a wide range of doubling times for this one tumour, some progressing very rapidly while others are apparently extremely slow growing. This applies not only to the primary tumour but also to its metastases, which may appear fifteen or even twenty years after treatment of the primary. Hence, although a majority of women who are going to die of breast cancer do so within five years of diagnosis, follow-up is necessary for twenty years or more before one can refer to a patient as 'cured'. Brinkley and Haybittle (1975) have shown how, even after survival curves of patients have become parallel to those of the general female population of the same age range, breast cancer continues to be a frequent cause of death. The disease may be bilateral and second primaries cannot always be ruled out as the originators of late metastases.

The early pre-invasive stages in the natural history of breast cancer are necessarily more obscure. The different histological groups of lesions shown in Fig. 8.2 can be demonstrated in the breast and appear to represent a continuum. In-situ carcinomas may be either lobular or intraductal, although some workers (e.g. Price and Gibbs, 1978) consider they are part of the same disease process. They tend to be bilateral, and lobular carcinomas-in-situ tend to occur in pre-menopausal women (possibly a reflection of their lead time) and in women with a particular genetic susceptibility. McDivitt et al. (1967) have followed up 50 women who have had areas of in-situ carcinoma excised but no subsequent mastectomy, for up to twenty years; 35 per cent developed an invasive cancer in the same breast and 25 per cent in the contralateral breast. Cunningham (1980) expressed concern that screening is leading to mastectomy for such lesions, which he argues are a benign manifestation of predisposition to carcinoma, not carcinoma itself. He considers that unilateral mastectomy is not only over-treatment but also inappropriate, since if the objective is to remove all the affected epithelium, the operation should be bilateral. Chamberlain (1978) has also pointed out that up to a third of so-called cancers detected at screening fall into this pre-invasive group. Whether their detection and removal is a benefit because it seems to offer cure before any spread has occurred, or a hazard because it may result in unnecessary mastectomies in women who would never have developed invasive cancer is a question which can only be resolved by a randomized controlled trial of alternative treatments.

Screening tests

The principal tests available for early detection of breast cancer are physical examination, either self-examination—or by a health worker, and x-ray mammography. Earlier hopes that thermography, a non-invasive technique which records the heat pattern emitted by the breast, might substitute for mammography have not been realized, while newer physical techniques such as ultrasound are not yet sufficiently developed for application as screening tests (Dodd, 1977).

X-ray mammography has improved considerably in recent years, in its safety, its sensitivity and its specificity. Lundgren (1979) developed the single oblique view to show all breast tissue including the axillary tail in the film, while at the same time halving radiation dose. With this technique he has achieved 93 per cent sensitivity in a population of Swedish women over the age of 35 years, the remaining 7 per cent presenting as interval cases within one year of a negative screening result.

As mammography has improved, the need for physical examination has diminished, although it contributed 6 per cent of the cancers detected at screening in the United States Breast Cancer Detection Demonstration Projects (Beahrs *et al.*, 1979). The overall sensitivity of the combined tests in this large study was lower than that of Lundgren, with 17 per cent of cancers diagnosed in one year presenting as interval cases after a negative screening result (sensitivity 83 per cent). This sensitivity is closer to that reported by Chamberlain *et al.* (1979) in a much smaller series of cancers from a British screening clinic.

No estimates are yet available of the sensitivity of self-examination of the breasts. It might be less than that of annual physical examination by health workers, although the latter is already very unsatisfactory at about 50 per cent, or it might be greater because of its greater frequency and the fact that the woman is more familiar with the feel of her own breasts and hence may be more likely to detect a divergence from normal.

The reproducibility of screening tests for breast cancer has already been discussed (Tables 8.3 and 8.4).

Specificity has received less attention in the literature about screening for breast cancer. Estimates of specificity (defining a false positive as a biopsy of a woman without cancer) from a number of studies range from 99.7 per cent (Lundgren, 1979) to 93.8 per cent (Chamberlain *et al.*, 1979); in all series, mammography is more specific than clinical examination. Presumably, some of the benign lesions detected by screening would eventually have presented with symptoms, so not all can be regarded as an extra burden generated by the screening programme; but in Britain it is estimated that initial screening increases the rate of benign biopsies by a factor of ten.

Acceptability

It has already been seen (p. 235) that in a general population of middle-aged women in Britain or North America, about two-thirds will accept an initial invitation to be screened, but that it may be difficult to keep up compliance with repeated annual rescreening above a level of about 50 per cent. Some of the factors influencing compliance with self-examination have been outlined on p. 235.

Hazards and costs

Similarly, the hazards and costs of screening for breast cancer have already been discussed in the general sections (pp. 245 and 249) on these aspects of screening for cancer.

Effectiveness

The trial by Shapiro (1977) provides evidence of the benefit of screening. Although started as long ago as 1963, it is still unique in the whole field of cancer screening as the only published randomized controlled trial of screening for cancer in a general unselected population. Sixty-two thousand women between the ages of 40 and 64 were randomly allocated either to a study group which was offered four successive annual screens by clinical examination and mammography, or to a control group offered no extra services for the diagnosis of breast cancer. The most important finding, confirming the benefit of screening, is shown in Table

9.2, which gives the number of deaths from breast cancer in study group and control group (which were of equal sizes) ten years after the start of the trial. There was a statistically significant reduction in deaths of about one-third in the study group as a whole. This was most marked in women aged 50–59, also occurred in older women (but did not reach a level of statistical significance), but was absent in the youngest age group. The absence of any effect in younger women applied whether the data were analysed by age at death, age at entry to the trial, or age at diagnosis.

Table 9.2 Mortality from breast cancer after ten years in study group offered screening and control group (from Shapiro, 1978)

Age at death (years)	Number of deaths from breast cancer	
	Study group	Control group
40–49	16	18
50–59	44*	71
60 and older	37	48
Total	97*	137

* p<0.05 for 50–59 year age group and for total.

Confirmation of the beneficial effect of screening comes from a comparison of case fatality rates of breast cancers diagnosed in this trial which, even after correcting for lead time, shows a significant reduction in cases detected by screening.

Because the mammography techniques used in this study are now outdated, and because of the disappointing result in the youngest age group, there is general agreement that further trials are needed to assess the impact of mammography apart from clinical examination, and to evaluate screening again for younger women; a number of such investigations have begun in several countries.

Conclusions

Breast cancer is unique in being the only cancer site for which there is experimental evidence that screening saves lives. Moreover, its already high incidence is still increasing and there is no immediate prospect of any method of primary prevention. Newer forms of therapy have probably contributed to reduced morbidity, but have so far made little or no impact on mortality, although the role of adjuvant chemotherapy is still under review. At present, therefore, screening seems to offer the best hope of controlling mortality from this most important disease—the commonest cancer in women and the commonest single cause of death of women between the ages of 30 and 59 years.

There are, however, a number of unresolved issues both on the benefits and the risks of screening. On the benefits side, it is not yet known if modern screening techniques can benefit women under the age of 50; the independent contributions of physical examination and mammography to lowered mortality are uncertain; nothing is known about the effectiveness of self-examination in reducing mortality; and the optimum frequency of rescreening is unknown. On the risks side, radiation hazard from mammography has now been reduced to such low levels that most workers consider that it is acceptable *if* mammography is contributing to reduced mortality and *provided that* dosage is closely monitored. But other risks, including physical and psychological damage resulting from false positives, and unnecessary mastectomies for non-malignant lesions, need further assessment. The resource costs are known to be large but an accurate cost–benefit assessment has not yet been done. A number of trials to answer these points are in progress and it is hoped that their results will give sufficient guidance to formulate a reasonable policy for provision of a service for early detection of breast cancer.

Cancer of the uterine cervix (ICD number 180)

Natural history

As outlined in Chapter 8, the natural history of the pre-invasive stages of cervical cancer has been extensively studied and would appear to fit the model shown in Fig. 8.2. However, the proportion of cases following each pathway is not known, nor is the average duration of time taken to progress from one stage to the next. On screening, many more women are found to have pre-invasive disease than would be expected to develop cancer later in life, suggesting that most pre-invasive lesions do not progress and implying that treatment of many early lesions detected at screening may be unnecessary. However, cross-sectional comparisons of age-specific incidence of pre-invasive and invasive cancer are unreliable because of the marked cohort effects in incidence of this disease, with today's young women showing a markedly higher incidence at each age than most previous cohorts (Beral, 1976). Moreover, the age-specific incidence of pre-invasive lesions detected at screening may be inflated by inclusion of cases which gave false negative results to earlier screens if the sensitivity of the test was low. A cohort study in British Columbia is attempting to overcome these difficulties, and to estimate the time sequence over which progression from carcinoma-in-situ to invasive cancer may occur (Walton Report, 1976). The modal age of onset of in-situ carcinoma in British Columbia in the mid-1970s was 25–29 years and the authors of the Walton Report estimate that the average period for progression to invasive carcinoma was thirty years, with the majority of patients progressing if left untreated.

The implication of this is that some of the in-situ cancers detected and removed from young women today will result in reduced incidence of invasive cancer in middle-aged women thirty years hence. However, invasive cancers occur from the age of 20 onwards and the cohort effect already referred to is demonstrated by increasing incidence rates of invasive cancer up to the age of 34 years. Presumably, the progression to invasion in these women follows a much more rapid course than that postulated above and has led to demands for concentrating screening on young women (e.g. Yule, 1978; Herbert, 1980). Nevertheless, out of all cervical cancer deaths, the proportion of those of young women is very small; in 1977 fewer than 0.5 per cent were of women under 25 and less than 15 per cent were of women aged 25–34 (British Medical Journal, 1980, b).

Both the age at which screening should start and the frequency with which it should be repeated continue to cause controversy, partly because such decisions must inevitably be taken in the light of the resources available, which vary between countries. In the United States, for example, a recent 'consensus development conference' (National Institutes of Health, 1980) recommended that screening should start when a woman first becomes sexually active, should be repeated after one year, and thereafter should be repeated at one- to three-yearly intervals until the age of 60. No numerical estimate of either effectiveness or resource costs was given in this statement. Similarly, the Walton Report in Canada (1976) recommended annual screening from age 18 years onwards.

By contrast, British recommendations, possibly with greater awareness of resource costs, have been more restricted. For example, Knox (1976) estimated that five-yearly screening from the age of 35 upwards could theoretically prevent three-quarters of the deaths from cervical cancer. Spriggs and Husain (1977) suggested that screening should start at 25 years of age for women attending clinics for contraception, pregnancy or venereal disease, and at 30 for other sexually active women. They recommended three- to five-yearly screening thereafter up to the age of 70, and estimated that in theory this could reduce deaths by over a half. Hakama (1978) reported that a five-yearly screening policy in Finland missed nearly 40 per cent of invasive cancers which presented in the intervals between successive screens; however, efforts to focus screening resources on a particularly high-risk group of women was judged to be impracticable because 70 per cent of the population would need to be included in the risk group in order to achieve the target of 90 per cent cancers detected by screening (Hakama *et al.*, 1979). Perhaps it needs to be emphasized once more that all the estimates of lives saved by alternative policies are necessarily based on unproven assumptions about the proportion of cancers which progress from one stage of epithelial change to another, and the time they take to do so. Firm evidence of the natural history is still lacking and likely to remain so.

Screening test

The screening test for cervical cancer is cytological examination of cells exfoliated from the squamo-columnar junction at the external os of the cervix. The cells are normally obtained at vaginal examination by scraping round the internal circumference of the os with a spatula and smearing the resulting specimen on a slide. An alternative method is a cytopipette which can be used by the woman herself to obtain cells, suspended in fluid in the pipette, from the posterior fornix. Various estimates of the sensitivity of the smear test range from 50 per cent (Coppleson and Brown, 1974)—based on interval cancers—to 82 per cent (Yule, 1973)— based on repeat testing after a three-month interval. The false negatives are thought to be more or less equally divided between laboratory error, faulty technique in taking the smear, and variation in the rate of exfoliation within the subject. It is generally accepted that the test is less sensitive for invasive lesions than for pre-invasive lesions. The cytopipette has a sensitivity of approximately 80 per cent that of the smear test (Husain, 1970).

As far as specificity is concerned, the cervical smear is one of the best cancer screening tests available, giving remarkably few false positive results. Yule (1973) reported that in a series of 96 678 women free from neoplasia of the cervix, only 63 had false positive screening results, from which it can be calculated that specificity was 99.9 per cent. However, the gynaecological examination which accompanies the taking of a cervical smear is far from specific, and may lead to identification of very large numbers of pelvic abnormalities, the great majority of which are probably of little importance. For example, Edwards (1974), in screening 2656 women, detected 4 carcinomas-in-situ (0.15 per cent) and 3 invasive cancers (0.11

per cent), but also uncovered 400 other conditions which she considered required treatment even though the patient had not sought care for them. This gives pelvic examination, as a test for cervical cancer, a specificity of only 85 per cent, implying that 15 per cent of women without cancer are subjected to further diagnostic and therapeutic measures. The predictive value of a positive pelvic examination as a screening test for cervical cancer is less than 2 per cent.

Edwards claims that the diagnosis of other conditions is of great value and argues from this that cervical cancer screening should be performed by gynaecologists rather than by less specialized medical or paramedical staff. She quotes some grateful patients in support of the notion that uncovering all this 'chronic ill health' is beneficial, but one wonders whether the 21 patients who defaulted from follow-up, out of 68 found to have pelvic tumours, felt that they had benefited, and the same must surely apply to the 86 with symptomless cervical polyps and the 2 with inoperable malignant pelvic tumours. As in the very similar situation found in stomach cancer screening, a rigorous assessment of the value of detecting unconnected diseases is required before it can be concluded that their diagnosis is beneficial.

Acceptability

From the studies quoted in Chapter 8, it is apparent that lack of acceptability is a major problem in cervical cancer screening. Those women at greatest risk are also those least likely to accept screening. Studies of response have mostly been based on invitations to be screened, but screening is usually merely provided as a service which women may seek out themselves if they are sufficiently aware, or which is carried out automatically (often without their knowledge) when they are having a vaginal examination for other reasons such as family planning. Such a system accentuates the inverse take-up between high- and low-risk women, and probably leads to unnecessarily frequent rescreening of those least at risk.

Adverse effects

The test itself, although uncomfortable and embarrassing for some women, is not physically harmful; the principle adverse effect of cervical cancer screening is the debatable one of 'over-treatment' of women with borderline results. In this category are included women with dysplasia, which some gynaecologists consider warrants treatment by cone-biopsy or even hysterectomy, and also young women with carcinoma-in-situ. In Finland, it is estimated that two-thirds of 'cases' detected at screening are treated unnecessarily (Hakama, 1978). Although cone-biopsy (which serves for both definitive diagnosis and treatment) is a relatively minor procedure, it may have adverse effects on subsequent pregnancies which the woman may have. A study of women below the age of 35 and with fewer than three children, who had had a cone-biopsy for treatment of carcinoma-in-situ detected at screening, and who had no other gynaecological abnormality, found that their subsequent fertility was lower than national fertility rates for women of the same age and parity. The difference in fertility, however, occurred only among women who already had two children. But in those women who did become pregnant, there was a higher incidence of spontaneous abortion, a higher rate of caesarean section and a higher rate of prematurity than national rates for women of the same age and parity. Uncertainty about the rate of progression of pre-invasive lesions in young women coupled with knowledge of increasing rates of invasive cancer in this age group lead gynaecologists to extirpative treatment as soon as possible. If the average lead time is as long as thirty years, the risk of invasion would be very small until the woman was well past her childbearing years, and more conservative treatment, e.g. by colposcopy and cryocautery or laser excision,would suffice in the early stages.

Effectiveness

The Papanicolaou test for identifying neoplastic cells obtained from the cervix was the first screening test developed for any form of cancer. Because it was capable of detecting pre-invasive disease, it seemed to offer a hope of eliminating invasive carcinoma of the cervix completely. Consequently, it was introduced on a wave of enthusiasm among gynaecologists, cytologists and the public, none of whom anticipated the difficulties and uncertainties which would subsequently arise. Many of these difficulties might have been avoided by a controlled trial to evaluate the effect of a cervical screening programme but, before this was realized, the service had been widely introduced and it was regarded as unethical to withhold it deliberately from a control or comparison group. Consequently, its evaluation has had to rely on correlation studies comparing incidence and mortality rates from cervical cancer in similar populations with differing screening intensities. Most of these studies have taken one particular area and examined the trends in incidence and mortality with the trend in proportion of women screened, e.g. in British Columbia (Boyes *et al.*, 1973), other Canadian provinces (Walton Report, 1976) and Aberdeen (Macgregor, 1976). The comparisons have been made more difficult by the fact that both incidence and mortality were in any case falling before the introduction of screening, and by confounding variables such as an increasing rate of hysterectomy for other reasons (Kinlen and Doll, 1973)—the rates of cervical cancer would be more appropriately expressed per uterus than per woman. Moreover, the populations concerned have been relatively small and hence the numbers of cancers variable from year to year. Also, accurate records of migrations in and out of the population, and of numbers of women who have had one, two or more screens, have not been kept. Iceland, however, is one place where most of these difficulties do not apply. This population, although small, is very stable with few migrations, few hysterectomies, a system of linking records of successive screens, a rising mortality rate from cervical cancer until 1970, and a screening service which started in 1964 and which had reached nearly 90 per cent of women aged 25–59 within ten years. Between 1970 and 1974, there was a more than twofold reduction in mortality from cancer of the cervix (Johannesson *et al.*, 1978). Although it cannot be concluded that this was entirely due to the screening service, this does seem the most plausible explanation of the sudden dramatic reversal of the previous mortality trend and provides the most definitive evidence yet available that screening for cervical cancer can be effective in reducing mortality. Taken together with the Icelandic findings, the evidence from other intensely screened areas such as Aberdeen and parts of Canada supports the view that cervical cancer screening is of benefit.

Conclusions

Screening for cervical cancer has been established as a service for longer than any other cancer screening programme and various lessons can be learned from the experience. These lessons include the need to delineate the period in the natural history of the disease at which screening should be aimed to provide control of the disease with the least over-treatment of borderline cases; the importance of achieving a good acceptance rate by subjects most at risk; the need for the screening test to have a high sensitivity; and the need to define an appropriate rescreening interval. Each of these can only be achieved by appropriate research investigations, which ideally should have been conducted before the screening service was introduced.

As practised in most of Great Britain today, and possibly in many other countries as well, screening for cervical cancer is extremely inefficient because no coherent policy is followed and the service is virtually unmonitored beyond a simple count of tests performed and positives found. It is used as a routine investigation by doctors in certain clinical situations, usually without thought or enquiry as to whether or not the patient is due for a screening test; and it is available for any women who are sufficiently motivated to seek it out for themselves whenever they wish. In most places, no effort is put into ensuring that high-risk women or women in the relevant age groups are screened, nor is any attempt made to identify false negatives to screening. It is probable that low-risk women are being repeatedly screened at too frequent intervals, while the service is not yet reaching those who really need it. Perhaps the most important lesson to be learnt from a public health point of view is that merely making the service generally available, without pursuing any predetermined policy, stands little chance of controlling mortality and is very wasteful of resources.

Choriocarcinoma (ICD number 181)

This tumour, arising from trophoblastic tissue in the placenta and invading the maternal host, is extremely rare but nevertheless possesses certain attributes which make it an ideal candidate for a screening programme. Such a programme has been in service in the UK for the past decade (Bagshawe *et al.*, 1973).

Definition of a high-risk group

Although the overall incidence is very low, a small group of women at exceptionally high risk can be identified. These are women who have had a hydatidiform mole pregnancy, which in Western societies probably occurs in around 1 in 12 000 pregnancies (Stevenson *et al.*, 1959; Yen and MacMahon, 1968). About 9 per cent of these pregnancies subsequently develop a choriocarcinoma, and this small high-risk group accounts for 45 per cent of the total incidence of invasive trophoblastic tumours. Not only is this high-risk group easily identifiable, but it has the additional advantage that, by definition, the women concerned are receiving obstetric care at the time. The need for screening can, therefore, be explained to them as part of the necessary follow-up of their condition and hence acceptance of screening is not a problem. An additional advantage is that the risk diminishes with time, and screening can be discontinued after two years. Thus, in contrast to screening programmes for other cancers, this one is aimed at a clearly defined, young, compliant population for a limited period of time.

Validity of the screening test

The test employed is serial measurement of human chorionic gonadotrophin (HCG), which is a biological marker of trophoblastic activity. The fact that serial measurements are needed, rather than a single measurement, is of course a disadvantage to the patient, but it is a rising titre that gives warning of tumour activity. Information on its sensitivity and specificity in screening is hard to find, but Bagshawe (1977) reported *no* false negatives and *no* false positives when using it to monitor recurrence in treated patients. It appears to have no physical disadvantages and its financial cost is not prohibitive, at £60 per woman screened over a two-year period (Bagshawe, 1978).

Effectiveness of treatment

One of the other remarkable features of choriocarcinoma is its susceptibility to chemotherapy. Although not all tumours respond, and some develop resistance, the majority now appear to be curable (Bagshawe, 1978). The lesser the total burden of tumour (as judged by HCG levels), the greater the chance of remission and presumed cure. This suggests that cases detected by screening have an excellent prognosis, although no data showing the results of treatment of screening-detected cases appear to have been published.

It is not possible from published data to say exactly how much of the improved prognosis for choriocarcinoma in the past decade has been due to the screening programme and how much has been due to the development of effective chemotherapy for symptomatic cases, since both the test and the therapy were developed at about the same time and controlled trials were not undertaken. It seems reasonable to assume, however, that the screening programme is contributing to the reduction in mortality from this previously lethal condition.

Cancer of the testis (ICD number 186)

The increasing incidence of testicular cancer in many Western countries (see Chapter 2), and the anatomical position of the testes have led to recent suggestions that screening for testicular cancer by self-examination might contribute to control of mortality from this cause (British Medical Journal, 1980, a; Lancet, 1980). Health education programmes to encourage self-examination by young men have been launched in the United States but, beyond anecdotal evidence of cases detected by this method (Garnick *et al.*, 1980), these programmes are still completely unevaluated. There is evidence that carcinoma-in-situ is common in undescended testes (Krabbe *et al.*, 1979), and boys with this condition constitute a particularly high-risk group. Whether similar multiple foci of pre-malignant histological changes will also be found in testicular swellings found by screening still remains to be seen; management of these lesions in young men could be problematical. The prospects for cure by surgery or radiotherapy are good in 'early' symptomatic cases of seminoma, but it is not known if screening-detected cases will behave in the same way. The situation is likely to be complicated by the diversity of pathological types of malignant tumours which may occur in the testis.

Cancer of the bladder (ICD number 188)

Recognition that certain carcinogenic chemicals used in rubber and in dye industries (Case *et al.*, 1954; Davies, 1965; see Chapter 6) were associated with an excess incidence of bladder cancer led to the introduction of a screening programme for workers who had been exposed to the chemicals before their withdrawal. Screening consists of cytological examination of a specimen of urine at a recommended frequency of six-monthly repeats. A system for tracing and offering the test to people who have retired from the relevant industry has been set up in Britain, but response is low (Wrighton, personal communication). Little is known of the sensitivity of cytology in detecting bladder cancer, but Turner *et al.* (1977) reported that only 2 out of 12 early cases of bladder cancer presenting with haematuria had positive cytology. Cases presenting in this way may only be a subset of all bladder cancer cases, but the implication is that the sensitivity of cytology is imperfect. Nothing is known of its specificity, and it is likely that this would prove difficult to assess, in view of the well-recognized borderline condition of bladder papillomas.

There is remarkably little evidence of the effectiveness of this screening programme. Fox and White (1976) studied prognosis in 27 men with bladder cancer registered as being workers in the rubber industry. They matched these cases (by age, area of residence and histological type of tumour) with 88 patients with bladder cancer, whose occupation was in other industries. The data were taken from routine registration statistics, and information on whether or not the cancers in rubber workers were diagnosed by the screening programme was not available. There was no difference in survival between the rubber workers and the controls, 33 per cent of the former and 38 per cent of the latter having survived five years. Cartwright *et al.* (1981) studied 88 men with bladder cancer from the workforce of a dye-manufacturing company and matched them by age and year of diagnosis with 88 bladder cancer patients from other industries, who were treated in the same hospital. The dye factory cases were subdivided into those diagnosed by screening and those presenting symptomatically. As expected, there was a higher proportion of early cases in those diagnosed by screening than in either the factory workers who presented symptomatically or the control hospital patients. Follow-up for up to twenty-five years showed that the cases detected by screening survived longer than the factory cases presenting with symptoms, but when the control patients were also taken into account, the difference in survival between screened and non-screened did not reach a level of statistical significance. Moreover, no allowance was made for lead time or length bias in screening-detected cases. At present, therefore, there does not seem to be any evidence that this industrial screening programme is effective.

General conclusions

In the absence of effective methods of primary prevention or effective treatments of symptomatically diagnosed tumours, screening offers the best hope of controlling mortality from some cancers. However, it cannot be assumed that early detection is an unequivocally good thing from which no harm can result. Rather, as Cole and Morrison (1980) point out, it is a double-edged sword and has inherent adverse effects as well as good.

The principal benefit it confers is on those individuals with early cancer who are detected by the test, with a lead time which is sufficiently long to alter the prognosis of their cancer but not so long as to subject them to unnecessary treatment. It may also be that screening confers the benefit of reassurance to some people without cancer who have negative results to the test, although this parti-cular form of benefit is hard to quantify.

Its adverse effects include the extra morbidity in some cases, induced by treatment which does not influence prognosis (e.g. resection of some lung cancers detected by screening but not cured by early treatment), over-treatment of borderline cases (e.g. mastectomy for some pre-neoplastic lesions of the breast), over-investigation with consequent worry, inconvenience and morbidity for people with false positive results, and inappropriate reassurance for people with false negative results which may lead them to delay in reporting subsequent symptoms. Moreover, each person screened suffers the inconvenience, discom-fort and very occasional risks associated with the screening test itself. Screening also puts a heavy burden on health service resources, both in the application of the test itself and in follow-up of positive results (most of which are usually false positives).

Because of all these factors, screening programmes should ideally be subjected to intensive rigorous research before being introduced as a public health service. The general aim of such research is to define a screening policy which will maximize the ratio of the benefit to adverse effect. Study of the period in the cancer's natural history at which early treatment will improve prognosis, balanc-ing the sensitivity against the specificity of the test, identifying those people at greatest risk and making the test acceptable to them, and determining the opti-mum rescreening interval are all important issues to be resolved.

The only convincing outcome by which the success of screening can be judged is a reduction in mortality from the cancer in question, and in order to prove that such a reduction can be attributed to screening, some form of controlled trial is required.

In practice, it is unlikely that all relevant information could ever be obtained without practising screening in a real-life service situation, so that research and development go together. This is now the case with screening for breast cancer (for which evidence of benefit is most clear-cut), and lung cancer (for which such evidence is markedly lacking). Colorectal cancer screening is now also being developed in the same manner. One hopes that these examples indicate a more realistic attitude on the part of both 'screeners' and public health authorities than that shown two decades ago when screening programmes for cervical cancer and stomach cancer were widely introduced on the assumption that each case detected was a life saved and that mortality from these causes could be drastically reduced in a very short time, and with no adverse effects. The inefficiency of most screening policies for cervical cancer (and the continuing debate about matters such as which groups to screen and how often) testify to the absence of evaluation at a time when it would have been ethically possible to conduct trials.

It is unrealistic to suppose that all deaths from cancer of a particular site could be prevented by screening, but nevertheless a worthwhile reduction (perhaps of the order of one-third to one-half) may be achieved by a programme which is accepted by a majority of those at risk and causes minimal hardship and cost to the public at large.

References

Archer, P. G., Koprowska, I., McDonald, J. R., Naylor, B., Papanicolaou, G. N. and Umiker, W. O. (1966). *Cancer Research* **26**, 2122.

Auerbach, O., Stout, A. P., Hammond, E. C. and Garfinkel, L. (1961). *New England Journal of Medicine* **265**, 253.

Bagshawe, K. D. (1977). *Proceedings of the Royal Society of Medicine* **70**, 303.

Bagshawe, K. D. (1978). *Annals of the Royal College of Surgeons* **60**, 36.

Bagshawe, K. D., Wilson, H., Dublon, P., Smith, A., Baldwin, M. and Kardana, A. (1973). *Journal of Obstetrics and Gynaecology of the British Commonwealth* **80**, 461.

Beahrs, O. H., Shapiro, S. and Smart, C. (1979). *Journal of the National Cancer Institute* **62**, 640.

Beral, V. (1976). *Lancet* **i**, 1037.

Boyes, D. A., Knowelden, J. and Phillips, A. J. (1973). *British Journal of Cancer* **28**, 105.

Brett, G. Z. (1969). *British Medical Journal* **4**, 260.

Brinkley, D. and Haybittle, J. L. (1975). *Lancet* **ii**, 95.

British Medical Journal (1976). **2**, 198.

British Medical Journal (1980, a). **280**, 961.

British Medical Journal (1980, b). **281**, 629.

Cartwright, R. A., Gadian, T., Garland, J. B. and Bernard, S. M. (1981). *British Journal of Epidemiology and Community Health* **35**, 35.

Case, R. A. M., Hosker, M. E., McDonald, D. B. and Pearson, J. T. (1954). *British Journal of Industrial Medicine* **4**, 75.

Chamberlain, J. (1978). In *Screening in Cancer*, pp. 158–82. Ed. by A. B. Miller. UICC Technical Report No. 40, Geneva.

Chamberlain, J., Clifford, R. E., Nathan, B. E., Price, J. L. and Burn, I. (1979). *Clinical Oncology* **5**, 135.

Clark, W. H., From, L., Bernardino, E. A. and Mihm, M. C. (1969). *Cancer Research* **29**, 705.

Cole, J. W. (1978). In *The Pathogenesis of Colorectal Cancer*, pp. 119–25. Ed. by B. C. Morson. Saunders, London.

Cole, P. and Morrison, A. S. (1980). *Journal of the National Cancer Institute* **64**, 1263.

Collins, W. T. and Gall, E. A. (1952). *Cancer* **5**, 62.

Coppleson, L. W. and Brown, B. (1974). *American Journal of Obstetrics and Gynecology* **119**, 953.

Correa, P. (1978). In *The Pathogenesis of Colorectal Cancer*, pp. 126–52. Ed. by B. C. Morson. Saunders, London.

Cunningham, L. (1980). *Lancet* **i**, 306.

Dales, L. G., Friedman, G. D., Ramcharan, S. and Collen, M. F. (1973). *Preventive Medicine* **2**, 221.

Davies, J. M. (1965). *Lancet* **ii**, 143.

Day, D. W. and Morson, B. C. (1978). In *The Pathogenesis of Colorectal Cancer*, pp. 58–71. Ed. by B. C. Morson. Saunders, London.

Dodd, G. D. (1977). *Cancer* **39**, 2796.

Edwards, D. (1974). *British Medical Journal* **4**, 218.

Fielding, J. W. L., Ellis, D. J., Jones, B. G., Paterson, J., Powell, D. J., Waterhouse, J. A. H. and Brookes, V. S. (1980). *British Medical Journal* **281**, 965.

Fontana, R. S., Sanderson, D. R., Woolner, L. B., Miller, W. E., Bernatz, P. E., Payne, W. S. and Taylor, W. F. (1975). *Chest* **67**, 511.

Fontana, R. S. and Taylor, W. F. (1978). In *Screening in Cancer*, pp. 233–53. Ed. by A. B. Miller. UICC Technical Report No. 40, Geneva.

Fox, A. J. and White, G. C. (1976). *Lancet* **i**, 1009.

Garnick, M. B., Mayer, R. J. and Richie, J. P. (1980). *New England Journal of Medicine* **302**, 297.

Gilbertson, V. A. and Nelms, J. M. (1978). *Cancer* **41**, 1137.

Gnauck, R. (1977). *Leber Magen Darm* **7**, 32.

Hakama, M. (1978). In *Screening in Cancer*, pp. 93–107. Ed. by A. B. Miller. UICC Technical Report No. 40, Geneva.

Hakama, M., Pukkala, E. and Saastamoinen, P. (1979). *Journal of Epidemiology and Community Health* **33**, 257.

Hanai, A. and Fujimoto, I. (1977). In *Epidemiology of Gastric Cancer*, pp. 21–33. Ed. by T. Hirayama. WHO–CC Monograph 1, Tokyo.

Hardcastle, J. D., Balfour, T. and Amar, S. S. (1980). *Lancet* **i**, 791.

Hebert, H. (1980). *The Guardian*, 29th September.

Hedley, D. W. (1979). *British Medical Journal* **1**, 550.

Hirayama, T. (1978). In *Screening in Cancer*, pp. 264–78. Ed. by A. B. Miller. UICC Technical Report No. 40, Geneva.

Husain, O. A. N. (1970). *American Journal of Obstetrics and Gynecology* **106**, 138.

Ichikawa, H. (1978). In *Screening in Cancer*, pp. 279–99. Ed. by A. B. Miller. UICC Technical Report No. 40, Geneva.

Johannesson, G., Geirsson, G. and Day, N. (1978). *International Journal of Cancer* **21**, 418.

Kinlen, L. and Doll, R. (1973). *British Journal of Preventive and Social Medicine* **27**, 146.

Knox, E. G. (1976). *British Journal of Cancer* **34**, 444.

Knut, M. (1977). *International Journal of Cancer* **20**, 477.

Krabbe, S., Stakkebaek, N. E., Berthelson, J. G., Eyben, F. V., Volsted, P., Mauritzen, K., Eldrup, J. and Nielsen, A. H. (1979). *Lancet* **i**, 999.

Lancet (1978). **ii**, 822.

Lancet (1980). **ii**, 1175.

Lilienfeld, A., Archer, P. G., Burnett, C. H., Chamberlain, E. W., Chazin, B. J., Davies, D., Davis, R. L., Haber, P. A., Hodges, F. J., Koprowska, I., Kordan, B., Lane, J. T., Lawton, A. H., Lee, L., MacCallum, D. B., McDonald, J. R., Milder, J. W., Naylor, B., Papanicolaou, G. N., Slutzker, B., Smith, R. T., Swepston, E. R. and Umiker, W. O. (1966). *Cancer Research* **26**, 2083.

Lilienfeld, A. M. and Kordan, B. (1966). *Cancer Research* **26**, 2145.

Lundgren, B. (1979). *Journal of National Cancer Institute* **62**, 799.

Macgregor, J. E. (1976). *Tumori* **62**, 287.

McDivitt, R. W., Hutter, R. V. P., Foote, F. W. and Stewart, F. W. (1967). *Journal of the American Medical Association* **201**, 96.

Morson, B. C. (1979). *Journal of the Royal Society of Medicine* **72**, 83.

Nash, F. A., Morgan, J. M. and Tomkins, J. G. (1968). *British Medical Journal* **2**, 715.

National Institutes of Health (1980). *British Medical Journal* **281**, 1264.

Office of Population Censuses and Surveys (1980). *Cancer Statistics—Survival*. Series MBI No. 3. HMSO, London.

Oshima, A., Sakagami, F., Hanai, A. and Fujimoto, I. (1977). In *Epidemiology of Gastric Cancer*, pp. 35–44. Ed. by T. Hirayama. WHO–CC Monograph 1, Tokyo.

Ostrow, J. D., Mulvaney, C. A., Hansell, J. R. and Rhodes, R. S. (1973). *American Journal of Digestive Diseases* **18**, 930

Price, J. L. and Gibbs, N. M. (1978). *Clinical Radiology* **29**, 447.

Schottenfeld, D., Winawer, S. J. and Miller, D. G. (1978). In *Screening in Cancer*, pp. 308–27. Ed. by A. B. Miller, UICC Technical Report No. 40, Geneva.

Shapiro, S. (1977). *Cancer* **39**, 2772.

Shapiro, S. (1978). In *Screening in Cancer*, pp. 133–57. Ed. by A. B. Miller. UICC Technical Report No. 40, Geneva.

Sherlock, P., Lipkin, M. and Winawer, S. J. (1975). *Advances in Internal Medicine* **20**, 121.

Sherlock, P. and Winawer, S. J. (1977). *Cancer* **40**, 2609.

Smith, A. J. (1979). *British Medical Journal* **1**, 253.

Sogo, J., Kobayashi, K., Saito, J., Fukimaki, M. and Muto, T. (1979). *World Journal of Surgery* **3**, 701.

Spratt, J. S. (1963). *Archives of Surgery* **86**, 283.

Spriggs, A. I. and Husain, O. A. N. (1977). *British Medical Journal* **2**, 1516.

Stevenson, A. C., Dudgeon, M. Y. and McClure, H. I. (1959). *Annals of Human Genetics* **23**, 395.

Swerdlow, A. J. (1979). *British Medical Journal* **2**, 1324.

Turner, A. G., Hendry, W. F., Williams, G. B. and Wallace, D. M. (1977). *British Medical Journal* **2**, 29.

Walton Report (1976). *Canadian Medical Association Journal* **114**, 2.

Wanebo, H. J., Woodruff, J. and Fortner, J. G. (1975). *Cancer* **35**, 666.

Weiss, W. (1971). *American Review of Respiratory Disease* **103**, 198.

Weiss, W. (1978). In *Screening in Cancer*, pp. 216–32. Ed. by A. B. Miller. UICC Technical Report No. 40, Geneva.

Yen, S. and MacMahon, B. (1968). *American Journal of Obstetrics and Gynecology* **101**, 126.

Yule, R. (1973). In *Cancer of the Uterine Cervix*, pp. 11–25. Ed. by E. C. Easson. Saunders, London.

Yule, R. (1978). *Lancet* **i**, 1031.

10

Delay in the diagnosis and treatment of cancer

Michael Calnan

For most people, it appears to be commonsense that the earlier cancer patients are diagnosed and treated the greater the chances of survival. However, professional and scientific opinions have not always supported this assumption, although much attention has been paid to the issue of delay. From an epidemiological point of view, information on the distribution of delay is important as it can be used to take into account the various components that might be linked to alteration in survival from malignant disease. For example, such delay data would be used to solve the debate about whether the relative improvement in the survival of patients treated in the 1970s compared with the 1960s in this country is due to patients attending with earlier stage disease or to improvement in results of therapy irrespective of stage distribution. (See Murcott (1981) for a sociological account of patient delay.)

Definitions

Delay in the diagnosis and treatment of cancer consists of two different components. Firstly, the delay between patients perceiving or experiencing a change in their body functioning and the first presentation of it to a doctor; secondly, the delay between the first presentation to a physician and the beginning of therapeutic action. Health care systems in some countries make it possible for the patient to be in touch with a hospital specialist on the occasion of the first presentation. In other countries, such as in the UK, the first presentation of the illness is usually to a general practitioner, which then can lead to referral to the appropriate hospital specialist. In this situation, there is an added intra-professional delay. So the delay within the health service in the UK could involve several components. First, there is the interval between a patient presenting a symptom to his general practitioner and referral to a specialist in an out-patient department. There is also the interval between first out-patient appointment and treatment. This period may be divided up into interval between first out-patient appointment and diagnostic tests, and diagnostic tests and treatment.

Antonovsky and Hartman (1974) suggest that this patient–physician dichotomy in definitions of delay is unsatisfactory. They state there is a need to include the stage between the point at which professional medical practitioners think a lay person should identify a symptom and the point at which the layman actually does. They devise an eight-stage model:

(i) a state of no pathology;

(ii) the existence of a pathology which is detectable by professional knowledge and skills available at any given time;

(iii) the existence of a pathology which is detectable by a layman who is as informed as can reasonably be expected at any time;

(iv) the actual definition of a condition by a given person as pathological;

(v) the first visit to a physician for purposes of enquiry about that condition;

(vi) the first visit to a cancer specialist;

(vii) the establishment of diagnosis and referral for appropriate treatment;

(viii) the initiation of therapy.

This appears to be a more comprehensive approach as it integrates both patient and medical delay into one model. A more sociological approach to delay was used by Kutner and Gordon (1961). They argued that patient delay can only be understood if it is defined in terms of the deviation from the normative pattern of behaviour in a given cultural group or population for a given symptom. Thus patient delay may vary according to different symptoms and for different populations. This approach is useful in that it highlights that the lay and scientific approaches may be different. Also, it highlights that the lengths of periods of delay or definitions of delay can vary between cultures and within cultures.

Extent of delay

A three-month dividing line is usually used to distinguish between those who are defined as patient delayers and non-delayers. This definition seems to be an arbitrary one but one which has been frequently adopted (for example, see Aitken-Swan and Paterson, 1959). Medical delay is usually defined as when more than one month elapses between the patient's consultation with the physician and the establishment of diagnosis or referral for appropriate treatment (Antonovsky and Hartman, 1974).

Antonovsky and Hartman (1974), in an extensive review of studies concerned with patient delay, suggested that at least three-quarters of patients delay visiting a doctor for at least one month after they have become aware of a symptom and that somewhere between 35 per cent and 50 per cent of the patients delay for over three months. For medical delay, their review led them to conclude that at least one month elapses in some 25 per cent of the cases between the first visit to a doctor and the initiation of appropriate treatment. In comparing the extent of patient delay with that of medical delay, Antonovsky and Hartman (1974) state:

> 'While the major source of delay in most cases seems to be with the patient, pointing to a great need for action in this regard, physician delay seems to pose a problem in itself.'

How far the extent of delay has changed over recent years is difficult to judge, although some writers claim that delay for some cancer sites has not been reduced over the last fifty years (Hackett et al., 1973).

Antonovsky and Hartman (1974) also raise a general methodological issue about the retrospective nature of much of this research. Accounts of delay are taken from patients who attend a cancer treatment centre. It is well known that people's recollections are coloured by present experience and thus it is feared that patients' accounts of the extent of delay will be coloured by this factor as well as memory loss. Certainly, interviews with patients that take place within a hospital setting may be coloured by patients' perceptions of moral judgements about how they should have behaved. Thus, delay may be denied. Another difficulty with retrospective studies is that it is often not possible to be certain that the remembered first symptoms were in fact attributable to the cancer. This is a particular problem when patients are asked to recollect non-specific symptoms, such as in colorectal cancer.

Research in this area has been predominantly concerned with patient as opposed to medical delay. These studies can be classified into five different types (Antonovsky and Hartman, 1974). They are:

(i)   sociodemographic approach;
(ii) rational-knowledge approach;
(iii) psychologistic approach;
(iv) sociocultural approach;
(v)   health care approach.

The sociodemographic factors that were found to be the most significant predictors of delay were age and socio-economic status. Both lower socio-economic status and low educational level are associated with delay, as is older age (Antonovsky and Hartman, 1974). Such an approach, whilst being useful in providing background information, cannot provide any explanation for such differences. No other firm generalizations can be made about other sociodemographic variables involved in delay.

The rational-knowledge approach refers to what Antonovsky and Hartman (1974) call the cancer-related variables. The emphasis in these studies is on knowledge about cancer and cancer treatment facilities. Antonovsky and Hartman (1974), in a summary of the findings from these types of study, suggest that having adequate knowledge to be able to interpret a disturbance in body function as a sign that something might be wrong is not enough to explain take-up of medical services. Good knowledge in itself may be related to delay, but so may be poor knowledge. Similarly, with regard to the part fear and anxiety play in delay, there is apparently contradictory evidence. Antonovsky and Hartman (1974) state:

'Fear apparently has various effects under different circumstances. The fear of being told the suspected truth may lead to delay, while non-delayers present their symptoms partly because they fear the consequences of further procrastination. The latter has been found particularly among those having the most knowledge about cancer.'

Fear about cancer may also be due to the implications of the disease for people's everyday lives. Certainly, there seems to be a felt stigma attached to cancer (Paterson and Aitken-Swan, 1954), although whether this is enacted, i.e. based on the way people actually respond to cancer sufferers, is difficult to judge. Fear and anxiety may also be due to feelings of guilt generated by the idea that cancer is self-inflicted. In the present climate, with emphasis on prevention and individuals being responsible for their health, such guilt feelings may become more common. Guilt feelings may particularly arise amongst smokers who suffer from cancer. The authors also make two important points about the relationship between effective reactions and cancer. They argue first that the effective state may be part of the overall make-up of the person and may reflect the way the person relates to reality in general and not to cancer specifically. Secondly, the effect may be related specifically to cancer or may be a generalized effect.

The psychological approaches have tended to focus on explanations which emphasize neuroticism, low intelligence, and styles of coping with fear and anxiety. No consistent relationships have been found between any of these variables and delay (Antonovsky and Hartman, 1974).

In the sociocultural approach to delay, the assumptions about the role of cultural background appear to involve an explanation which is essentially deterministic. For example, it is argued (Antonovsky and Hartman, 1974) that the culture provides the individual with orientations towards health in three different ways. The first way is that cultural values and social structure may provide the individual with values which put an emphasis on deferred gratification, planning, mastery of the world, and other factors which are conducive to the uptake of health services; on the other hand, the culture may provide the individual with values which generate fatalism which is not conducive to uptake of services. Secondly, the culture provides the individual with knowledge about health relative to other values and an understanding of good health habits. Finally, the culture provides individuals with recipes about how to respond to specific situations.

These authors fail to find a study which specifically utilizes such a framework to explain delay/non-delay in respect to cancer, although the marked socioeconomic differences in behaviour may suggest the importance of cultural background.

The problem with this type of approach is that, in an attempt to get away from the psychologism or individualism of other models, the image of the lay person is as one who is seen predominantly as a product of his or her culture. This person is portrayed as a 'cultural dope'.

The final set of studies examine delay/non-delay in the context of an individual's general orientation towards health care. Apart from the economic barriers involved in fee for service payments, and the geographic barriers causing lack of accessibility to services, Antonovsky and Hartman (1974) argue that there are even more subtle barriers. For example, tension and strain caused by breakdown in communication in the doctor–patient relationship may invoke delay in the patient. The patient may have lost faith in the doctor or in the value of medicine in general and thus may delay in seeking medical care.

Antonovsky and Hartman (1974) conclude by suggesting that, because of the multiplicity of factors involved in explaining delay/non-delay, further investment in the area may be of limited value.

It is evident that there is a lack of conclusive and useful findings which adequately explain delay—which is surprising given the vast amount of research carried out in this area (Antonovsky and Hartman, 1974). It may be due to the complicated nature of the topic but it may also be due to the theoretical approach adopted in much of this research. The assumptions in this approach are that patients should not delay and should conform to organizationally defined rules. The assumption is that patients or laymen should passively respond to doctors' orders or officially prescribed rules and, when they do not, there is a need to find out why. The explanation of 'why delay' is couched in terms of laymen being deviant or being rule breakers because they do not conform to the solutions that have been officially recommended. Assuming that patients should comply with these rules, the assumption is that patients who do not are in some way idiosyncratic or irrational. Thus, explanations have emphasized either individuals' intrinsic traits which are pathological, such as poor coping styles and neuroticism, or studies have identified some deficiency or pathologies within the culture in which the individual lives. For example, having a culture which does not reinforce the value of deferred gratification is one factor used to explain delay. One reason for the failure of these research studies to adequately explain patient delay might be because of this assumption about the passive position of the patient in the doctor–patient relationship. If the patient is seen to be active and critical, and not necessarily sharing the views of the medical profession, then delay can be explained in terms not of some idiosyncratic characteristic of the patient but in terms of the patient's rational action. Thus, patients may have 'good' reasons for delaying, one of which may be their beliefs about the value of medical treatment. So the question of why patients delay should be reversed to 'why do some patients go immediately?' (Stimson, 1974).

Antonovsky and Hartman (1974) suggest that variations in delay occur with the cancer site. So the following section is divided according to cancer site.

Specific malignancy sites

Bladder cancer

Wallace and Harris (1965) assessed the sources of delay for patients with bladder tumour in the South London area. They showed quite clearly that there was relatively little patient delay, with half the patients attending their family doctor within a week and about three-quarters within a month of onset of symptoms. Family doctors see many patients with haematuria for every one with a bladder neoplasm; in general, they refer such patients very quickly to hospital. There was a certain degree of delay—e.g. treating patients for urinary infection. However, they identified the major component of delay as due to the hospital system; this was partly due to the appointments system but also to inadequate investigation when first seen and then having to wait for admission and definitive investigation. A follow-up to this paper (Turner et al., 1977) described the opening of a haematuria diagnostic service at the same hospital. Over a three-year period, nearly 100 patients attended the hospital, where they could be seen on the day of referral without an appointment for preliminary investigation. The authors describe how 65 per cent of the patients were admitted within two weeks for final investigation and, out of the 95 patients, 12 new cases of cancer of the bladder were identified (also 1 with cancer of the kidney and 1 cancer of the penis). They suggest that all the patients, who had relatively early stage cancers, were probably being diagnosed more speedily than they would have been without such a special service.

Breast cancer

Many studies have attempted to explain why patients delay with symptoms of breast cancer (see Green and Roberts, 1974, for review). As with other areas, there has been a multiplicity of approaches which has resulted in markedly contrasting findings (Humphrey, 1978). For example, Cameron and Hinton (1968) found that 20 per cent of patients waited over three months. Those who delayed were more likely to say they felt little or no anxiety over the tumour, to be more introverted, to be unfamiliar with hospital and to have less education.

The authors conclude:

'There is a complex interplay of knowledge, suspicion, denial, anxiety and apparent indifference contributing to delay. Appropriate anxiety hastens consultation. Patients who deny concern or who are mistakenly reassured by a physician may delay seeking treatment for years.'

On the other hand, Margarey and Todd (1976) tend to adopt a more psychoanalytical explanation. They argue that conscious fears, including that of mastectomy, were found to have no significant influence on the time that a woman takes to report the presence of a breast lump to her doctor, or to commence the practice of breast self-examination. The length of delay is determined by unconscious, non-rational processes, and other factors beyond her control. The problem with the adoption of this approach is the difficulty in testing it. Finally, Williams *et al.* (1976), in their study of delay, found that absence of pain, ignorance of the possible severity of the condition and, conversely, the fear of the consequences if cancer was diagnosed, all were crucial factors in influencing delay.

There are obvious difficulties in assessing the relative value of these three studies in that it is not clear as to which model of behaviour each of the studies is using in explaining patient delay. A set of explicit theoretical propositions about patient behaviour is required, which can be used as the basis for understanding and evaluating results.

Studies of medical delay in the diagnosis and treatment of breast cancer are less frequent. However, Bywaters and Knox (1976), in a study of the organization of breast cancer services in the West Midlands region of the UK, identified delays which were attributable to patients, general practitioners, hospital doctors and administrative processes. Whilst emphasizing the need to reduce patient delay, these authors were also concerned about the behaviour of doctors, both general practitioners and specialists, who failed to detect breast lumps. The form in which the data were recorded did not permit resolution of this cumulative delay into its component parts and the authors found a number of cases where opportunities for earlier diagnosis were apparently missed. They quote four cases which were discovered at out-patient clinics, whither the patients had been referred by their general practitioners for other conditions without discovery of their breast lumps, and two cases where the patients were admitted to hospital and underwent major surgery without discovery of breast lumps which they themselves knew to be present at the time. These two patients were not treated until twelve and thirteen months later. Bywaters and Knox (1976) showed that, of 243 patients, there was a delay of over six months between onset of symptoms to first out-patient appointment in 33 cases.

The intervals between the first out-patient appointment and treatment showed a delay of over four weeks in 33 of the 243 patients. Most of the delay between first out-patient appointment and treatment occurred before biopsy rather than between biopsy and treatment. Less than half of those biopsied were admitted within two weeks of their outpatient appointment.

Colorectal cancer

Rowe-Jones and Aylett (1965) analysed information from 100 patients with colon and 100 patients with rectal cancer attending their clinic. For the colon cases, the average duration of symptoms was seven months and for the rectal cases over ten months before attending for general practitioner advice. Over a fifth of the patients were further delayed before a diagnosis was made. In general, the delay after contacting the health service was in the hospital diagnosis in the colon cancer patients and the general practitioner as far as the rectal cancers were concerned. There was no apparent delay between definitive diagnosis and institution of treatment. They concluded that the delay did result in advanced stage disease and consequently influenced prognosis. Holliday and Hardcastle (1979) reviewed the delay to diagnosis in colorectal cancer patients attending the Nottingham hospitals. Most of the delay occurred outside the hospital and was equally attributable to the patient and the family doctor. Patients seemed to be unaware of the importance of bowel symptoms, whilst the family doctors in particular failed to examine patients with rectal cancer, and did not recognize symptoms suggestive of colon cancer. There was some degree of hospital delay, which was predominantly due to waiting for investigation, poor quality x-rays, and inadequate sigmoidoscopy.

The lack of knowledge about colorectal cancer amongst lay people is exemplified by an Australian study (Dent and Goulston, 1978). The authors conclude that despite the extent of the population's personal experience with colorectal cancer compared with other cancers, objective knowledge about colorectal cancer is poor. Knowledge is significantly less and uncertainty significantly greater than for other forms of cancer, and knowledge about colorectal cancer is not consistent or organized into a coherent system.

A study by Dent et al. (1978) on the knowledge of and attitudes towards colorectal cancer by gastroenterologists concluded that there was: 'a surprising ignorance of recent developments in colorectal cancer'. These authors also suggest that delay in the diagnosis of colorectal cancer occurs in 20 per cent to 50 per cent of patients. While over half the cases of delay may be due to patient delay, medical delay may be more important. They state:

> 'Medical delay may have more serious consequences, destroying the patient's confidence in his or her physician; ignorance of recognised high-risk groups may not only delay diagnosis but result in failure to take simple measures to prevent colorectal cancer.'

Conclusions

This brief review suggests that the extent of delay in diagnosis and treatment of cancer might be large. The evidence suggests that patient delay as opposed to medical delay accounts for the greater part, although medical delay may be longer for certain specific cancer sites and may have more serious implications.

There has been a plethora of studies attempting to explain patient delay. Apart from their methodological weaknesses, the studies generally lack theoretical coherence. Future research should move away from the assumption that patients who delay are in some way idiosyncratic and move towards an approach that sees the patient as being rational and critical, with good reasons for not going to the doctors immediately symptoms are perceived. To understand patient delay, it is necessary to understand immediate patient uptake of health services. If such an approach is adopted, the focus shifts away from use of services towards attempts to understand the way lay people interpret and evaluate disturbances in body functioning. Thus the response of going immediately to the health services is seen as one form of action amongst various alternatives. The adoption of this approach might bring a better understanding of why patients vary in their evaluations of symptoms. Models of illness behaviour, which have adopted this perspective, are available although they have yet to be adequately tested in empirical research (Fabrega, 1974).

References

Aitken-Swan, J. and Paterson, R. (1959). *British Medical Journal* **1**, 708.

Antonovsky, A. and Hartman, H. (1974). *Health Education Monograph* **2**(2), 98.

Bywaters, J. L. and Knox, E. G. (1976). *Lancet* **i**, 849.

Cameron, A. and Hinton, J. (1968). *Cancer* **21**, 1121.

Dent, O., Bassett, M. and Goulston, K. (1978). *The Australian and New Zealand Journal of Surgery* **48**(3), 331.

Dent, O. and Goulston, K. (1978). *Community Health Studies* **12**(1), 20.

Fabrega, H. (1974). *Disease and Social Behavior: An Interdisciplinary Perspective*. Massachusetts Institute of Technology.

Green, L. W. and Roberts, B. J. (1974). *Health Education Monograph* **2**(2), 129.

Hackett, T. P., Cassem, N. H. and Raker, J. W. (1973). *New England Journal of Medicine* **289**, 14.

Holliday, H. W. and Hardcastle, J. D. (1979). *Lancet* **i**, 309.

Humphrey, M. (1978). In *Breast Cancer*, pp. 57–66. Ed. by P. A. Van Keep and P. C. Brand. MTP Press, New York.

Kutner, B. and Gordon, G. (1961). *Journal of Health and Human Behaviour* **2**, 171.

Margarey, C. J. and Todd, P. B. (1976). *New Zealand Journal of Surgery* **46**, 391.

Murcott, A. (1981). In *Medical Work, Realities and Routines*, pp. 128–40. Ed. by P. Atkinson and C. Heath. Gower, London.

Paterson, R. and Aitken-Swan, J. (1954). *Lancet* **ii**, 857.

Rowe-Jones, D. C. and Aylett, S. O. (1965). *Lancet* **ii**, 973.

Stimson, G. (1974). *Social Science and Medicine* **8**(2), 97.

Turner, A. G., Hendrey, W. F., Williams, G. B. and Wallace, D. M. (1977). *British Medical Journal* **2**, 29.

Wallace, D. and Harris, D. (1965). *Lancet* **ii**, 332.

Williams, E. M., Baum, M. and Hughes, L. E. (1976). *Clinical Oncology* **2**, 327.

Index